Handbook of Neurodevelopmental Disorders

Handbook of Neurodevelopmental Disorders

Edited by Ella Keller

AMERICAN
MEDICAL PUBLISHERS
www.americanmedicalpublishers.com

American Medical Publishers,
41 Flatbush Avenue,
1st Floor, New York,
NY 11217, USA

Visit us on the World Wide Web at:
www.americanmedicalpublishers.com

ISBN: 978-1-63927-296-9

Cataloging-in-Publication Data

Handbook of neurodevelopmental disorders / edited by Ella Keller.
p. cm.
Includes bibliographical references and index.
ISBN 978-1-63927-296-9
1. Developmental disabilities. 2. Central nervous system--Diseases. 3. Neurodevelopmental treatment.
4. Developmental neurobiology. 5. Pediatric neuropsychology. I. Keller, Ella.
RJ506.D47 H36 2022
616.858 8--dc23

Table of Contents

Preface

The group of disorders that affect the development of the nervous system are known as neurodevelopmental disorders. It leads to abnormal brain function due to which emotion, learning, self-control and memory get affected. The different types of neurodevelopmental disorders are intellectual disability, autism spectrum disorders, motor disorders, traumatic brain injury, down syndrome, etc. The factors causing neurodevelopmental disorders can be genetic disorders, immune dysfunction, infectious diseases like meningitis or encephalitis, metabolic diseases and physical trauma. The treatment of neurodevelopmental disorders depends on the condition and can vary accordingly. It can include interventions such as medication, therapy and surgery. This book aims to shed light on some of the unexplored aspects of neurodevelopmental disorders and recent researches related to them. From diagnosis to treatment, case studies related to all contemporary topics of relevance to such disorders have been included herein. With state-of-the-art inputs by acclaimed experts of neurology, this book targets students and professionals.

Significant researches are present in this book. Intensive efforts have been employed by authors to make this book an outstanding discourse. This book contains the enlightening chapters which have been written on the basis of significant researches done by the experts.

Finally, I would also like to thank all the members involved in this book for being a team and meeting all the deadlines for the submission of their respective works. I would also like to thank my friends and family for being supportive in my efforts.

Editor

1

ADHD medication in offspring of immigrants — does the income level of the country of parental origin matter?

Arzu Arat[1,2*], Viveca Östberg[2], Bo Burström[3] and Anders Hjern[1,2]

Abstract

Background: Child psychiatric treatment facilities vary greatly worldwide and are virtually non-existent in many low-income countries. One of the most common psychiatric disorders in childhood is ADHD, with an estimated prevalence of 3–5% in Sweden. Previous studies have shown a similar prevalence of ADHD in minority and majority children in Sweden and the UK. However, clinical studies demonstrated that children from immigrant families living in Sweden received less psychiatric care than those of native-born parents. We tested the hypothesis that the consumption of child psychiatric care in immigrant families would be determined by the availability of such treatment in the parents' country of origin. Patterns of medication for attention-deficit hyperactivity disorder (ADHD) were studied as a proxy for child psychiatric care.

Methods: This was a register study of dispensed stimulant medication during 2013–2014 in Swedish national birth cohorts from 1995–2009. The study population, consisting of nearly 1.4 million children, was divided by national income of the parental country of origin and whether the parents were native Swedes, European immigrants, non-European immigrants or a mixture. Logistic regression was used to calculate the odds ratios of having been dispensed at least one ADHD drug during 2013, with adjustments for gender, family status indicating whether the child is living with both parents, household income and area of residence.

Results: Having parents born in low-income (OR [95% confidence interval] 0.27 [0.24–0.29]) or middle-income (European: OR 0.23 [0.20–0.26], non-European: OR 0.39 [0.34–0.41]) countries was associated with lower ADHD treatment levels than having parents born in high-income countries (European: OR 0.60 [0.54–0.66], non-European: OR 0.68 [0.59–0.79]), when compared to children of parents born in Sweden. In families with a background in low or middle income countries, there was no significant association between household income and ADHD medication, while in children with Swedish and mixed backgrounds high level of disposable income was associated with lower levels of ADHD medication.

Conclusion: The use of child psychiatric care by immigrant families in Sweden was largely associated with the income level of the country of origin.

Keywords: Attention-deficit hyperactivity disorder, Child mental health services, Health inequalities, Immigrant families, Income levels

* Correspondence: arzu.arat@chess.su.se
[1]Department of Medicine, Karolinska Institute, 171 76, Stockholm, Sweden
[2]Centre for Health Equity Studies (CHESS), Stockholm University/Karolinska Institute, 106 91 Stockholm, Sweden
Full list of author information is available at the end of the article

Background

As with all Nordic welfare societies, Sweden aims to provide equitable access to healthcare for all its citizens, regardless of their gender, socioeconomic situation, region of residence and ethnic, cultural and religious background [1]. The increasing number of immigrants in the country has inspired a number of studies about whether they receive the same equitable access to healthcare as Swedish-born citizens. A recent Danish study found that adult immigrants, their descendants and native Danes did receive equitable access to free healthcare [2], as did a study carried out in Sweden during the 1990s [3].

A clinical study in Sweden however demonstrated differences in the consumption of child psychiatric care between native and immigrant families [4]. Adolescents with immigrant parents from low-income countries were shown to have lower odds of receiving outpatient and inpatient psychiatric care than those with Swedish-born parents. An earlier study led by the same researcher showed that migrant background also played an important role in the referral patterns of adolescents to psychiatric clinics. Children with Swedish parents were more likely to be referred by their own families, whereas children with Asian or African backgrounds were more likely to be referred by social or legal agencies [5].

One of the most common psychiatric disorders in childhood in Western countries is attention-deficit hyperactivity disorder (ADHD), with an estimated prevalence of 3–5% in Swedish school children [6]. Studies in Sweden [7] and Great Britain [8] have shown clear social gradients for ADHD, with a higher prevalence in families with a low socioeconomic status (SES). In contrast, the large national study in Great Britain [8] and a small Swedish population-based study [9] showed that children with a minority background had a very similar prevalence of ADHD to the majority of the population. Interestingly, both a regional Swedish study [10] and national studies in the United States [11] and New Zealand [12] found that minority children were less likely to be diagnosed with ADHD and receive ADHD medication.

Parents play an important role in referring children to psychiatric clinics. Therefore, parental health beliefs, as well as their attitudes, knowledge and experience of mental health services, influence consumption patterns [4, 13, 14]. An analysis of worldwide resources for child and adolescent psychiatry carried out by the World Health Organization (WHO), described huge differences between different global regions [15]. In low-income countries, such resources were often virtually non-existent and they were also scarce in many middle-income countries. This means that immigrant parents from these regions of the world could be expected to have very little experience of such care in their country of origin.

The aim of this study was to test the hypothesis that the developmental level of the parental country of origin, operationalized as low, middle and high-income countries, would be an important determinant of the consumption patterns of child and adolescent psychiatry care by immigrant families in Sweden.

Methods

This study was based on Swedish national register data held by the National Board of Health and Welfare and Statistics Sweden. A unique identity number with 10 digits is given to all Swedish residents at birth or immigration and this number can be used to link information on those individuals from different register sources.

We tested our hypothesis after controlling for family socio-demographic characteristics. The analysis was further elaborated on by analysing the link between household income and ADHD medication within immigrant background groups.

Study population

The study population consisted of Swedish born birth cohorts from 1995 to 2009 who were still Swedish residents on 31 December 2012. We excluded individuals who had a diagnosis of narcolepsy in the patient discharge register, because they are prescribed the same medication as children with ADHD. Individuals were also excluded if information on their county of residence, household income, family status or maternal country of birth were missing. A total of 14,405 individuals were excluded, leaving 1,385,397 Swedish born-children in the final study population.

Immigrant background classification

Table 1 describes the immigrant categories in the study, based on the parental country of birth obtained from the Swedish Register of Total Population. Children having two Swedish parents were recorded as having Swedish background. A mixed category was constructed for children with one Swedish and one foreign-born parent. The rest of the categorization was based on maternal country of birth. The countries were first categorised as European or non-European and then further classified based on gross national income per capita into low, middle and high-income countries [16].

Outcome variable: ADHD medication

The Swedish Prescribed Drug Register has unique patient identifiers for all drugs prescribed and dispensed to the whole Swedish population since July 2005. The quality of the register has been evaluated and found to be excellent [17]. The first-time purchase of at least one prescription of a drug with an anatomical therapeutic chemical code of N06BA01- N06BA04 between 1 January 2013 and 30 June 2014, was used to create the ADHD medication variable.

Table 1 Nationalities in the immigrant categories in the study

Immigrant Category	Major Nationalities
Sweden (Both parents)	Sweden (100%)
Mixed (One foreign born parent)	European (21,4%), non-European (23,1%)
High income European country	Northern Europe (38%), Eastern Europe (30%), Western Europe (11%), Southern Europe (8%)
Middle income European country	Former Yugoslavia (84%), Romania (7%)
High income non-European country	Chile (49%), Arabian peninsula (13%), North America (11%), South Korea and Japan (8%), Argentina and Uruguay (6%).
Middle income non- European country	Iraq (39%), Turkey (17%), Lebanon (16%), Iran (14%)
Low income non- European country	Somalia (21%), Syria (18%), Ethiopia/Eritrea (17%), South Asia (16%), South East Asia (9%), Northern Africa (7%).

Socio-demographic variables

Socio-demographic variables were created by using the Swedish Longitudinal Integration Database for Health Insurance and Labor Market studies. The unique ID number was used to link information on parental variables from the Swedish Multi-Generation Register. A disposable household income was calculated based on all taxed income and transfers minus taxes paid divided by the number of consumer units in the household. Disposable income of the household is created by Statistics Sweden according to an algorithm that includes all incomes in the household reported to Swedish Tax Agency, subtracted by taxes and divided by consumer units. This variable was then presented in quintiles based on the total sample. Family status was constructed as a dichotomous variable for a child living with a single parent or both parents. Both variables reflected the information when the child was four years old. This was a choice made to prevent inverse causality.

The National Board of Health and Welfare [18] has reported considerable regional differences in the consumption of ADHD medication. Due to the absence of any obvious demographic or geographical patterns in these regional differences, it was assumed that this pattern mirrored varying practices in diagnosis and prescription in different counties rather than variations in the prevalence of ADHD. To account for these differences, the counties were classified into four categories according to the proportion of children prescribed, and whose parents purchased, the ADHD medication during 2013: high prescription (>3.0%), moderate prescription (2.3–3.0%), low prescription (2.1–2.3%) and very low prescription (≤2.0%).

Statistical analysis

Logistic regression was used to calculate odds ratios (OR) with 95% confidence intervals (CIs) as estimates of effects, with at least one retrieved prescription of ADHD medication as the outcome variable. Two models were used to investigate the association between immigrant background and the incidence of ADHD medication. In Model 1, we entered gender and the child's age in 2013, broken down into three categories: 4–8, 9–14 and 15–18 years. In Model 2, we added household income, family status and the county of residence, categorised as explained above. In order to estimate the possible effects of child's gender, an interaction analysis was performed with the immigrant background variable in a logistic regression model that included age and county of residence.

The interaction effects of household income were analysed by calculating odds ratios for ADHD medication in a regression model stratified by household income. Mean length of time spent in Sweden by the parent was calculated for all immigrant backgrounds.

The mean age when ADHD medication was dispensed was calculated to investigate the differences between children with Swedish and immigrant backgrounds. A selection was performed for those who were residents in Sweden on 31 December 2005.

A sensitivity analysis was used to analyse the diagnosis of ADHD in specialist care during 2013. Details on these results are provided in Additional file 1. All statistical analyses were performed using SAS version 9.4 for Windows (SAS Institute Inc., Cary, NC, USA).

Results

The register entries for the study population, showed that 36,564 children (2.6%) had at least one ADHD drug dispensed to them during the study period, with boys being more likely to receive ADHD medication than girls (3.7% versus 1.7%).

Table 2 presents the study population stratified by immigrant categories. Children from a middle-income European (0.7%) and low income country immigrant background (1.1%) were the least likely to receive medication, compared with children with Swedish (2.8%), mixed (2.9%) or high-income non-European immigrant backgrounds (3.0%).

It was more common for a child in the Swedish category to belong to one of the two highest income quintiles (49.1%) than immigrant or mixed backgrounds. The percentage declined considerably in children in the non-European middle-income (13.7%) and low-income (14.5%)

Table 2 Socio-demographic characteristics of the study population: Swedish, Mixed, European (Euro) and Non-European (Non Euro)

	Sweden	Mixed	Euro High	Euro Middle	Non Euro High	Non Euro Mid	Non Euro Low	Total
N	1,058,422	161,924	18,961	30,364	6,996	63,768	44,962	1,385,397
	%	%	%	%	%	%	%	%
Gender								
Boy	51.5	51.3	51.4	51.7	51.4	50.9	51.4	51.4
Girl	48.5	48.7	48.6	48.3	48.6	49.1	48.6	48.6
Age								
15–18	32.0	28.1	28.7	30.1	31.2	26.3	26.4	31.0
9–14	32.8	31.8	26.9	31.0	32.0	30.7	29.6	32.4
4–8	35.2	40.2	44.4	38.9	36.8	43.0	44.0	36.6
Household Income Quintiles								
Lowest	9.7	19.2	29.5	32.5	34.9	54.2	50.7	29.4
2nd	19.2	20.7	21.3	27.5	23.1	22.4	24.0	17.0
3rd	22.0	18.0	15.2	18.6	14.7	9.7	10.9	11.9
4th	23.2	19.0	15.6	13.1	12.8	7.2	7.5	13.3
Highest	25.9	23.2	18.4	8.3	14.6	6.5	7.0	28.4
Single parent								
	11.3	18.8	19.7	15.7	29.5	14.6	26.7	13.2
Years spent in Sweden by parent (mean)								
	-	23.6	19.1	17.2	22.5	17.0	16.7	19.5
ADHD Diagnosis								
	2.1	2.1	1.6	0.5	2.1	1.1	1.0	2.0
ADHD Medication								
	2.8	2.9	2.1	0.7	3.0	1.4	1.1	2.6

country categories. Single parenthood was more common in families with immigrant parents and particularly common in those born in high and low-income countries outside Europe (Table 2).

Table 3 presents the incidence of ADHD medication dispensed to boys and girls. Both boys and girls in the European middle-income category had the lowest ADHD medication levels. With regard to children in single parent households, the incidence of ADHD medication was higher for children in the Swedish, mixed or high-income categories.

Table 4 shows the results of the multiple logistic regression analyses. Compared to Sweden, children in the European middle-income category had the lowest odds for ADHD medication (OR 0.28), followed by Non-European low-income (OR 0.39) and middle-income countries (OR 0.49). Children in the families with one foreign born parent (OR 1.05) and high-income (OR 0.76) categories had similar odds for ADHD medication as the Swedish category. Adjusting for county of residence and household income (SES) in Model 2 only marginally changed these effects.

Table 5 presents the odds ratios for ADHD medication dispensed by income quintiles in the parental country of birth categories. Swedish children and children with a mixed background who lived in a household with higher income were less likely to receive ADHD medication compared to children with same background living in households with lower income. This stepwise social gradient was absent in all other immigrant background groups.

In a sensitivity analyses that had an ADHD diagnosis in specialised care as the outcome, the multiple logistic regression gave similar results as the medication outcome (Additional file 1: Table S1). Compared to children with native parents, children in the European middle-income category had the lowest odds of receiving an ADHD diagnosis (OR [95%CI]: 0.32 [0.28–0.37]), followed by the non-European low (0.52 [0.47–0.57]) and middle- income countries (0.59 [0.55–0.64]). Children of families with one parent foreign country background and European and non-European high-income categories had similar odds for ADHD diagnosis as the Swedish category with ORs of 1.10 [1.0–1.14] and 0.87 [0.78–0.98] respectively. When adjusted for county of residence and disposable income (SES) in Model 2, the odds were only marginally changed. The lower figures for diagnosis compared to medication levels was due to

Table 3 Gender stratified socio-demographic indicators and incidence (%) of ADHD medication dispensed by origin

	Swedish	Mixed	Euro High	Euro Middle	Non-Euro High	Non-Euro Mid	Non-Euro Low	Total
BOYS (n)	544,583	83,114	9,758	15,702	3,596	32,453	23,086	712,292
	%	%	%	%	%	%	%	%
Age								
15–18	5.4	6.1	4.8	1.7	5.7	2.7	1.9	5.2
9–14	5.3	5.5	3.9	1.3	5.2	3.1	2.7	5.1
4–8	1.2	1.2	0.9	0.3	1.4	0.7	0.7	1.1
Household Income Quintiles								
Lowest	6.2	5.0	2.6	1.1	3.9	1.9	1.5	4.4
2nd	4.4	4.0	2.5	0.9	3.7	1.9	1.4	4.0
3rd	3.6	3.6	3.0	1.0	2.7	2.1	1.9	3.5
4th	3.4	3.8	2.9	1.1	5.7	2.3	1.5	3.4
Highest	3.4	3.4	3.2	1.0	4.2	2.2	2.0	3.4
Single Parent								
	8.6	7.3	6.1	2.1	5.4	3.3	2.2	7.5
All	3.9	3.9	2.8	1.0	4.0	2.0	1.6	3.7
GIRLS (n)	513,839	78,810	9,203	14,662	3,400	31,315	21,876	673,105
	%	%	%	%	%	%	%	%
Age								
15–18	3.0	3.8	2.8	0.8	3.2	1.3	1.1	2.9
9–14	1.8	1.8	1.5	0.4	2.7	0.9	0.8	1.7
4–8	0.4	0.4	0.2	0.1	0.4	0.2	0.2	0.3
Household income quintiles								
Lowest	2.8	2.0	1.4	0.4	1.4	0.6	0.5	1.9
2nd	1.8	1.7	1.1	0.3	2.2	0.6	0.5	1.6
3rd	1.5	1.7	1.3	0.4	3.3	1.0	0.8	1.5
4th	1.4	1.8	1.9	0.8	1.8	1.3	0.8	1.5
Highest	1.5	1.7	0.6	0.5	2.2	1.0	1.0	1.4
Single parent								
	3.9	3.4	2.1	0.8	4.1	1.4	0.9	3.4
All	1.7	1.8	1.3	0.4	2.1	0.7	0.6	1.6

Table 4 Logistic regression of ADHD medication dispensed

		Model 1	Model 2
	(%)	OR (95% CI)	OR (95% CI)
Sweden	76.4	1	1
Mixed	11.7	1.05 (1.02–1.08)	0.90 (0.88–0.93)
European high	1.4	0.76 (0.68–0.84)	0.60 (0.54–0.66)
European middle	2.2	0.28 (0.25–0.32)	0.23 (0.20–0.26)
Non-European high	0.5	1.00 (0.86–1.14)	0.68 (0.59–0.79)
Non- European middle	4.6	0.49 (0.46–0.53)	0.39 (0.36–0.41)
Non- European low	3.3	0.39 (0.36–0.43)	0.27 (0.24–0.29)

Model 1 is adjusted for age and gender
Model 2 is adjusted for age, gender, income, county of residence and lone parenthood

the prescriptions by practitioners who do not report to the Swedish Patient Register.

The mean age for first ADHD diagnosis and first medication was calculated for all immigrant backgrounds and for both genders and no major differences were observed between the populations (data not shown). The mean of length of stay of parent was calculated for all migrant groups. Since length of stay of the mother was strongly nested with the child's age, there was large variation in the number of years spent in Sweden (data not shown). Mean length of stay was 19.5 years and figures were only slightly different across groups (Table 2).

Table 5 Logistic regression for ADHD medication by household income level within each immigrant category

	Lowest Income	2nd Income Quintile	3rd Income Quintile	4th Income Quintile	Highest Income
		OR (95% CI)	OR (95% CI)	OR (95% CI)	OR (95% CI)
Sweden	1	0.88 (0.85–0.91)	0.74 (0.72–0.78)	0.65 (0.62–0.67)	0.51 (0.49–0.53)
Mixed	1	0.97 (0.88–1.06)	0.85 (0.78–0.94)	0.81 (0.74–0.89)	0.61 (0.56–0.67)
European high	1	0.99 (0.73–1.33)	1.07 (0.78–1.48)	1.06 (0.78–1.44)	0.78 (0.58–1.07)
European middle	1	0.98 (0.68–1.41)	1.12 (0.76–1.65)	1.23 (0.83–1.84)	0.73 (0.43–1.22)
Non-European high	1	1.16 (0.79–1.70)	1.06 (0.68–1.65)	1.18 (0.77–1.83)	0.89 (0.58–1.38)
Non- European middle	1	1.13 (0.95–1.35)	1.20 (0.96–1.50)	1.17 (0.92–1.50)	0.91 (0.70–1.19)
Non- European low	1	0.97 (0.77–1.23)	1.21 (0.92–1.60)	0.87 (0.62–1.23)	0.96 (0.70–1.34)

Model is adjusted for age, gender, county of residence and lone parenthood

Discussion

This register-based study of nearly 1.4 million Swedish children demonstrates that children whose parents were born in countries where there were few child psychiatric resources, namely the non-European low and middle-income countries, were less likely to receive ADHD medication than children with parents born in Sweden or other high-income countries. For the children of Swedish-born and mixed parents, ADHD medication levels were higher for children in households with low level of disposable income, where as in families with an origin in low or middle income countries, there was no such gradient between household income and ADHD medication.

The observed pattern of ADHD medication and diagnosis by immigrant categories is likely to reflect the facilities available for child and adolescent psychiatry in the parents' country of origin. According to a report by the WHO [15] child and adolescent mental health care is scarce in countries that are in the lowest World Bank income categories. It seems very probable that the presence, or absence, of child psychiatry in the country of origin influences parental belief systems around mental health and behaviour in children and consequently their attitudes towards seeking help. The influences of parental country of origin on attitudes towards behavioural disorders have been covered by several previous studies. One study found that immigrant parents from Morocco, Turkey and Suriname who were living in The Netherlands had lower sensitivity, but higher specificity, for ADHD detection rates, than Dutch parents [14]. This suggests that a higher degree of deviance was present before ADHD was considered by these immigrant parents. Another study found that Pakistani women living in the UK were less likely to access mental health services for conditions judged as mild or moderate [19].

Compared to Swedish-born and mixed families, we expected a reversed social gradient in families in the low-income and middle-income countries with respect to household income and ADHD medication levels. This would fit a cross-cultural pattern, where a higher education, and consequently higher income, often leads to more familiarity with the belief systems associated with Western child psychiatry [20]. Also, higher income indicates more stable integration into the job market, leading to higher knowledge of the Swedish healthcare system and of ways to seek help for children's health problems. Absence of this social gradient in our study population underlines the importance of availability of child psychiatry services in the country of origin for use of child psychiatry services in Sweden.

We cannot exclude the possibility of a healthy migrant effect behind the lower rates of ADHD diagnosis and medication consumption in children with an immigrant background. Family, twin and adoption studies provide robust evidence for strong genetic influences on ADHD [21, 22], which makes a low prevalence of parental ADHD a possible mechanism for a healthy migrant effect that carries over to the next generation. However, the clear patterns observed related to gross national income per capita in the parental country of birth and parental socioeconomic status in Sweden cannot easily be explained by a healthy migrant effect. Therefore, this points to a more structural explanation.

Strengths and limitations

To the best of our knowledge, this is the first study that has tested the hypothesis that the availability of child psychiatric services in the country of origin was an important determinant of consumption of such care after migration. This was made possible by our large national cohort, where foreign-born parents could be divided into categories based on the developmental level of their country of origin and these categories could be further divided by their income level in Sweden.

The study has several limitations. According to national guidelines for ADHD medication, specialists are only advised to prescribe stimulants in cases where other interventions have failed. Therefore, only the more severe cases of ADHD are captured by medication levels. However, a sensitivity analysis of children diagnosed in specialised care confirmed the pattern found for medication in our study, making it improbable that this bias would have had a major impact on our study.

At the time of the study medication was not free for children, as it is today. This might be expected to explain the differences in levels of medication dispense between lower and higher household income, for the children with migrant low and middle income country background. However, sensitivity analysis with diagnosis levels shows this to be less likely since there were no costs for medical visits for children.

Teachers play an important role in referring children with behavioural problems, like ADHD, to child psychiatrists, since the symptoms of ADHD often interfere with school work. Labelling child behavioural problems in the school setting can easily be influenced by preconceptions about the children's ethnic background, leading to biased referral patterns. Our study showed a clear gradient of consumption of care by the gross national income per capita of the parental country of origin. This gradient also existed between children in families with a non-European heritage, such that children in the non-European high income category had higher medication levels compared to low and middle income country backgrounds. Thus, preconceptions about children with a non-European background seem unlikely to explain this pattern.

Conclusions

The observed pattern of ADHD medication and diagnosis by immigrant categories might reflect the facilities available for child and adolescent psychiatry in the parents' country of origin, and thus their familiarity with child psychiatric services. Child psychiatric services need to find ways of reaching out to immigrant families with this background in order to provide equitable child psychiatric care.

Abbreviations

ADHD: Attention-deficit hyperactivity disorder; CI: Confidence interval; OR: Odds ratio; SES: Socioeconomic status; WHO: World Health Organization

Acknowledgements

Not applicable.

Funding

This study received funding from the European Commission through the Horizon 2020 Framework under the grant agreement number: 634,201.

Authors' contributions

AA. Substantial contributions in design of the study, preparation, analysis and interpretation of data as well as drafting and revising the manuscript. VÖ. Major contributions in design of the study. Substantial input in interpretation of the data and key contributions in improving the manuscript by providing thorough revisions. BB. Major contributions in conception and design of the study. Actively involved in revising the manuscript. AH. Substantial contributions in conception and design of the study. Active involvement in preparation of data set and provision of expertise regarding the data source. Major help in analysis and interpretation of data as well as drafting and revising the manuscript. All authors read and approved the final manuscript.

Consent for publication

Not applicable.

Competing interests

The authors declare that they have no competing interests.

Author details

[1]Department of Medicine, Karolinska Institute, 171 76, Stockholm, Sweden. [2]Centre for Health Equity Studies (CHESS), Stockholm University/Karolinska Institute, 106 91 Stockholm, Sweden. [3]Department of Public Health Sciences, Karolinska Institute, 171 77 Stockholm, Sweden.

References

1. Wiking E: Health care on equal terms for immigrants in Sweden: Inst för neurobiologi, vårdvetenskap och samhälle/Dept of neurobiology, care sciences and Society; 2012.
2. Nielsen SS, Hempler NF, Waldorff FB, Kreiner S, Krasnik A. Is there equity in use of healthcare services among immigrants, their descendents, and ethnic Danes? Scand J Public Health. 2012;40(3):260–70.
3. Hjern A, Haglund B, Persson G, Rosen M. Is there equity in access to health services for ethnic minorities in Sweden? Eur J Pub Health. 2001;11(2):147–52.
4. Ivert AK, Merlo J, Svensson R, Levander MT. How are immigrant background and gender associated with the utilisation of psychiatric care among adolescents? Soc Psychiatry Psychiatr Epidemiol. 2013;48(5):693–9.
5. Ivert AK, Svensson R, Adler H, Levander S, Rydelius PA, Torstensson Levander M. Pathways to child and adolescent psychiatric clinics: a multilevel study of the significance of ethnicity and neighbourhood social characteristics on source of referral. Child Adolesc Psychiatry Ment Health. 2011;5(1):6.
6. Mossler K, Kadesjö B, Hellgren L. Kort om ADHD hos barn och vuxna En sammanfattning av Socialstyrelsens kunskapsöversikt. Socialmedicinsk tidskrift. 2014;81(2):164–6.
7. Hjern A, Weitoft GR, Lindblad F. Social adversity predicts ADHD-medication in school children–a national cohort study. Acta Paediatr. 2010;99(6):920–4.
8. Green H, McGinnity Á, Meltzer H, Ford T, Goodman R: Mental health of children and young people in great Britain, 2004. In: Basingstoke: Palgrave Macmillan; 2005.
9. Holmberg K, Hjern A. Health complaints in children with attention-deficit/hyperactivity disorder. Acta Paediatr. 2006;95(6):664–70.
10. Jablonska B, Kosidou K, de Leon AP, Wettermark B, Magnusson C, Dal H, Dalman C. Neighborhood socioeconomic characteristics and utilization of ADHD medication in schoolchildren a population multilevel study in Stockholm County. J Atten Disord. 2016:1087054716643257.
11. Morgan PL, Staff J, Hillemeier MM, Farkas G, Maczuga S. Racial and ethnic disparities in ADHD diagnosis from kindergarten to eighth grade. Pediatrics. 2013;132(1):85–93.
12. Ghosh M, Holman CAJ, Preen DB. Exploring parental country of birth differences in the use of psychostimulant medications for ADHD: a whole-population linked data study. Aust N Z J Public Health. 2015;39(1):88–92.

13. Olaniyan O, Garriett V, Mychailyszyn MP, Anixt J, Rowe PC, Cheng TL. Community perspectives of childhood behavioral problems and ADHD among African American parents. Ambul Pediatr. 2007;7(3):226–31.
14. Zwirs BW, Burger H, Buitelaar JK, Schulpen TW. Ethnic differences in parental detection of externalizing disorders. Eur Child Adolesc Psychiatry. 2006;15(7): 418–26.
15. World Health Organization: Mental health atlas 2005: World Health Organization. Dept. of mental health and Substance Abuse; 2005.
16. How does the World Bank classify countries? - World bank data helpdesk [https://datahelpdesk.worldbank.org/knowledgebase/articles/378834-how-does-the-world-bank-classify-countries].
17. Wettermark B, Hammar N, Fored CM, Leimanis A, Otterblad Olausson P, Bergman U, Persson I, Sundstrom A, Westerholm B, Rosen M. The new Swedish prescribed drug register–opportunities for pharmacoepidemiological research and experience from the first six months. Pharmacoepidemiol Drug Saf. 2007;16(7):726–35.
18. Salmi P, Bergman GJ. Användningen av centralstimulantia vid ADHD Utvecklingen regionalt och i riket. In: Socialstyrelsen. 2015;
19. Stein SM, Christie D, Shah R, Dabney J, Wolpert M. Attitudes to and knowledge of CAMHS: differences between Pakistani and white British mothers. Child Adolesc Mental Health. 2003;8(1):29–33.
20. Bussing R, Zima BT, Gary FA, Garvan CW. Barriers to detection, help-seeking, and service use for children with ADHD symptoms. J Behav Health Serv Res. 2003;30(2):176–89.
21. Wallis D, Russell HF, Muenke M. Review: genetics of attention deficit/ hyperactivity disorder. J Pediatr Psychol. 2008;33(10):1085–99.
22. Freitag CM, Retz W. Family and twin studies in attention-deficit hyperactivity disorder. In: *Attention-Deficit Hyperactivity Disorder (ADHD) in Adults. Volume 176*. Basel: Karger publishers; 2009. p. 38–57.

2

Attention-deficit hyperactivity disorder and nonsuicidal self-injury in a clinical sample of adolescents: the role of comorbidities and gender

Judit Balázs[1,2*], Dóra Győri[1], Lili Olga Horváth[1,3], Gergely Mészáros[2,4] and Dóra Szentiványi[1,3]

Abstract

Background: The aim of the present study was to investigate the possible association between attention-deficit hyperactivity disorder (ADHD) and non-suicidal self-injury (NSSI) with special focus on the role of comorbidities and gender in a clinical sample of adolescents with both a dimensional and a categorical approach to psychopathology.

Methods: Using a structured interview, the Mini International Neuropsychiatric Interview Kid and a self-rated questionnaire, the Deliberate Self-Harm Inventory, the authors examined 202 inpatient adolescents (aged: 13–18 years) in the Vadaskert Child and Adolescent Psychiatric Hospital and Outpatient Clinic, Budapest, Hungary. Descriptive statistics, Mann–Whitney U test, chi-square test and mediator model were used.

Results: Fifty-two adolescents met full criteria for ADHD and a further 77 showed symptoms of ADHD at the subthreshold level. From the 52 adolescents diagnosed with ADHD, 35 (67.30%) had NSSI, of whom there were significantly more girls than boys, boys: $n = 10$ (28.60%), girls: $n = 25$ (71.40%) (($\chi^2(1) = 10.643$ $p < .001$ $\varphi = .452$). Multiple mediation analyses resulted in a moderated mediation model in which the relationship between symptoms of ADHD and the prevalence of current NSSI was fully mediated by the symptoms of comorbid conditions in both sex. Significant mediators were the symptoms of affective and psychotic disorders and suicidality in both sexes and the symptoms of alcohol abuse/dependence disorders in girls.

Conclusions: ADHD symptoms are associated with an increased risk of NSSI in adolescents, especially in the case of girls. Our findings suggest that clinicians should routinely screen for the symptoms of ADHD and comorbidity, with a special focus on the symptoms of affective disorders and alcohol abuse/dependence psychotic symptoms to prevent NSSI.

Keywords: Attention-deficit hyperactivity disorder, ADHD, Non-suicidal self-injury, NSSI, Comorbidities, Gender, Clinical sample, Adolescents, Dimensional, Categorical approach

Background

Attention-deficit hyperactivity disorder (ADHD) –the main symptoms of which are inattention, hyperactivity and impulsivity (American Psychiatric Association, 2013) – is one of the most common psychiatric disorders, with a prevalence of 4-6% in children and adolescents [1, 2] and up to two-thirds of them have impairment in adulthood as well [3]. Several studies highlighted that people with ADHD have a significantly lower quality of life than people without ADHD [4–6]. More than two-thirds of ADHD cases have at least one comorbid psychiatric diagnosis, which can be both externalizing and/or internalizing disorders [7–9]. Moreover, it has recently become clear that ADHD is related to high suicidality in all age groups, both in girls and boys [10–14] and comorbid conditions mediate this association [15].

* Correspondence: balazs.judit@ppk.elte.hu; judit.agnes.balazs@gmail.com
[1]Institute of Psychology, Eötvös Loránd University, Izabella str. 46, Budapest 1064, Hungary
[2]Vadaskert Child and Adolescent Psychiatry Hospital, Budapest, Hungary

During the last decades, several clinicians and researchers suggested that besides categorical diagnosis of psychiatric disorders, dimensional approaches should be taken into account both in clinical work and research [16–20]. Recently our research group completed a systematic review on subthreshold ADHD [21]. We found that different definitions of subthreshold ADHD exist, the common point being that the definition of subthreshold ADHD does not fulfil the required criteria of the threshold ADHD definition (according to the classification systems)in children and adolescents [21]. We concluded that the prevalence rate of subthreshold ADHD is wide-ranging (0.8–23.1%), the comorbidity of subthreshold ADHD is high, up to 7% of people with subthreshold ADHD had at least one comorbid disorder, and there are several areas where subthreshold ADHD has a meaningful impact on functioning – for example, children with subthreshold ADHD had a significantly increased risk of grade retention and graduation failure, had fewer friends, more negative reputations and reported lower levels of friendship quality than children without subthreshold ADHD [21]. Moreover our previous results highlighted that even subthreshold ADHD increases the prevalence of suicidality in children and adolescents [15].

Non-suicidal self-injury (NSSI) became an individual diagnosis for the first time in the Diagnostic and Statistical Manual of Mental Disorders 5th Edition (DSM-5), under Section III. 'Conditions for Further Study' [22]. The definition of NSSI in DSM-5 emphasizes the deliberate, non-suicidal purpose of self-injury, which is not a culturally sanctioned behaviour. The prevalence of NSSI in an adolescent population sample was found to be 13–45% [23, 24], while it was 4% in adults [25] and 40–80% in a clinical sample of adolescents [26, 27]. It is also well known today that NSSI is often comorbid with both internalizing and externalizing disorders [28, 29]. Recently, several researchers have focused on the connection between self-injurious behaviours and suicide and found that the two phenomena often overlap [26, 30, 31], and share comorbid conditions, such as borderline personality disorder [32], depression and/or anxiety [33], and/or alcohol dependence [34], and/or ADHD (see below). However, several factors seem to distinguish suicide and NSSI, such as the frequency and methods of self-injuring and specific comorbid and personality disorders [32, 35].

Researchers have been recently a growing interest in a possible association between ADHD and self-injury, including NSSI – already two systematic review papers have summarized the results and found a strong association between ADHD and self-injury [28, 29]. One of the common traits of the two phenomena is poor response inhibition, which is associated with impulsivity [36, 37]. A further question is whether there is a direct association between the symptoms of ADHD and the prevalence of NSSI or whether comorbid conditions mediate this association. Swanson et al. [38] found, in a sample of girls with ADHD, aged 6–12, that the association between ADHD and NSSI is mediated by impulsivity and other symptoms of externalizing disorders. Taylor et al. [39] found, in an adult normal population, that there are significant associations between ADHD symptom severity and self-injury and suicidal behaviour (including ideation and attempts) and they are mediated by comorbidities, such as affective, anxiety, drug, and alcohol abuse disorders and emotion-focused coping style. Based on a 10-year follow-up study of girls aged 6–12, with and without ADHD, and the onset of self-injury in their adulthood, Meza et al. [37] suggested that childhood response inhibition predicted young-adult suicidality, including ideation, suicide attempts and NSSI, and peer victimization in adolescence emerged as a significant partial mediator of young-adult response inhibition and NSSI linkage.

According to our knowledge, there is no previous study that has investigated,in both adolescent girls and boys, whether there is a direct association between their symptoms of ADHD and the prevalence of NSSI or whether comorbidity between ADHD and NSSI conditions mediate this association. Therefore, the objective of the current cross-sectional study was to investigate the prevalence of NSSI in an inpatient clinical sample of adolescent girls and boys, either with the symptoms or with a full diagnosis of ADHD. Although, the cross-sectional nature of the analyses preclude causal inferences, we planned to examine whether there is a direct association between ADHD symptoms (fulfilling or not the diagnostic threshold) and the prevalence of NSSI and how the symptoms of comorbid psychiatric conditions influence this, and whether there is a difference between girls and boys at this age.

Methods

Ethics

The Ethical Committee of the Medical Research Council, Hungary (ETT-TUKEB) approved the study. The parents of all adolescents included in the study, and adolescents older than 14 years provided written informed consent after the nature of the study had been explained. There was no economic or any other type of compensation provided to the participants.

Subjects

Adolescents, who were inpatients in the Vadaskert Child and Adolescent Psychiatric Hospital and Outpatient Clinic, Budapest, Hungary between 25.02.2015 and 09.05.2016, were included in the study. Inclusion criteria were that the adolescent had to be aged between 13 and 18 years and he/she had to be psychiatric inpatient. Exclusion criterion was mental retardation in the medical history.

Measures

Psychiatric symptoms and disorders with both subthreshold and fulfilling diagnostic criteria of the classification systems were evaluated by the Hungarian version of the modified Mini International Neuropsychiatric Interview Kid (M.I.N.I. Kid) 2.0 [40–43]). The M.I.N.I. Kid is a structured diagnostic interview for the assessment of major child/adolescent psychiatric disorders, such as affective disorders (i.e. major depressive episode, dysthymic disorder, hypo/manic episode, anxiety disorders (i.e. panic disorder, agoraphobia, separation anxiety disorder, social anxiety disorder, specific phobia, post-traumatic stress disorder (PTSD), generalized anxiety disorder (GAD)), obsessive-compulsive disorder (OCD), substance-related dependence/abuse (e.g. alcohol abuse/dependence and psychoactive substance abuse/dependence), Tourette's disorder, ADHD, Conduct Disorder (CD), oppositional defiant disorder (ODD), eating disorders (e.g. anorexia nervosa, bulimia nervosa), adjustment disorder, psychotic disorders and suicidality. The interviewer posed the questions of the M.I.N.I. Kid to the adolescent. In its original form, the structure of the M.I.N.I. Kid is branching, which means, if the core symptoms of a disorder are not present, the additional questions on the symptoms of that disorder should not be asked. However, in the current study we used the modified version of the M.I.N.I. Kid, which means we excluded the 'branching logic' and in this way the M.I.N.I. Kid evaluated all the possible symptoms of a disorder. To ensure inter-rater reliability, all interviewers participated in a training course before the study and during the study interviewers were regularly supervised.

Self-injuries were evaluated by the Deliberate Self-Harm Inventory (DSHI) [44]. DSHI is a self-rated questionnaire, which assesses whether people engage in direct self-injury behaviour, self-inflicted damage of the surface of an individual's body by self-cutting, self-burning, self-hitting, self-biting and skin damage by other methods. The questionnaire contains 17 items. The questions on the method of self-injury should be answered by a 'yes' or 'no'. DSHI comprises facets on frequency, severity and duration of self-injury. The DSHI is branching, which means, if all questions on the method of self-injury are answered with 'no,' the additional questions should not be asked. However, if there is at least one 'yes' answer, then the following questions on the age onset, frequency, duration and severity of self-injury should be asked.

Diagnostic definitions

The definition of psychiatric disorders, including ADHD and all comorbid diagnoses, were based on DSM-IV [45]. The definition of subthreshold ADHD required the presence of more than five symptoms of ADHD [15].

Current suicidality was defined as having any suicidal ideations and/or suicide attempt with direct desire to end one's life currently and/or in the past month. The presence of current suicidality was noted if the child answered 'yes' to any of the following questions: In the past month did you: Wish you were dead?;, Want to hurt yourself?; Think about killing yourself?; Think of a way to kill yourself?; Attempt suicide? [40–43].

NSSI was defined according to DSM-5 [22] as a: deliberate, non-suicidal purpose of the self-injurious act, which is not socially sanctioned. It is important to distinguish it from drug overdoses, culturally sanctioned behaviours (e.g. piercings), and repetitive, stereotypical forms among people with developmental disorders. Self-injurious acts should have occurred on at least 5 occasionsin the past year. Moreover, the individual who engages in NSSI must have the aim of achieving a better emotional state after the action [22].

Statistics

Data were analysed using IBM SPSS Statistics 22.0. Descriptive statistics, Mann–Whitney U test, Chi-square test and mediator model were used. In our survey we used bootstrapping procedure (5000 bootstrap sample) in mediator model. Mann-Whitney U test was used in order to show the age difference between gender, and Chi-square test was used to analyze gender differences among adolescents with both ADHD and NSSI. Those M.I.N.I. Kid [40–43] diagnoses that were comorbid with ADHD and had a prevalence of3% or more, were included in comparative and mediator model analyses. According to this the following diagnoses were not included in the statistical analyses: Tourette's syndrome, tic disorder, anorexia nervosa, bulimia nervosa, adjustment disorder, autism spectrum disorder.

In the case of Chi-square and Mann–Whitney U test analyses, the data of those adolescents who had a diagnosis of ADHD according to the M.I.N.I. Kid were included. The data of those adolescents who had no ADHD diagnosis but who had other diagnoses were excluded.

While dichotomous variables cannot be used in a mediator model and only 10 variables can be handled in the model, we added the number of symptoms of the M.I.N.I. Kid diagnoses, and these continuous variables were involved in the model. Thus, in the case of the mediator model we enrolled the whole group of adolescents (n = 202): both those who had an ADHD diagnosis according to M.I.N.I. Kid and those who did not have an ADHD diagnosis, but had more than five ADHD symptoms (subthreshold ADHD), and also those who had fewer than five ADHD symptoms. In the mediator model, the independent variable was the amount of ADHD symptoms and the outcome variable was the number of self-harm-forms according to the DSHI [40], and gender was included as covariate. NSSI variable is based on sum of all 17 Deliberate Self-Harm Inventory (DSHI) items. It means that this variable is created as a sum of YES answers of occurred types of self-harming behavior, because many individuals who self injure use more than one method [44]. In order to show the gender differences, we used gender as the moderator variable in the moderated mediator model.

Mediator variables were the following grouped diagnoses: a) affective disorders: major depressive episode, dysthymic disorder, hypo/manic episode; b) anxiety disorders: panic disorder, agoraphobia, separation anxiety disorder, social anxiety disorder, specific phobia, PTSD, GAD; c) OCD; d) CD and ODD; e) alcohol abuse and dependence; f) psychoactive substance abuse and dependence; g) psychotic disorder; h) suicidality.

The study is asserting statistical mediation with cross-sectional data.

Results

Subjects

The study population included 202 psychiatric inpatient adolescents, 99 (49%) boys and 103 (51%) girls. Mean age of the whole study population was 14.87 years (SD = 1.38), the mean age of boys was 14.8 years (SD = 1.43), while the mean age of girls was 14.94 years (SD = 1.35). There was no significant difference between the mean age of boys and girls (U = 4771.000 z = –.806 $p > .05$).

Altogether 52 (25.7%) adolescents fulfilled the diagnosis of ADHD according to M.I.N.I. Kid, 23 (44.2%) boys and 29 (55.8%) girls. The mean age of adolescents diagnosed with ADHD was 14.75 years (SD = 1.25). The mean age of boys with ADHD was 14.95 years (SD = 1.29), and the mean age of girls was 14.58 years (SD = 1.21). There was no significant difference between the mean age of boys and girls diagnosed with ADHD (U = 290.000 z = –.832 $p > .05$).

Additionally, there were 77 (38.1%) adolescents who had more than five ADHD symptoms – which was the threshold for subthreshold ADHD – but less than the required criteria according to the DSM-IV. The mean age of these adolescents was 14.88 years (SD = 1.53). The 77 adolescents with subthreshold ADHD included 40 boys (52%) and 37 girls (48%). The mean age of boys was 15 years (SD = 1.55), and of girls it was 14.76 years (SD = 1.52). There was no significant difference between the mean age of boys and girls with subthreshold ADHD (U = 675.500 z = –.673 $p > .05$).

Of the 52 adolescents diagnosed with ADHD, 35 (67.30%) had NSSI – 10 (28.60%) boys and 25 (71.40%) girls. There were significantly more girls than boys among the adolescents 'with both ADHD and NSSI($\chi^2(1) = 10.643$ $p < .001$ $\phi = .452$).

Table 1 presents the prevalence of the most common comorbid mental disorders of adolescents with ADHD and NSSI ($n = 35$).

Figure 1. shows the mediation model including path A and path B and the direct pathway/effect between ADHD and NSSI (C′). Path A presents the effect of the symptoms of ADHD (independent variable) on comorbid mental disorders (mediating factors). The symptoms of ADHD predict significantly the symptoms of all measured comorbid mental disorders. Path B presents the effect of comorbid mental disorders on the prevalence of NSSI. Alcohol abuse and dependence, psychotic disorder, suicidal behaviour significantly predict the appearance of NSSI. Gender was included as covariate.

Figure 2. shows the indirect pathway/effect between ADHD and NSSI via mediating factors (path A* path B). The linkage between ADHD and NSSI was fully mediated by comorbid mental disorders. Mediating factors were affective disorders, alcohol abuse and dependence, psychotic disorder and suicidal behaviour. There was no evidence of a statistically significant direct pathway (direct effect (C′) from the symptoms of ADHD to the prevalence of NSSI.

The association among ADHD, NSSI and comorbid mental disorders was analysed with Spearman correlation separately for boys and girls ($N = 202$). According to this result moderated mediation model contains direct and the significant indirect effects by gender (Fig. 3). There was no evidence of a statistically significant direct pathway from the symptoms of ADHD to NSSI either in boys or in girls. The association between the symptoms

Table 1 The prevalence of the most common comorbid mental disorders of adolescents diagnosed with ADHD and NSSI ($n = 35$)

Mental disorders	Prevalence %	n
Suicidality	94	33
ODD	66	23
GAD	63	22
Psychotic disorder	60	21
Mania	51	18
Social anxiety disorder	49	17
OCD	46	16
Major Depressive Episode	43	15
Dysthymia	34	12
Panic disorder	31	11
Separation anxiety disorder	26	9
CD	23	8
Agoraphobia	23	8
Psychoactive substance dependence	23	8
Hypomania	20	7
Specific phobia	20	7
Alcohol abuse /dependence	20	7
Psychoactive substance abuse	20	7
PTSD	17	6

CD Conduct Disorder, *GAD* Generalized Anxiety Disorder, *OCD* Obsessive Compulsive Disorder, *ODD* Oppositional Defiant Disorder, *PTSD* Posttraumatic Stress Disorder

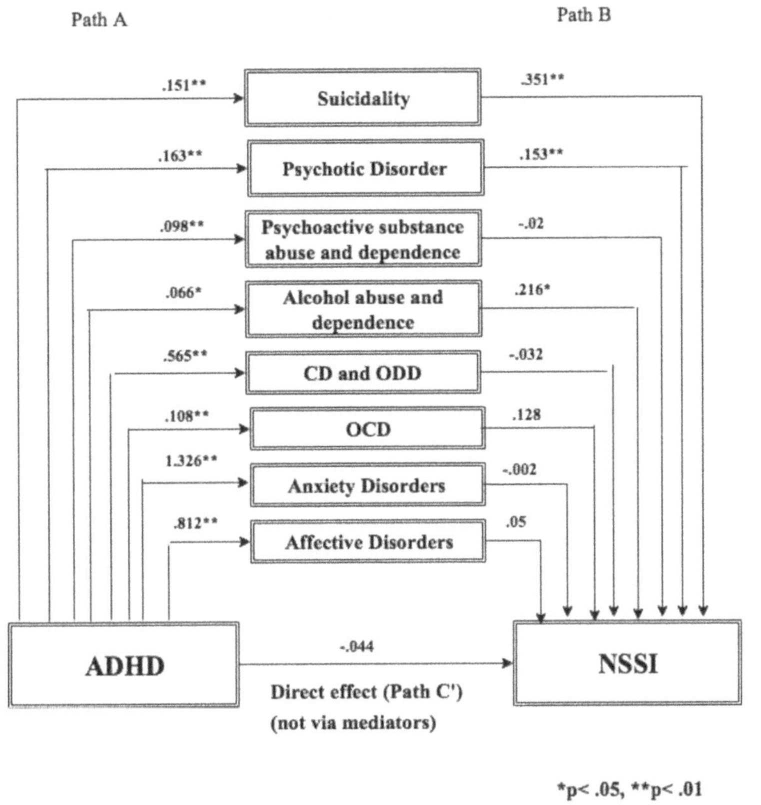

Fig. 1 Mediation model including path A, path B and the direct pathway/effect between ADHD and NSSI (C'). Path A: The effect of the symptoms of ADHD on comorbid mental disorders. Path B: The effect of the comorbid mental disorders on prevalence of NSSI. CD: Conduct Disorder, OCD: Obsessive Compulsive Disorder, ODD: Oppositional Defiant Disorder

of ADHD and the prevalence of NSSI was mediated – indirect effect – by comorbid mental disorders. Mediating factors were for both genders: affective disorders, psychotic disorder, and suicidal behaviour. In addition to these, alcohol abuse and dependence were mediating factors only for girls.

Discussion

Although there has recently been a growing interest in a possible association between ADHD and NSSI [29, 46], to the best of our knowledge this is the first study to have investigated, in an adolescent clinical sample including both girls and boys, whether there is a direct effect of the symptoms of ADHD on NSSI or 'whether comorbidities mediate between these conditions and whether there is an effect of gender on this association.

Although the main focus of the current study was not on the prevalence data, first of all we would like to highlight that based on the self-rated screening tool, more than two-thirds of the adolescents with ADHD had NSSI. Similar to earlier findings [23, 47, 48], in our ADHD subsample gender had a significant effect on NSSI: we found that more than two-thirds of the adolescents with ADHD and NSSI were girls, that is to say that less than half of the boys and more than 85% of the girls had NSSI. Later, we will come back to the discussion of the gender differences found in ADHD and NSSI. All these results have high clinical significance: clinicians should screen for the risk factors of NSSI in their patients with ADHD, with a special focus on girls.

Our results are in line with those previous studies that stated that people with ADHD have a higher risk than those without of developing comorbid psychiatric problems, both externalizing and internalizing ones [7–9]. Focusing on comorbidity of those adolescents with ADHD, who had NSSI as well, in the current study the most common comorbidity next to ADHD and NSSI was suicidality followed by the symptoms of ODD, GAD and psychotic disorders, all of which were present in more the two-thirds of patients with ADHD and NSSI. Almost half of the patients with ADHD and NSSI had comorbid symptoms of manic episode, social phobia and OCD, and one-third of them had the symptoms of comorbid alcohol abuse /dependence, dysthymic and panic disorder, while one-quarter of them had the symptoms of comorbid separation anxiety, agoraphobia, conduct or substance use disorder.

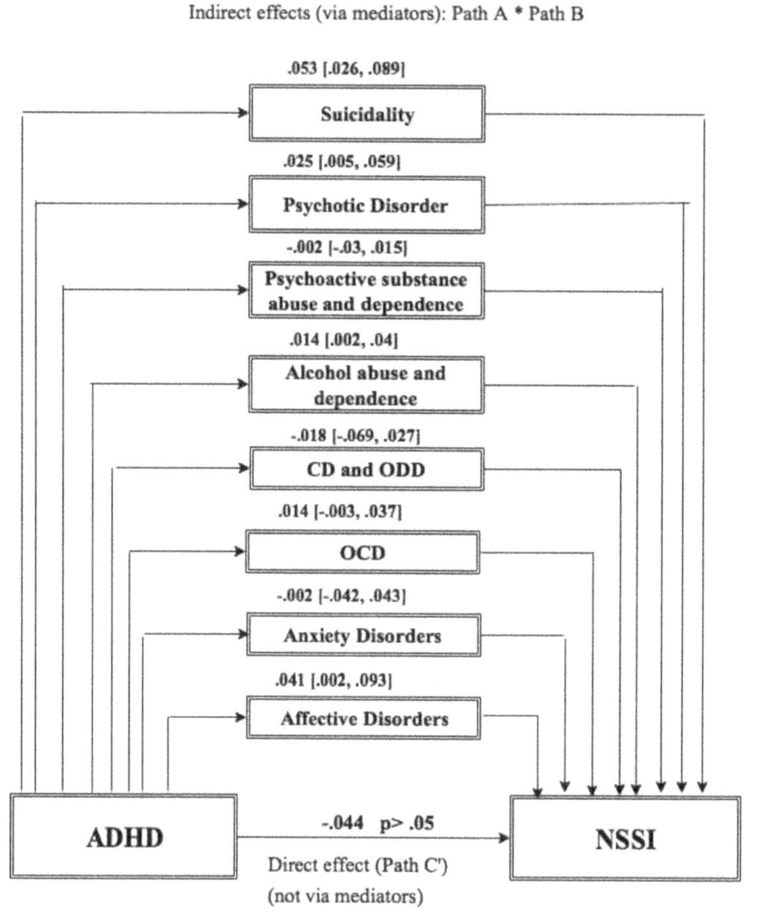

Fig. 2 Mediation model including the indirect pathway/effect via mediating factors (Path A* Path B), and the direct pathway/effect (C') between ADHD and NSSI. *CD:* Conduct Disorder, OCD: Obsessive Compulsive Disorder, ODD: Oppositional Defiant Disorder. Bootstrap-method, BootLLCI-BootULCI: 95% confidence interval: confidence interval not containing 0 implies that there is statistically significant effect

Coming to the discussion of the main focus of the current study, we found that there is no direct association between the symptoms of ADHD and the prevalence of NSSI in a clinical sample of adolescents in any sex. Comorbidities fully mediate the association between these conditions. In both sexes the symptoms of affective disorders, suicidality and psychotic disorders were significant mediators between the symptoms of ADHD and NSSI, while in the case of girls so too were the symptoms of comorbid alcohol abuse/dependence.

There is increasing evidence that NSSI is most often used to attempt to avoid, regulate, reduce or escape from negative emotions, such as anxiety, sadness, or guilt [27, 28, 49]. Even the criterion of NSSI in DSM-5 includes that the individual who engages in NSSI must have the aim of achieving a better emotional state after the action [22]. Moreover the symptoms of ADHD have several negative impacts in everyday life, such as the adolescent cannot pay attention during task sat school or in homework, often has conflict with parents, teachers and peers due to hyperactivity and impulsivity, again the DSM-5 definition includes this criterion as well [22]. All these can all lead to low self-esteem, frustration and depressed mood. This mechanism may explain the mediator role of the symptoms of depression between the symptoms of ADHD and NSSI.

We would like to draw attention to the fact that based on this ADHD inpatient adolescent study population our result supports those recent studies that suggested a strong connection between self-injurious behaviours and suicide [5, 30, 31]: almost all (94%) of our inpatient adolescents with ADHD and NSSI had comorbid suicidality.

Interestingly, an internationally new result in this study is the high comorbidity of the symptoms of psychotic disorder with ADHD and NSSI. The reason for this high psychotic symptom comorbidity may be that the population of the current study included inpatients with ADHD, who may have been admitted to a psychiatric unit not only – or possibly often not – due to the consequences of ADHD, but also because of the presence of

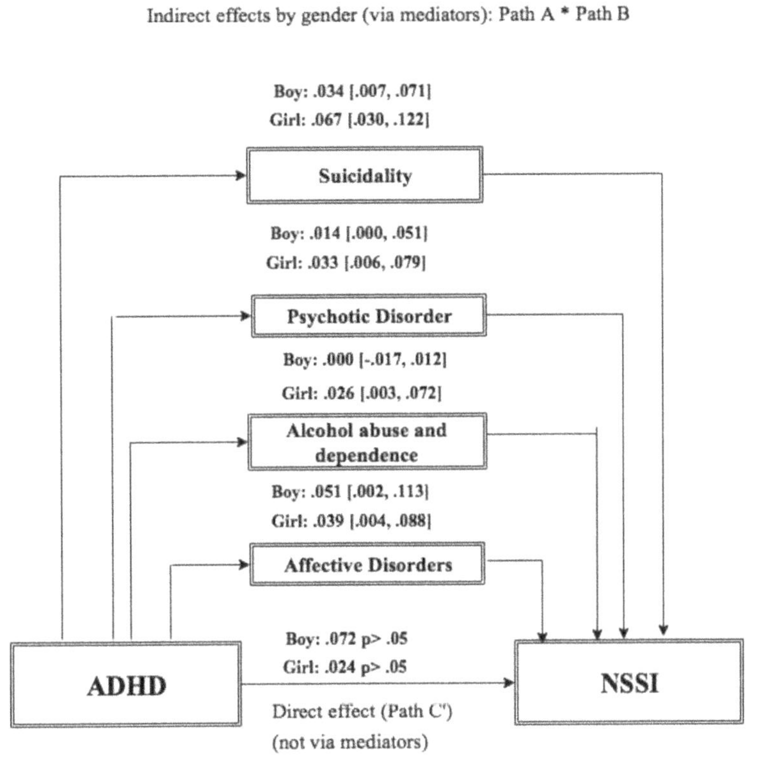

Fig. 3 Mediation model including the significant indirect pathway/effect via mediating factors (Path A* Path B), and the direct pathway/effect between ADHD and NSSI (C') by gender. Bootstrap-method, BootLLCI-BootULCI: 95% confidence interval: confidence interval not containing 0 implies that there is statistically significant effect

severe comorbidities, such as psychotic symptoms. A possible explanation for this new result could be that what Hafner et al. [50] found based on their overview from 1996 to 2016, comparing people with schizophrenia who were in the prodrome at first admission to those with unipolar depression and with healthy controls and then analysed the medium-term (5-year) and long-term (12-year) data. They found that the prodromal stages of schizophrenia and depression were very similar until positive symptoms appeared. The most frequent symptom in schizophrenia is depressed mood [50].

Our results are consistent with those studies that found high comorbidity of NSSI and alcohol abuse/dependence [51] and ADHD and alcohol abuse/dependence [52]. Moreover, Fulwiler et al. [51] did not find differences in the prevalence of alcohol abuse/dependence in the case of people with self-injurious and suicidal behaviour, which could be another explanation of our result on the connection of self-injurious behaviours and suicidality, as described above. Lam et al. [53] also suggest that alcohol and other substance abuse/dependence comorbidity of ADHD could be the link between self-injury and suicidality. Izutsu et al. (2006), focusing on adolescents, found that the prevalence of childhood ADHD is higher among those adolescents with self-injury behaviour, who had comorbid substance use. Furthermore, Hurtig et al. [33] found in their longitudinal cohort study that substance abuse/dependence comorbidity, including alcohol, significantly predicts later NSSI (next to CD and family conflicts) in patients with ADHD.

Previous results on the influence of sex on the pattern and course of comorbid psychopathological conditions 'concurrent with ADHD are still controversial [54–58]. In the current study, besides with the symptoms of psychotic disorders, we found gender differences – again a higher prevalence of girls than boys – in the case of alcohol abuse/dependence and major depressive episode in the comorbidity of ADHD and NSSI, however the differences were only tendencies. One-third of girls with ADHD and NSSI had alcohol dependence as well, while only 10 % of the boys with ADHD and NSSI had this comorbidity. Our result supports those previous researches that found that girls with ADHD have a higher risk of having substance use, including alcohol, than boys [59–63]. The higher prevalence of the comorbidity of psychotic symptoms with ADHD and NSSI in girls needs further research, while previous data supported that in the general population the lifetime prevalence of psychotic symptoms is equal in girls and boys, however the onset of this disorder is earlier in boys [64]. Moreover, examining that part of our ADHD subsample who had no NSSI, we did not find differences in the comorbidity between girls and boys, only that there was a tendency in the case of separation anxiety disorder (again it was higher in girls than in boys). This result supports those previous studies that found that gender does not have an effect on the prevalence of comorbidity with ADHD [65, 66].

Limitations of these findings include their being cross-sectional, therefore no causal relationship was revealed among the investigated factors, we cannot ensure that the mediator (i.e., comorbid diagnoses/ symptoms) came after ADHD symptoms and before the NSSI, moreover mediator variables may temporally occur in between the predictors and the criterion measures. Our data are based self-reported NSSI, which can be biased, i.e., it can be an underestimation, why adolescents may want to deny it. Moreover, we could not use age at which NSSI first occurred in our analyses because there were too many missing and inappropriate data among answers related to this question. Finally, as described the study population are inpatients with ADHD, which suggests that these patients belonged to the more severe end of the spectrum, and in addition the reason for hospitalization could have been comorbid diagnoses, which can be severe comorbidities as well.

Conclusions

In conclusion, the high prevalence of NSSI, especially in the case of girls, and its overlap with suicidality among adolescents with the symptoms of ADHD, calls to the attention of clinicians the importance of screening routinely for the risk factors of NSSI and suicidality in this population, with a special focus on girls. While the symptoms of comorbid conditions of ADHD, such as affective disorders, suicidality, alcohol abuse/dependence and psychotic disorders, fully mediate the relation between the symptoms of ADHD and NSSI, the early recognition and treatment of the symptoms of ADHD and these conditions can be important in the prevention of NSSI.

Abbreviations

ADHD: Attention-Deficit Hyperactivity Disorder; CD: Conduct Disorder; DSHI: Deliberate Self-Harm Inventory; DSM-5: Diagnostic and Statistical Manual of Mental Disorders 5th Edition; ETT-TUKEB: Ethical Committee of the Medical Research Council, Hungary; GAD: Generalized Anxiety Disorder; M.I.N.I. Kid: Mini International Neuropsychiatric Interview Kid; NSSI: Non-Suicidal Self-Injury; OCD: Obsessive-Compulsive Disorder; ODD: Oppositional Defiant Disorder; PTSD: Post-Traumatic Stress Disorder

Acknowledgements

For the careful data collection and entry, we thank Eszter Berényi, Fanni Csepely, Csilla L. Csernitzky, Mária Fehér, Bianka Gyepes, Sára Hawartheh, Gabi Hegedűs, Dalma Jánosi, Krisztina Kerepesi, Norbert Kutor, Rita Margetán, Balázs Mayer, Ádám Nagy, Vera Nemesbüki, Krisztina Pék, Eszter Szabó, Inez Anna Szilágyi, Tímea Tóth, Eszter Varga.

Funding

This work was supported by the Hungarian Scientific Research Fund (Hungarian abbreviation: OTKA, No: K-108336). OTKA grant supported part time research job of Ms. Horvath and Ms. Szentivanyi, who participated in the collection, analysis, and interpretation of the data.
Judit Balazs was supported by the János Bolyai Research Scholarship of the Hungarian Academy of Sciences. Bolyai Research Scholarship supported a part time research job of Dr. Balázs, who participated in designing of the study and in interpretation of data and in writing the manuscript.

Authors' contributions

JB designed the study and wrote the protocol and wrote the first draft of the manuscript. GM was the coordinator of the study. LOH. and DSz. were responsible for the data entry and data collection. DGy made the analyses and participated in the writing the first draft of the manuscript. All authors contributed to and have approved the final manuscript.

Consent for publication

Not applicable.

Competing interests

The authors declare that they have no competing interests.

Author details

[1]Institute of Psychology, Eötvös Loránd University, Izabella str. 46, Budapest 1064, Hungary. [2]Vadaskert Child and Adolescent Psychiatry Hospital, Budapest, Hungary. [3]Doctoral School of Psychology, Eötvös Loránd University, Budapest, Hungary. [4]Semmelweis University, School of Ph.D. Studies, Budapest, Hungary.

References

1. Brown RT, Freeman WS, Perrin JM, Stein MT, Amler RW, Feldman HM, Pierce K, Wolraich ML. Prevalence and assessment of attention-deficit/hyperactivity disorder in primary settings. Pediatrics. 2001;107:E43.
2. Scahill L, Schwab-Stone M. Epidemiology of ADHD in school-age children. Child Adolesc Psychiatr Clin N Am. 2000;9:541–55.
3. Faraone SV, Biederman J, Mick E. The age-dependent decline of attention deficit hyperactivity disorder: a meta-analysis of follow-up studies. Psychol Med. 2006;36(2):159–65.
4. Danckaerts M, Sonuga-Barke EJS, Banaschewski T, Buitelaar J, Döpfner M, Hollis C, Santosh P, Rothengerger A, Sergeant J, Streinhausen HC, Taylor E, Zuddas A, Coghill D. The quality of life of children with attention deficit/hyperactivity disorder: a systematic review. Eur Child Adolesc Psychiatry. 2009;19:83–105.
5. Velő S, Keresztény Á, Szentiványi D, Balázs J. Quality of life of patients with attention-deficit/hyperactivity disorder: systematic review of the past 5 years. (in Hungarian: Figyelemhiányos-hiperaktivitás zavar diagnózisú gyermekek és felnőttekéletminősége: az elmúlt öt év vizsgálatainak szisztematikus áttekintő tanulmánya.). Neuropsychopharmacol Hung. 2013;15:73–82.
6. Gy D, Miklósi M, Keresztény A, Sz V, Szentiványi D, Gádoros J, Balázs J. Self- and parent-rated quality of life of a treatment Naïve sample of children with ADHD: the impact of age, gender, type of ADHD, and Comorbid psychiatric conditions according to both a categorical and a dimensional approach. J Atten Disord. 2017;21:721–30.
7. Balázs J, Gádoros J. Komorbiditás a gyermekpszichiátriában: Valóban olyan gyakori a mániás epizód - ADHD együttes jelentkezése? Psychiatr Hung. 2005;20:293–8.
8. Biederman J, Newcorn J, Sprich S. Comorbidity of attention deficit hyperactivity disorder with conduct, depressive, anxiety, and other disorders. Am J Psychiatry. 1991;148:564–77.
9. MTA Cooperative Group. A 14-month randomized clinical trial of treatment strategies for attention-deficit/hyperactivity disorder. Arch Gen Psychiatry. 1999;56:1073–86.

10. Biederman J, Ball SW, Monuteaux MC, Mick E, Spencer TJ, McCreary M, Cote M, Faraone SV. New insights into the comorbidity between ADHD and major depression in adolescent and young adult females. J Am Acad Child Adolesc Psychiatry. 2008;47:426–34.
11. Chronis-Tuscano A, Molina BS, Pelham WE, Applegate B, Dahlke A, Overmyer M, Lahey BB. Very early predictors of adolescent depression and suicide attempts in children with attention-deficit/hyperactivity disorder. Arch Gen Psychiatry. 2010;67:1044–51.
12. Galéra C, Bouvard MP, Encrenaz G, Messiah A, Fombonne E. Hyperactivity-inattention symptoms in childhood and suicidal behaviors in adolescence: the youth Gazel cohort. Acta Psychiatr Scand. 2008;118:480–9.
13. Manor I, Gutnik I, Ben-Dor DH, Apter A, Sever J, Tyano S, Weizman A, Zalsman G. Possible association between attention deficit hyperactivity disorder and attempted suicide in adolescents - a pilot study. Europ Psychiatry. 2010;25:146–50.
14. Balázs J, Keresztény A. Attention-deficit/hyperactivity disorder and suicide: a systematic review. World J Psychiatry. 2017;7:44–59.
15. Balazs J, Miklosi M, Kereszteny A, Dallos G, Gadoros J. Attention-deficit hyperactivity disorder and suicidality in a treatment naive sample of children and adolescents. J Affect Didord. 2014;152-154:282–7.
16. Balazs J, Miklosi M, Kereszteny A, Hoven CW, Carli V, Wasserman C, Apter A, Bobes J, Brunner R, Cosman D, Cotter P, Haring C, Iosue M, Kaess M, Kahn JP, Keeley H, Marusic D, Postuvan V, Resch F, Saiz PA, Sisask M, Snir A, Tubiana A, Varnik A, Sarchiapone M, Wasserman D. Adolescent subthreshold-depression and anxiety: psychopathology, functional impairment and increased suicide risk. J Child Psychol and Psychiatry. 2013;54:670–7.
17. Bertha EA, Balazs J. Subthreshold depression in adolescence: a systematic review. Europ Child Adolesc Psychiatry. 2013;22:589–603.
18. Lecrubier Y. Refinement of diagnosis and disease classification in psychiatry. Eur Arch Psychiatry Clin Neurosci. 2008;258(Suppl. 1):6–11.
19. Möller HJ. Systematic of psychiatric disorders between categorical and dimensional approaches: Kraepelin's dichotomy and beyond. Eur Arch Psy Clin N. 2008;258(Suppl 2):48–73.
20. Okasha A. Would the use of dimensions instead of categories remove problems related to subthreshold disorders? Eur Arch Psy Clin N. 2009; 259(Suppl 2):129–33.
21. Balázs J, Keresztény A. Subthreshold attention deficit hyperactivity in children and adolescents: a systematic review. Europ Child Adolesc Psychiatry. 2014;23:393–408.
22. American Psychiatric Association. Diagnostic and statistical manual of mental disorders fifth edition. Washington, DC, London, England: American Psychiatric Association; 2013.
23. Brunner R, Kaess M, Parzer P, Fischer G, Carli V, Hoven C, Wasserman C, Marchiapone M, Apter A, Balazs J, Bobes J, Cosman D, Haring C, Iosue M, Kahn JP, Keeley H, Marusic D, Meszaros G, Resch F, Saiz P, Varnik A, Wasserman D. Life-time prevalence and psychosocial correlates of adolescent direct self-injurious behavior: a comparative study of findings in 11 European countries. Europ Child Adolesc Psychiatry. 2013;55:337–48.
24. Nock MK. Self-injury. Ann Rev Clin Psychol. 2010;6:339–63.
25. Briere J, Gil E. Self-mutilation in clinical and general population samples: prevalence, correlates, and functions. Am J Orthop. 1998;68:609–20.
26. Jacobson CM, Muehlenkamp JJ, Miller AL, Turner JB. Psychiatric impairment among adolescents engaging in different types of deliberate self-harm. J Cli Child Adolesc Psychology. 2008;37:275–363.
27. Nock MK, Prinstein MJ. A functional approach to the assessment of self-mutilative behavior. J Consult Clin Psy. 2004;72:885–90.
28. Bentley KH, Cassiello-Robbins CF, Vittorio L, Sauer-Zavala S, Barlow DH. The association between nonsuicidal self-injury and the emotional disorders: a meta-analytic review. Clin Psychol Rev. 2015;37:72–88.
29. Meszaros G, Horváth LO, Balazs J. Self-Injury and externalizing pathology: a systematic literature review. BMC Psychiatry. 2017;17:160.
30. Darke S, Török M. Childhood physical abuse, non-suicidal self-harm and attempted suicide amongst regular injecting drug users. Drug Alcohol Depend. 2013;133:420–6.
31. Nock MK, Joiner TE Jr, Gordon KH, Lloyd-Richardson E, Prinstein MJ. Non-suicidal self-injury among adolescents: diagnostic correlates and relation to suicide attempts. Psychiatry Res. 2006;144:65–72.
32. Garcia-Nieto R, Blasco-Fontecilla H, de Leon-Martinez V, Baca-Garcia E. Clinical features associated with suicide attempts versus suicide gestures in an inpatient sample. Archives of Suicide Research. 2014;18:419–31.
33. Hurtig T, Taanila A, Moilanen I, Nordstrom T, Ebeling H. Suicidal and self-harm behaviour associated with adolescent attention deficit hyperactivity disorder-a study in the northern Finland birth cohort 1986. Nord J Psychiatry. 2012;66:320–8.
34. Ilomaki E, Rasanen P, Viilo K, Hakko H. Suicidal behavior among adolescents with conduct disorder–the role of alcohol dependence. Psych Res. 2007;150:305–11.
35. Fulwiler C, Forbes C, Santangelo SL, Folstein M. Self-mutilation and suicide attempt: distinguishing features in prisoners. JAm Acad Psych Law. 1997;25:69–77.
36. Hinshaw SP, Owens EB, Zalecki C, Huggins SP, Montenegro-Nevado AJ, Schrodek E, Swanson EN. Prospective follow-up of girls with attention-deficit/hyperactivity disorder into early adulthood: continuing impairment includes elevated risk for suicide attempts and self-injury. J Cons Clin Psychology. 2012;80:1041–51.
37. Meza J, Owens EB, Hinshaw SP. Response inhibition, peer preference and victimization, and self-harm: longitudinal associations in young adult women with and without ADHD. J Abnor Child Psychol. 2016;44:323–34.
38. Swanson EN, Owens EB, Hinshaw SP. Pathways to self-harmful behaviors in young women with and without ADHD: a longitudinal examination of mediating factors. J Child Psychol Psychiatry. 2014;55:505–15.
39. Taylor MR, Boden JM, Rucklidge JJ. The relationship between ADHD symptomatology and self-harm, suicidal ideation, and suicidal behaviours in adults: a pilot study. ADHD Attent Deficit Hyperact Disord. 2014;6:303–12.
40. Balazs J, Biró A, Lefkovics E, Tamás Z, Nagy P, Gádoros J. A Gyermek M.I.N.I. kérdőív magyar nyelvű változatának ismertetése. Psychiatria Hungarica. 2004;19:358–64.
41. Lecrubier Y, Sheehan DV, Weiller E, Amorim P, Bonora L, Sheehan KH, Janavs J, Dunbar GC. The MINI international neuropsychiatric interview (M. I. N. I.). A short diagnostic structured interview: reliability and validtiy according the CIDI. Eur Psychiat. 1997;12:224–31.
42. Sheehan DV, Lecrubier Y, Sheehan KH, Amorim P, Janavs J, Weiller E, Hergueta T, Baker R, Dunbar GC. The Mini-international neuropsychiatric interview (M.I.N.I.): the development and validation of a structured diagnostic psychiatric interview for DSM-IV and ICD-10. J Clin Psychiatry. 1998;59(Suppl. 20):22–33. 34-57
43. Sheehan DV, Sheehan KH, Shytle RD, Janavs J, Bannon Y, Rogers JE, Milo KM, Stock SL, Wilkinson B, Wilkinson B. Reliability and validity of the Mini international neuropsychiatric interview for children and adolescents (MINI-KID). J Clin Psychiatry. 2010;71:313–26.
44. Gratz KL. Measurement of deliberate self-harm: preliminary data on the deliberate self-harm inventory. J Psychopathol Behav Assess. 2001;23:253–63.
45. American Psychiatric Association. Diagnostic and statistical manual of mental disorders fourth revied edition. Washington, DC: American Psychiatric Association; 1994.
46. Allely CS. The association of ADHD symptoms to self-harm behaviours: a systematic PRISMA review. BMC Psychiatry. 2014;14:133.
47. Bresin K, Schoenleber M. Gender differences in the prevalence of nonsuicidal self-injury: a meta-analysis. Clin Psychol Review. 2015;38:55–64.
48. Csorba J, Dinya E, Plener P, Nagy E, Páli E. Clinical diagnoses, characteristics of risk behaviour, differences between suicidal and non-suicidal subgroups of Hungarian adolescent outpatients practising self-injury. Europ Child Adoles Psychiatry. 2009;18:309–20.
49. Klonsky ED. The functions of deliberate self-injury: a review of the evidence. Clin Psychol Rev. 2007;27:226–39.
50. Häfner H, Maurer K, an der Heiden W. ABC schizophrenia study: an overview of results since 1996. Soc Psychiatry Psychiatr Epidemiol. 2013;48:1021–31.
51. Fulwiler C, Forbes C, Santangelo S, Folstein M. Self-mutilation and suicide attempt: distinguishing features in prisoners. Am Acad Psych Low. 1997;25(1):69–77.
52. Biederman J, Carter RP, Monuteaux MC, Fried R, Byrne D, Mirto T, Spencer T, Wilens TE, Faraone SV. Adult psychiatric outcomes of girls with attention deficit hyperactivity disorder: 11-year follow-up in a longitudinal case-control study. Am J Psychiatry. 2010;167:409–17.
53. Lam T. Attention deficit disorder and hospitalization owing to intra- and interpersonal violence among children and young adolescents. J Adolesc Health. 2005;36:19–24.

54. Izutsu T, Shimotsu S, Matsumoto T, Okada T, Kikuchi A, Kojimoto M, Noguchi H, Yoshikawa K. Deliberate self-harm and childhood hyperactivity in junior high school students. Europ Child Adolsc Psychiatry. 2006;15:172–6.
55. Biederman J, Monuteaux MC, Mick E, Spencer T, Wilens TE, Silva JM, Snyder E, Faraone SV. Young adult outcome of attention deficit hyperactivity disorder: a controlled 10-year follow-up study. Psychol Med. 2006;36:167–79.
56. Keresztény A, Dallos G, Miklósi M, Róka A, Gádoros J, Balázs J. A gyermek- és serdülôkori figyelemhiányos-hiperaktivitás zavar komorbiditásainak összehasonlítása. [comparing the comorbidity of attention-deficit/hyperactivity disorder in childhood and adolescence]. Psychiatr Hung. 2012;27:165–73.
57. Lewinsohn PM, Rohde P, Seeley JR. Adolescent psychopathology: III the clinical consequences of comorbidity. J Am Acad Child Adolesc Psychiatry. 1995;34:510–9.
58. Willcutt EG, Pennington BF, Chhabildas NA, Friedman MC, Alexander J. Psychiatric comorbidity associated with DSM-IV ADHD in a nonreferred sample of twins. J Am Acad Child Adolesc Psychiatry. 1999;38:1355–13621.
59. Gittelman R, Mannuzza S, Shenker R, Bonagura N. Hyperactive boys almost grown up. I. Psychiatric Status. Arch Gen Psychiatry. 1985;42:937–47.
60. Biederman J, Monuteaux MC, Mick E, Spencer T, Wilens TE, Klein KL, Price JE, Faraone SV. Psychopathology in females with attention-deficit/hyperactivity disorder: a controlled, five-year prospective study. Biol Psychiatry. 2006;60:1098–105.
61. Biederman J, Mick E, Faraone SV, Braaten E, Doyle A, Spencer T, Wilens TE, Frazier E, Johnson MA. Influence of gender on attention deficit hyperactivity disorder in children referred to a psychiatric clinic. Am J Psychiatry. 2002; 159:36–42.
62. Matuszka B, Bácskai E, Czobor P, Egri T, Gerevich J. Associations between concurrent use of tobacco and alcohol and symptoms of attention-deficit hyperactivity disorder among ninth grader students. (In Hungarian: A dohányzás és az alkoholfogyasztás együttes előfordulásának összefüggései a figyelemhiányos hiperaktivitás-zavar tüneteivel kilencedik osztályos tanulók körében.). Orv Hetil. 2015;156:1750–7.
63. Ottosen C, Petersen L, Tidselbak Larsen J, Dalsgaard S. Gender differences in associations between attention-deficit/hyperactivity disorder and substance use disorder. J Am Acad Child Adolesc Psychiatry. 2016;55:227–34.
64. Häfner H, Maurer K, Löffler W. An der Heiden W, Munk-Jørgensen P, Hambrecht M, Riecher-Rössler a. The ABC schizophrenia study: a preliminary overview of the results. Soc Psychiatry Psychiatr Epidemiol. 1998;33:380–6.
65. Biederman J, Kwon A, Aleardi M, Chouinard VA, Marino T, Cole H, Mick E, Faraone SV. Absence of gender effects on attention deficit hyperactivity disorder: findings in nonreferred subjects. Am J Psychiatry. 2005;162:1083–9.
66. Novik TS, Hervas A, Ralston SJ, Dalsgaard S, Pereira RR, Lorenzo MJ. Influence of gender on attention-deficit/ hyperactivity disorder in Europe – ADORE. EuropChild. Adolesc Psychiatry. 2006;15:I/15–24.

3

Education and employment status of adults with autism spectrum disorders in Germany

Fabian Frank[1,2*], Martina Jablotschkin[1,3], Tobias Arthen[1], Andreas Riedel[1], Thomas Fangmeier[1], Lars P. Hölzel[1,4] and Ludger Tebartz van Elst[1]

Abstract

Background: Adults with autism spectrum disorders (ASD) experience challenges in participating in the labour market and struggle to achieve and maintain appropriate professional positions, possibly due to impairments of communication and social interaction. Studies have shown high rates of unemployment as well as evidence of inadequate employment. As knowledge on the participation in the German labour market is scarce, the aim of our study was to examine employment status, type of occupation and inadequate employment in a sample of clinically mostly late-diagnosed and most likely not intellectually disabled adults with ASD in Germany.

Methods: We conducted a cross-sectional-survey in clinically mostly late-diagnosed adults with ASD. Employment status, type of occupation, and the level of formal education and training were examined through a postal questionnaire. Inadequate employment regarding participants' current and longest practised occupation was assessed by transforming participants' information into skill levels of the "Classification of Occupations 2010" of the German Federal Employment Agency, and comparing these with participants' level of formal education and training.

Results: The response rate was 43.2% ($N = 185$ of $N = 428$ potential participants). 94.6% were first-time diagnosed when being 18 years of age or older. 56.8% held a general university entrance-level qualification and 24.9% had obtained a Masters' or diploma degree as their highest vocational qualification. 94.1% had been employed at some time. Of these, 68.4% reported being currently employed, 13.5% being currently unemployed and 17.0% being retired for health reasons. Regarding the longest-practised and the current occupation, the highest proportion of participants was found in the occupational area "health and social sector, teaching and education" (22.4% and 23.3%, respectively). With respect to inadequate employment, 22.1% were found to be overeducated in relation to their longest-practised occupation and 31.3% in relation to their current occupation. This is significantly higher than the percentage of overeducation in the general population.

Conclusions: Despite largely high formal qualifications, the clinically mostly late-diagnosed adults with ASD represented in our sample are disadvantaged regarding their participation in the German labour market, especially with respect to rates of unemployment, early retirement and overeducation. Employment support programs should be developed to improve employment outcomes.

Keywords: Autism, Asperger syndrome, High functioning, Employment, Education, Adults

* Correspondence: fabian.frank@uniklinik-freiburg.de
[1]Department of Psychiatry and Psychotherapy, Medical Center – University of Freiburg, Faculty of Medicine, University of Freiburg, Hauptstraße 5, 79104 Freiburg, Germany
[2]Department of Social Work, Protestant University of Applied Sciences Freiburg, Bugginger Straße 38, 79114 Freiburg, Germany
Full list of author information is available at the end of the article

Background

Autism spectrum disorders (ASD) are associated with qualitative impairment in using and contextualizing communication for social purposes and the capacity to process socially relevant information, and with restrictive repetitive behaviour patterns [1, 2]. Given that the capacity to process socially relevant information and to interact in a socially suitable manner are essential requirements in occupational environments, everyday work processes can pose major challenges for adults with ASD [3], as most workplaces require adherence to social norms and decorum. With respect to social and sensory issues interfering with their job performance [4] as well as potential problems regarding their ability to manage social and interactional aspects of work [5, 6], earlier studies revealed challenges in obtaining, securing and maintaining employment in adults with ASD [7–9]. Furthermore, successful participation in the labour market can be hindered by differences with employers, for example regarding the understanding of productivity requirements or required support in work [10], and by possible ASD-related problems, for example prioritization and self-organization of work-tasks.

Even in adults with ASD and no co-occuring intellectual disability, studies show high rates of unemployment up to 60% [4, 5, 8, 9, 11–14]. In this context, it is important to recognize that adults with ASD are often high educational achievers in terms of school and university qualifications [12, 13] and therefore apparently have good prerequisites for adequate participation in the labour market. However, a recent Australian study by Baldwin et al. [15] showed that 46.2% of employed adults with ASD were inadequately employed or overeducated, meaning that their highest level of formal education and training exceeded the occupational skill level needed for their current occupation. These findings indicate that even though individuals with ASD often possess high levels of formal education and training [12, 15] and desire to work [16], adults with ASD often struggle to participate in the labour market or to achieve and maintain appropriate professional positions.

Apart from studies reporting rates of 60% not-working (employable age, but no occupation due to i.e. being retired for health reasons, being homemaker or being unemployed) [12] or of 36.0% being unemployed [4] knowledge on the participation of adults with ASD in the German labour market in terms of adequate employment is scarce. Therefore, the aim of our study was to examine, by means of a cross-sectional-survey, the integration of a sample of clinically mostly late-diagnosed and most likely not intellectually disabled adults with ASD in the German labour market in terms of employment status, type of occupation and, in particular, regarding adequate or inadequate employment in terms of over- or undereducation.

Methods

Design and sample

The study population of the present postal cross-sectional-survey consists of a sample of clinically mostly late-diagnosed and most likely not intellectually disabled individuals with ASD who attended the "specialised outpatient assessment clinic for ASD in adulthood" (Spezialsprechstunde für Autismus-Spektrum-Störungen im Erwachsenenalter) of the Medical Center – University of Freiburg for diagnostic analysis between September 2009 and March 2014. Clinically late-diagnosed means, that ASD was first time diagnosed when individuals were in adult age of 18 years or older. Diagnostic analysis was based on a structured clinical examination following ICD-10 and DSM-IV criteria, the NICE-Guidelines [17] and the German S3-Guidelines for diagnosing ASD [18]. A detailed description of the diagnostic approach and of the procedures and measures used is provided elsewhere [12, 19]. All individuals aged 18 years or older diagnosed with ASD during this consultation between September 2009 and March 2014, who did not object to being contacted for research purposes, were included in the study. Formal IQ-testing was not part of the diagnostic process in all of these individuals. Of those individuals who have undergone formal IQ-testing, no individual possessed an IQ-score below 70. Furthermore, based on the educational performance and other assessments, we do not except any of the diagnosed individuals to be ranged as intellectually disabled. Therefore, it is most likely, that there are no individuals with co-occuring intellectual disability represented in our initial sample. Between September 2009 and March 2014, $N = 485$ individuals were diagnosed with ASD. $N = 57$ objected being contacted for research purposes. Therefore, the potential study population comprised $N = 428$ adults with ASD. In October 2015 these individuals received information on the study and a questionnaire by post. A post-paid and post-addressed return envelope was enclosed, and a reminder letter was sent to all potential participants after two weeks, as these measures are associated with an increased response rate [20]. The survey was conducted with full anonymity and participation was voluntary. The study was approved by the Ethics Review Committee of the Medical Centre – University of Freiburg (number: 288/15).

Measures and procedures

Regarding the level of formal education and training, the employment status, the type of occupation, and the occupational skill level, the following measures were obtained or derived from participants.

Employment status

Initially, participants were asked whether they had ever been employed (yes/no). Thereupon, participants who had ever been employed were asked whether they were employed at present (yes/no) and, if so, how many hours they usually worked per week and whether their employment was located in a sheltered environment (yes/no). Additionally, participants who had ever been employed were asked whether they rated themselves as currently unemployed (yes/no), for how many months they had been unemployed within the last five years, and whether they had already retired (yes/no), and for which reasons (age, early retirement, health reasons).

Type of occupation

To classify the occupation type for the current and the longest practised occupation, the survey asked participants to record (a) their professional activity, (b) their subject area, and (c) their economic sector within short open-ended questions for both, the current and the longest practised occupation. This information was used to assign each participant to an occupational grouping according to the "Classification of Occupations 2010" (Klassifikation der Berufe 2010; KldB) of the German Federal Employment Agency [21]. The KldB codes all jobs and occupations in the German labour market by means of a five-digit documentation code. The first digit describes the occupational area, the second indicates the major occupational group, the third represents the sub-major occupational group, the fourth shows the minor occupational group, and the fifth describes the occupational skill level [21]. To ensure a consistent transformation of participants' occupational information into the KldB classification, an online database of the German Federal Employment Agency was used [22]. The occupational information recorded by the participants was entered into this database and automatically transformed into the five-digit documentation code of the KldB. Additionally the derived KldB five-digit documentation codes of every participant were manually reviewed for plausibility and adjusted if necessary. An explanatory example for the transformation of participants' information into KldB five-digit documentation codes – in this case the documentation code for a medical specialist in psychiatry – is given in Table 1.

To assess differences from the general population, participants' data regarding the occupational area (first digit of the KldB five-digit documentation codes) of the current occupation was compared to data from the German Federal Employment Agency [23].

Occupational skill level and level of formal education

The fifth digit of each occupation listed within the KldB describes the occupational skill level. The KldB comprises four skill levels, which are differentiated as follows: level 1 – assistant or semi-skilled occupational activities; level 2 – professional oriented occupational activities; level 3 – complex specialist occupational activities; level 4 – highly complex occupational activities [23]. According to the Institute for Employment Research (Institut für Arbeitsmarkt- und Berufsforschung) of the German Federal Employment Agency skill levels are primarily defined by the required level of formal education and training [24], as shown in Table 2.

For each participant, the occupational skill level was recorded based on the previously derived KldB five-digit documentation code. To assess inadequate employment, i.e. over- or undereducation in relation to the current and the longest-practised occupation, we compared the skill level of the related KldB documentation code with the skill level derived from the level of formal education and training. Inadequate employment in terms of overeducation is assumed if a lower KldB skill level is accompanied by a higher KldB level of formal education and training. Conversely, undereducation is indicated if a higher KldB skill level is accompanied by a lower KldB level of formal education and training. Overeducation and undereducation were examined for both the longest-practiced occupation and the occupation pursued at the time of the survey. To assess differences compared to the general population, participants' data regarding over- or undereducation with respect to the current occupation was compared to data derived from the employment statistics of the German Federal Employment Agency [25].

Table 1 Example for transformation of participants' information into KldB codes

Description of occupation within the survey					
survey Item	professional activity	subject area		economic sector	
example	physician	psychiatry		health care system	
Transformation in 5-digit documentation code of the KldB [21, 22]					
structure	occupational area	occupational group			occupational skill level
		major	sub-major	minor	
5-digit code	8	1	4	6	4
explanation	health and social sector	medical health	human and dental medicine	psychiatric consultant	highly complex occupational activities

Table 2 Formal level of education and training transferred to KldB

Formal level of education	KldB occupational skill level	
Master's degree or Diploma university	4	highly complex occupational activities
Master's degree or Diploma university of applied sciences		
Bachelor's degree: university or university of applied sciences/technical college	3	complex specialist occupational activities
Apprenticeship II: technical school, master school or vocational academy		
Apprenticeship I: dual system of vocational and educational training within vocational schools and/or companies	2	professional orientated occupational activities
Other vocational qualification	1	assistant or semi-skilled occupational activities
No vocational qualification		

Sociodemographic and clinical variables

Sociodemographic data (age, sex, marital and relationship status, school-leaving qualification) and presence of comorbidities were collected using the German Health Interview and Examination Survey for Adults [26]. Additional clinical variables (ASD diagnosis, age at first-time ASD diagnosis) were collected using self-constructed items.

Pretest

Since individuals with ASD often have peculiarities in their understanding and use of language [27], impairment of linguistic pragmatics was considered in the construction of the questionnaire. Therefore, the endeavor was to use comprehensible and unequivocal formulation, which was examined within a pretest in five adults diagnosed with ASD using think-aloud methodology [28]. The questionnaire was then adapted linguistically and visually based on the results of this pretest. The final version of the questionnaire is available in German as a supplementary file (see Additional file 1).

Statistical analysis

Descriptive data analysis was performed using IBM SPSS Statistics for Windows, version 21. Comparisons of participants' data with data from the general population were conducted using Chi-square tests.

Results

The response rate was 43.2% (N = 185 of N = 428 potential participants). Participants' sociodemographic and clinical characteristics are summarized in Table 3.

The majority of the participants is male (61.6%) and the mean age of the sample was 39.5 (SD 11.3) years (c.f. Table 3). 36.6% were in a long-term relationship. The most frequent self-reported ASD diagnosis was asperger's syndrome (78.9%), while the mean age at first-time diagnosis of any ASD was 34.7 (SD 12.5) years. 94.6% were 18 years of age or older at first-time diagnosis of any ASD and hereby can be classified as clinically late-diagnosed. The most frequent self-reported comorbidity was depression, at 48.9% (c.f. Table 3).

Level of formal education and training

Regarding the general education level, 11.9% of the participants held a certificate of basic secondary education (German: Hauptschulabschluss; 9 years school attendance; lower secondary level), 28.6% had a general certificate of secondary education (German: Realschulabschluss; 10 years school attendance; lower secondary level), 56.8% had a general university entrance-level qualification (German: Hochschulreife; 12 or 13 years school attendance; upper secondary level), and 2.7% had no school-leaving certificate or had a qualification that was not further specified (missing data N = 0).

With regard to the level of formal education and training according to the KldB, 13.3% of the participants were assigned to skill level 1 (10.5% no vocational qualification; 2.8% other vocational qualification), 43.1% to skill level 2 (43.1% apprenticeship I), 12.7% to skill level 3 (8.8% apprenticeship II; 3.9% Bachelor's degree), 24.9% to skill level 4 (8.8% Master's or diploma degree from university of applied sciences; 16.0% Master's or diploma degree from university), and 6.1% were still in vocational education and training, meaning that their skill level was not specified within the KldB classification (missing data N = 4).

Employment status

Regarding the employment status, 94.1% (N = 174) of the participants reported having ever been employed (missing data N = 0). Of these, 68.4% (N = 119) reported being employed at present, with an average number of 33.3 h worked per week (SD 12.1; missing data N = 6) and 8.0% reported working in a sheltered workshop (missing data N = 6). Regarding the current employment situation of participants who had ever been employed, 17.0% were in early retirement for health reasons (missing data N = 3) and 13.5% stated that they were unemployed (missing data N = 3). Of those who had ever been employed, 49.0% reported no periods of unemployment in the five years prior to this survey (missing data N = 17). Participants with periods of unemployment within this time frame (N = 80) reported an average of 24.4 (SD 20.0; Range 0.50 to 60.00) months of unemployment in the last five years (missing data N = 0).

Type of occupation

Apart from the occupational area "armed forces", all KldB occupational areas were represented in the study sample (c.f. Table 4).

Table 3 Sociodemographic and clinical characteristics

Sociodemographic Characteristics			
Gender (N = 185)		Family status (N = 183)[d]	
male[a]	61.6	unmarried[a]	71.0
Age (N = 185)		married[a]	22.4
mean (SD)[b]	39.5 (11.3)	divorced[a]	6.6
minimum[c]	21	Relationship status (N = 183)[d]	
maximum[c]	64	long-term relationship > 6 months[a]	36.6
Clinical Characteristics			
Primary Diagnosis (N = 185)		Comorbidities[a,e,f] (N = 184)	70.1
asperger[a]	78.9	Depression[a]	48.9
atypical[a]	9.7	orthopedic diseases[a]	19.0
infantile[a]	4.3	OCD[a]	13.0
not specified / unknown[a]	7.1	respiratory diseases[a]	11.4
Age when diagnosed I (N = 184)[e]		Age when diagnosed II (N = 184)[e,g]	
mean (SD)[b]	34.7 (12.5)	≥ 18 years of age[a]	94.6
minimum[c]	3	≤ 18 years of age[a]	5.4
maximum[c]	60		

[a]in percent
[b]means and standard deviation
[c]years of age
[d]missing data N = 2
[e]missing data N = 1
[f]just the four most stated comorbidities are listed
[g]being ≥18 years of age at first-time diagnosis is classified as late-diagnosed

Regarding the longest-practised and the current occupation, the highest proportion of participants was found in the occupational area "health and social sector, teaching and education" (22.4% and 23.3%, respectively) followed by "corporate organization, accounting, legal and administrative sectors" (19.3% and 19.4%, respectively). A comparison of participants' distribution across the various occupational areas (regarding their current occupation) with data from the German Federal Employment Agency [23] revealed a significant difference between the study sample and the general population ($Chi^2 = 54.0$; df 8; $p < .001$). In particular, the proportion of participants working in the field of "natural sciences, geography and computer science" was higher than in the general population (c.f. Table 4).

Table 4 Occupational area by KldB

Occupational area by KldB	longest- practiced occupation (N = 161)[b]	current occupation (n = 103)[c]	occupation general population [23][d]
Agricultural, forestry and horticulture sector[a]	1.2	1.0	1.5
Commodity extraction, production and manufacturing[a]	16.1	12.6	22.5
Construction, architecture, surveying[a]	2.5	3.9	5.8
Natural sciences, geography and informatics[a]	13.7	15.5	3.6
Traffic, logistics, protection and security[a]	9.3	9.7	13.2
Commercial services, commodity trading, sale, tourism[a]	9.3	8.7	12.1
Corporate organization, accounting, legal and administrative sectors[a]	19.3	19.4	20.6
Health and social sector, teaching and education[a]	22.4	23.3	17.7
Linguistics, literature, humanities, social and economic sciences, media, art, culture and design[a]	6.2	5.8	2.7

[a]in percent
[b]missing data N = 6; not classifiable N = 7
[c]missing data N = 7; not classifiable N = 9
[d]no data available for the occupational area "armed forces"

Occupational skill level, inadequate employment and overeducation

To assess inadequate employment in terms of over- or undereducation in participants who had ever been employed (N = 174) not including education and training (N = 9), a vocational orientation phase (N = 1), or a so-called one-euro-job (N = 1; one-euro jobs are public services jobs that pay at least one euro per hour and do not affect unemployment benefits in individuals who are registered as unemployed), the KldB skill levels with respect to the longest-practised occupation were compared with participants' highest level of formal education and training according to the KldB skill levels (missing data N = 9). Likewise, for participants who were employed at the time of the survey (N = 119), not including education and training (N = 8), retraining (N = 1) or an internship (N = 1), the KldB skill levels with respect to the current occupation were also compared with participants' highest level of formal education and training according to the KldB skill levels (missing data N = 10).

In Table 5, the column "all" shows the distribution of participants across KldB skill levels regarding their longest-practised and their current occupation. For both, the majority of participants were situated in skill level 2 (50.6% and 41.4%, respectively). The following columns in Table 5 sort participants into three categories relating to the match or mismatch between the skill level of their longest-practised respectively current occupation and their level of formal education and training according to the KldB. In total, 62.3% were found to be at parity regarding the skill requirements of their longest-practised occupation, 15.6% were undereducated, meaning that their skill levels of formal qualification were below the occupational skill requirements, and 22.1% were classified as overeducated (c.f. Table 5). With respect to the current occupation 54.5% were found to be in parity, 14.1% were undereducated and 31.3% were classified as overeducated, meaning that their formal qualifications exceeded the skill requirements needed for the current occupation (c.f. Table 5).

According to data from the employment statistics of the German Federal Employment Agency, 63.0% of the general population in Germany are at parity, 22.0% are undereducated and 15.0% are overeducated in their

Table 5 Occupational skill level, overeducation and undereducation

skill level longest-practiced job[a]		all	parity	undereducated	overeducated
1	n	16	4	–	12
	%	10.4	25.0	–	75.0
2	n	78	56	7	15
	%	50.6	71.8	9.0	19.2
3	n	21	6	8	7
	%	13.6	28.6	38.1	33.3
4	n	39	30	9	–
	%	25.3	76.9	23.1	–
column total	n	154	96	24	34
	%	100	62.3	15.6	22.1
skill level current job[b]		all	parity	undereducated	overeducated
1	n	17	3	–	14
	%	17.2	17.6	–	82.4
2	n	41	26	2	13
	%	41.4	63.4	4.9	31.7
3	n	11	1	6	4
	%	11.1	9.1	54.5	36.4
4	n	30	24	6	–
	%	30.3	80.0	20.0	–
column total	n	99	54	14	31
	%	100	54.5	14.1	31.3

[a]N = 154; missing data N = 9; excluded because of being in education and training N = 9, excluded because of stating the longest practiced occupation being a vocational orientation phase N = 1 or a so-called one-euro-job N = 1

[b]N = 99; missing data N = 10; excluded because of being in education and training N = 8, excluded because of stating the present practiced occupation being retraining N = 1 or an internship N = 1

employment [25]. In this regard, there is a significant difference between the general population and the study sample with respect to under- and overeducation regarding the current occupation (Chi^2 = 21.0; df 2; p < .001).

Discussion

This study aimed to examine the participation of clinically mostly late-diagnosed and most likely not intellectually disabled adults with ASD in the German labour market by means of a postal cross-sectional survey in former patients of the "specialised outpatient assessment clinic for ASD in adulthood" of the Medical Center – University of Freiburg.

A sufficient response rate of 43.2% was achieved. However, as not all potential participants replied, the critical issue is the representativeness of this sample. It remains unclear whether individuals with, for instance, higher psychosocial functioning or better opportunities and achievements in the labour market were more likely to participate in this survey, which might have biased the results. It is most probable that the employment rate and appropriate occupational positions were overestimated, as it is well known in research that individuals are more likely to report positive aspects than negative aspects [29].

Although the majority of our sample was male, the proportion of women was higher than in the typical male-to-female ratio in ASD [30]. However, this ratio is in accordance with comparable studies, which showed higher proportions of women among late-diagnosed adults with ASD [12, 13, 31]. This might be explained by gender specific compensation strategies [32], for example imitation learning, which lead for example to a better social adjustment and therefore a later identification of ASD. Thus, the late first-time diagnosis in 94.6% of the participants in this sample can be deemed as a specificity of this study. Our sample probably represents a subsample of adults with ASD comprising more able individuals with comparatively good adaptive and compensatory social skills. This is also reflected in the specificity of our study design and sample, addressing adults with clinically mostly late-diagnosed ASD and most likely no co-occuring intellectual disability. As a consequence, this might also explain the high proportion of participants who were married or in a long-term relationship compared to other studies on psychosocial outcomes in adults with ASD [13, 33, 34]. However, high rates of self-reported comorbidities were found, comparable to those reported in other studies [13, 33], which might also influence participants' employment situation. All participants were at an employable age, with an age range of 21 to 64 years, and therefore represent the relevant target group of this survey.

Regarding the general level of education, the sample considerably exceeds the educational attainment of the general population, with 56.8% of participants possessing university entrance-level qualifications, compared to 29.5% within the general population in Germany in 2015 [35]. In Germany the university graduate ratio was 32.0% in 2014 [36], and 14.8% of the general population possessed a Masters' or diploma degree as their highest vocational qualification in 2015 [35] and would therefore be assigned to skill level 4 of the KldB in terms of the level of formal education and training. This falls well below the percentage of study participants in our sample assigned to skill level 4 (24.9%). As the proportion of participants with no qualifications (10.5%) or a not further specified qualification (2.8%) who can therefore be assigned to KldB skill level 1, is also below that of individuals with no vocational qualifications in the general population in Germany (16.8%) in 2015 [35], our sample shows a comparatively high level of formal education and training in adults with late-diagnosed ASD, which potentially leads to promising chances in the labour market. In this respect – at first glance – participants' participation in the labour market seems satisfactory, as only 5.9% had never been employed. However, only 68.4% of those who had ever been employed were currently employed at the time of the survey. Moreover, a self-reported unemployment rate of 13.5% was found, which considerably exceeds the current unemployment rate in Germany, which lay at 6.4% in 2015 [37]. It appears that – despite partly high formal qualifications and a share of 49.0% of participants having never experienced times of unemployment – adults with ASD often experience problems in maintaining stable employment relationships. In this regard, international studies suggest, that challenges in maintaining employment in adults with ASD can be explained by social and sensory issues interfering with their job performance as well as their ability to manage interactional aspects of work [4–6]. In view of the fact that 17.0% of those participants who had ever been employed later retired early for health reasons, and taking into account the reported high prevalence of comorbidities, it would appear that employment support is necessary that takes into account the specific characteristics of ASD regarding social and sensory issues, as well as further health-related aspects regarding the ability to work.

Although we found a strong trend towards occupations within the area "natural sciences, geography and computer sciences" compared to the general population [23], adults with ASD cover a broad range of occupational areas. In particular, the occupational area "health and social sector, teaching and education" was represented by a high proportion of our sample. This result does not tie in with the stereotype that adults with ASD are only found in more technically orientated, and not socially orientated, professions. These findings are in line with a study by Baldwin et al. [15] who also found that adults with ASD are employed in a wide variety of different occupational environments.

Even though the proportion of participants who were inadequately employed and overeducated was lower than that found in similar studies [12, 15], a significant difference emerged compared to the general population regarding the current occupation, with 31.3% of participants being inadequately employed in terms of overeducation. Moreover, the proportion of participants who were overeducated in their current profession was higher than the proportion of participants who were overeducated in their longest practised profession (22.1%). Thus, it appears that adults with ASD are partly unable to maintain professional positions in accordance with their level of formal qualification. This finding can be linked to studies, showing that differences with employers, i.e. regarding the understanding of productivity requirements and self-organization of work tasks, or possible ASD-related issues, i.e. impaired ability to handle social aspects, can hinder successful participation in the labour market [5–10].

According to our findings, while adults with ASD as seen in our specialised outpatient clinic have above-average levels of formal education and training, at least in part, they experience problems and challenges to establish themselves in the German labour market and/or to sustain professional positions that are appropriate to their level of formal education and training. This is alarming and in need of explanation. It can be assumed that the constraints associated with ASD are better compensated in educational contexts, as potentially impaired executive and soft-skills meet with higher tolerance, and individuals with ASD experience more assistance than is provided in working environments. Furthermore, greater flexibility and autonomy for individuals to utilize their own style of learning and working, with reduced impact of social difficulties, may also be a factor in the higher attainment of individuals with ASD in educational context compared with their employment status. This underlines the need for a better integration and improved support of adults with ASD in occupational settings, and demonstrates that potential strengths associated with ASD, such as honesty, efficiency or precision [38], should be identified and reinforced. This is of particular relevance since support programs for adults with ASD, addressing, e.g., work preparation and communication with employers, proved to be effective in increasing employment rates [39, 40]. A promising approach to meet the support requirements of adults with ASD could be "training-on-the-job" measures, as the most important issue does not seem to lie in obtaining professional positions, but rather in maintaining them. For the development and implementation of such measures, further research on the experience of employment situations in adults with ASD is needed, i.e. expectations regarding workplace design, challenges in professional transitions or experiences with ASD related sensory and interactional difficulties in occupational environments as well as support needs concerning these matters.

Conclusions

Despite an above-average level of general education in terms of school-leaving qualifications and a high level of formal education and training, even exceeding the level within the general population, adults with late-life diagnosis of ASD are at a disadvantage regarding their participation in the labour market in Germany. Consequently, there are high rates of unemployment and early retirement for health reasons represented in our sample. Furthermore, adults with ASD seem to struggle to maintain professional positions that are appropriate to their formal qualifications and are often inadequately employed in terms of overeducation. Based on the results of our study, and on previous studies demonstrating good outcomes from employment support programs, the development of "training-on-the-job" interventions seems particularly promising to enhance the labour market participation of adults with ASD.

Abbreviations

ASD: Autism spectrum disorder; DSM-IV: Diagnostic and Statistical Manual of Mental Disorders 4th Revision; ICD-10: International Statistical Classification of Diseases and Related Health Problems 10th Revision; IQ: Intelligence quotient; KldB: Classification of occupation 2010; NICE: National Institute for Health and Care Excellence

Acknowledgements

The article processing charge was funded by the German Research Foundation (DFG) and the Albert-Ludwigs-University Freiburg in the funding programme Open Access Publishing. We thank Sarah Mannion for copyediting the manuscript.

Funding

Not applicable.

Authors' contributions

FF coordinated the study, participated in formulating the research question, participated in designing the study and the questionnaire, performed the statistical analyses and wrote the paper. MJ participated in the coordination of the study, participated in designing the study and the questionnaire, performed the data acquisition and data management and supported the statistical analyses. TA substantially supported data management as well as the statistical analyses and edited various drafts of the paper. AR and TF participated in formulating the research question, contributed substantially to designing the study and the questionnaires and supported data acquisition. LPH and LTvE formulated the research question, conceptualized the study design and supervised the study. All authors revised the manuscript critically for important intellectual content and read and approved the final manuscript.

Consent for publication

Not applicable.

Competing interests

The authors declare that they have no competing interests.

Author details

[1]Department of Psychiatry and Psychotherapy, Medical Center – University of Freiburg, Faculty of Medicine, University of Freiburg, Hauptstraße 5, 79104 Freiburg, Germany. [2]Department of Social Work, Protestant University of Applied Sciences Freiburg, Bugginger Straße 38, 79114 Freiburg, Germany. [3]Department of Oncological Rehabilitation – UKF Reha gGmbH, Medical Center – University of Freiburg, Breisacher Straße 117, 79106 Freiburg, Germany. [4]Parkklinik Wiesbaden Schlangenbad, Rheingauer Straße 47, 65388 Schlangenbad, Germany.

References

1. Wing L. The autistic spectrum: a guide for parents and professionals. 2nd ed. London: Robinson; 2003.
2. American Psychiatric Association. Diagnostic and statistical manual of mental disorders: DSM-5. Washington, D.C: American Psychiatric Association; 2013.
3. Fried R, Joshi G, Kotte A, Kagan E, Biederman J. Toward developing a simulated workplace laboratory for adults with high functioning autism spectrum disorders. Open J Psychiatr. 2013; https://doi.org/10.4236/ojpsych.2013.33032.
4. Kirchner JC, Dziobek I. Towards successful employment of adults with autism: a first analysis of special interests and factors deemed important for vocational performance. Scand J Child Adolesc Psychiatry Psychol. 2014;2:77–85.
5. Vogeley K, Kirchner JC, Gawronski A, Tebartz van Elst L, Dziobek I. Toward the development of a supported employment program for individuals with high-functioning autism in Germany. Eur Arch Psychiatry Clin Neurosci. 2013;263:197–203.
6. Lawer L, Brusilovskiy E, Salzer MS, Mandell DS. Use of vocational rehabilitative services among adults with autism. J Autism Dev Disord. 2009; 39:487–94.
7. Barnhill GP. Outcomes in adults with Asperger syndrome. Focus Autism Dev Disabil. 2007;22:116–26.
8. Howlin P. Social disadvantage and exclusion: adults with autism lag far behind in employment prospects. J Am Acad Child Adolesc Psychiatry 2013;52(9):897.
9. Barnard J, Harvey V, Potter D, Prior A. Ignored or ineligible?: the reality for adults with autism spectrum disorders. London: National Autistic Society; 2001.
10. Scott M, Falkmer M, Girdler S, Falkmer T. Viewpoints on factors for successful employment for adults with autism spectrum disorder. PLoS One. 2015; https://doi.org/10.1371/journal.pone.0139281.
11. Theunissen G, Kulig W, Leuchte V, Paetz H. Handlexikon Autismus-Spektrum: Schlüsselbegriffe aus Forschung, Theorie, Praxis und Betroffenen-Sicht. Stuttgart: Kohlhammer Verlag; 2014.
12. Riedel A, Schröck C, Ebert D, Fangmeier T, Bubl E, Tebartz van Elst L. Überdurchschnittlich ausgebildete Arbeitslose – Bildung, Beschäftigungsverhältnisse und Komorbiditäten bei Erwachsenen mit hochfunktionalem Autismus in Deutschland. Psychiatr Prax. 2016;43:38–44.
13. Hofvander B, Delorme R, Chaste P, Nydén A, Wentz E, Ståhlberg O, et al. Psychiatric and psychosocial problems in adults with normal-intelligence autism spectrum disorders. BMC Psychiatry. 2009;9:35.
14. Barneveld PS, Swaab H, Fagel S, van Engeland H, de Sonneville LMJ. Quality of life: a case-controlled long-term follow-up study, comparing young high-functioning adults with autism spectrum disorders with adults with other psychiatric disorders diagnosed in childhood. Compr Psychiatry. 2014;55: 302–10.
15. Baldwin S, Costley D, Warren A. Employment activities and experiences of adults with high-functioning autism and Asperger's disorder. J Autism Dev Disord. 2014;44:2440–9.
16. Hendricks D. Employment and Adults with autism spectrum disorders: challenges and strategies for success. J Vocat Rehabil. 2010;32:125–34.
17. National Institute for Health and care Excellence. Autism: guidance and guidelines. 2014. https://www.nice.org.uk/guidance/qs51 22137029. Accessed 9 Mar 2018.
18. DGKJP, DGPPN. S3-Leitlinie Autismus-Spektrum-Störungen im Kindes-, Jugend- und Erwachsenenalter: Teil 1: Diagnostik. 2016. http://www.awmf.org/leitlinien/detail/ll/028-018.html. Accessed 9 Mar 2018.
19. Tebartz van Elst L, Maier S, Fangmeier T, Endres D, Mueller GT, Nickel K, et al. Disturbed cingulate glutamate metabolism in adults with high-functioning autism spectrum disorder: evidence in support of the excitatory/inhibitory imbalance hypothesis. Mol Psychiatry. 2014;19:1314–25.
20. Edwards P, Roberts I, Clarke M, DiGuiseppi C, Pratap S, Wentz R, et al. Methods to increase response rates to postal questionnaires. Cochrane Database Syst Rev. 2007; https://doi.org/10.1002/14651858.MR000008.pub4.
21. Bundesagentur für Arbeit. Klassifikation der Berufe 2010. Nürnberg: Bundesagentur für Arbeit; 2011.
22. Bundesagentur für Arbeit: Dokumentationskennziffern. https://berufenet.arbeitsagentur.de/berufenet/faces/index;BERUFENETJSESSIONID=igMKTSoAdFmegFtRNTwCb3Kwlhc4-oXDsRKl0X0YeiEdtbfttsCa!-1293359102?path=null; 2015. Accessed 9 Mar 2018.
23. Bundesagentur für Arbeit. Berichterstattung nach Berufen: ausgeübte berufliche Tätigkeit. 2016. https://statistik.arbeitsagentur.de/Statistikdaten/Detail/201603/iiia6/beschaeftigung-berufe-sektoren/berufe-sektoren-12-0-201603-xlsx.xlsx. Accessed: 30 Mar 2017.
24. Paulus W, Matthes B. FDZ-Methodenreport 08/2013 Klassifikation der Berufe 2010: Struktur, Codierung und Umsteigeschlüssel. Nürnberg: Bundesagentur für. Arbeit. 2013;
25. Reichelt M, Vicari B. IAB-Kurzbericht 25/2014 Ausbildungsinadäquate Beschäftigung in Deutschland. Nürnberg: Institut für Arbeitsmarkt- und Berufsforschung; 2014.
26. Scheidt-Nave C, Kamtsiuris P, Gößwald A, Hölling H, Lange M, Busch MA, et al. German health interview and examination survey for adults (DEGS) - design, objectives and implementation of the first data collection wave. BMC Public Health. 2012;12:730.
27. Riedel A, Suh H, Haser V, Hermann I, Ebert D, Riemann D, et al. Freiburg questionnaire of linguistic pragmatics (FQLP): psychometric properties based on a psychiatric sample. BMC Psychiatry. 2014;14:374.
28. Someren MW, Barnard YF, Sandberg JAC. The think aloud method: a practical guide to modelling cognitive processes. London: Academic Press; 1994.
29. Fadnes LT, Taube A, Tylleskär T. How to identify information bias due to self-reporting in epidemiological research. IJE. 2009;7(2)
30. Fombonne E, Quirke S, Hagen A. Prevalence and Interpretation of recent trends in rates of pervasive developmental disorders. Mcgill J Med. 2009;12:73.
31. Lehnhardt FG, Gawronski A, Volpert K, Schilbach L, Tepest R, Vogeley K. Das psychosoziale Funktionsniveau spätdiagnostizierter Patienten mit Autismus-Spektrum-Störungen – eine retrospektive Untersuchung im Erwachsenenalter. Fortschritte Neurol Psychiatr. 2012;80:88–97.

32. Dworzynski K, Ronald A, Bolton P, Happé F. How different are girls and boys above and below the diagnostic threshold for autism spectrum disorders? J Am Acad Child Adolesc Psychiatry. 2012;51:788–97.
33. Howlin P. Outcome in adult life for more able individuals with autism or Asperger syndrome. Autism. 2000;4:63–83.
34. Engström I, Ekström L, Emilsson B. Psychosocial functioning in a group of Swedish adults with Asperger syndrome or high-functioning autism. Autism. 2003;7:99–110.
35. Statistisches Bundesamt. Bildungsstand: Bevölkerung nach Bildungsabschluss in Deutschland. 2015. https://www.destatis.de/DE/ZahlenFakten/GesellschaftStaat/BildungForschungKultur/Bildungsstand/Tabellen/Bildungsabschluss.html. Accessed 6 Apr 2017.
36. Autorengruppe Bildungsberichterstattung. Bildung in Deutschland 2016: Ein indikatorengestützter Bericht mit einer Analyse zu Bildung und Migration. Bielefeld: W. Bertelsmann Verlag; 2016.
37. Bundesagentur für Arbeit. Arbeitslosenquote in Deutschland im Jahresdurchschnitt von 1995 bis 2017. 2017. https://de.statista.com/statistik/daten/studie/1224/umfrage/arbeitslosenquote-in-deutschland-seit-1995/. Accessed 6 Apr 2017.
38. Müller E, Schuler A, Burton BA, Yates GB. Meeting the vocational support needs of individuals with Asperger syndrome and other autism spectrum disabilities. J Vocat Rehabil. 2003;18:163–75.
39. Mawhood L, Howlin P. The outcome of a supported employment scheme for high-functioning adults with autism or Asperger syndrome. Autism. 1999;3:229–54.
40. Wehman PH, Schall CM, McDonough J, Kregel J, Brooke V, Molinelli A, et al. Competitive employment for youth with autism spectrum disorders: early results from a randomized clinical trial. J Autism Dev Disord. 2014;44:487–500.

4

Computer-assisted cognitive remediation therapy increases hippocampal volume in patients with schizophrenia

Tsubasa Morimoto[1], Yasuhiro Matsuda[1*], Kiwamu Matsuoka[1], Fumihiko Yasuno[1], Emi Ikebuchi[2], Hiroyuki Kameda[3], Toshiaki Taoka[4], Toshiteru Miyasaka[5], Kimihiko Kichikawa[5] and Toshifumi Kishimoto[1]

Abstract

Background: Cognitive remediation therapy (CRT) effectively reduces neurocognitive impairment in patients with schizophrenia, but few studies have used structural neuroimaging methods to assess its neuroanatomical effects. We investigated these effects, as well as the association between changes in cortical volume and neurocognitive performance.

Method: Between August 2013 and September 2016, we performed a randomized controlled study comprising a CRT group (16 individuals) and a treatment-as-usual (TAU) group (15 individuals) of patients with schizophrenia. CRT participants engaged in twice-weekly computer-assisted CRT sessions and weekly group meetings for 12 weeks. T1-weighted magnetic resonance imaging was performed before and after the intervention period, and whole-brain voxel-based morphometric analysis was used to detect significant cortical gray matter volume changes. We also assessed the correlation between cortical volume changes and CRT-derived neurocognitive improvements.

Results: The CRT group exhibited significantly greater improvements than the TAU group in verbal fluency ($P = 0.012$) and global cognitive scores ($P = 0.049$). The CRT group also exhibited significantly greater increases in right hippocampal volume than the TAU group ($P < 0.001$). Changes in verbal fluency scores and right hippocampal volumes were positively correlated ($r = 0.53$, $P = 0.001$).

Conclusion: We found that CRT significantly increased right hippocampal volumes and that these enhancements were positively correlated with changes in verbal fluency scores. Our results indicate that CRT induces cognitive improvement through hippocampal plasticity.

Keywords: Cognitive remediation, Rehabilitation, Structural neuroimaging, Hippocampus, Schizophrenia, Jcores

Background

Kraeplin referred to schizophrenia as "dementia praecox" and described it as a progressive neurodegenerative disease resulting in cognitive deficits [1]. Indeed, studies addressing progressive neuropsychological changes in schizophrenia indicate that patients experience gradual decline in neurocognitive function [2]. Several structural magnetic resonance imaging (MRI) studies have reported progressive gray matter (GM) loss in the brain of individuals with schizophrenia. These findings were supported by a recent meta-analysis of 19 trials including 813 patients, which discovered significantly accelerated whole-brain GM volume loss in individuals with schizophrenia [3].

Cognitive impairment is an important aspect of schizophrenia. Therefore, possible means of alleviating cognitive deficits are of interest to clinicians and researchers. Because antipsychotics do not improve neurocognitive function as much as previously hoped [4, 5], researchers

* Correspondence: yasu-matsuda@naramed-u.ac.jp
[1]Department of Psychiatry, Nara Medical University School of Medicine, 840 Shijo-cho, Kashihara, Nara 634-8522, Japan
Full list of author information is available at the end of the article

are considering alternative approaches such as cognitive remediation therapy (CRT) [6, 7], an evidence-based non-pharmacological treatment intended to improve functions related to daily tasks, including those related to school, work, social interactions, and independent living [8]. A meta-analysis of 26 randomized, controlled trials of CRT for schizophrenia treatment (totaling 1151 patients) reported that CRT has a medium effect size (0.41) on cognitive performance [9].

Over the last 15 years, investigators have been developing and optimizing computer-assisted CRT for individuals with schizophrenia [10]. We developed a program called the Japanese Cognitive Rehabilitation Program for Schizophrenia (Jcores). Recent studies have shown that a 12-week CRT program using Jcores (Vocational Cognitive Ability Training by Jcores [VCAT-J]) improves neurocognitive performance [11].

Nonetheless, it remains unknown how CRT mediates neuroanatomical changes. To date, two randomized, controlled studies have used structural neuroimaging to test the effect of CRT on individuals with schizophrenia. Penadés et al. [12] reported that, compared to social skills training, paper-and-pencil task CRT produces significantly greater improvements in the fractional anisotropy index of white matter in the corpus callosum and the right posterior thalamic radiation. Eack et al. [13] showed that computer-assisted CRT protects against GM loss in the hippocampus, parahippocampal gyrus, and left fusiform gyrus, as evidenced by a 2-year follow-up study that compared patients with and without CRT.

While the interventions developed by Penadés et al. [12] and Eack et al. [13] require over 4 months and 2 years, respectively, VCAT-J requires only 12 weeks. In the current study, we examined whether the VCAT-J could affect the brain structures of individuals with schizophrenia. We hypothesized that the VCAT-J intervention would induce changes in specific brain regions, especially the hippocampus—the volume of which is associated with various types of cognitive performance [14] and wherein activity-dependent neuroplasticity has repeatedly been observed [13, 15–18]. We also searched for associations between post-intervention regional cortical volume and neurocognitive functional changes, as assessed through scores on the Japanese version of the Brief Assessment of Cognition in Schizophrenia (BACS-J).

Methods

Participants and procedure

We recruited patients from one university hospital and two private hospitals by posters placed in the outpatient department and the day-treatment unit. Overseeing medical professionals have declared that all participants were capable of providing consent for themselves. To meet the selection criteria of the study, participants were required to: be of outpatient status, meet the criteria for schizophrenia established by the Diagnostic and Statistical Manual of Mental Disorders-Fourth Edition (Text Revision), and be aged between 20- and 60-years-old at the time of registration. Patients were excluded if they exhibited evidence of an organic central nervous system disorder, a history of drug or alcohol abuse, or intellectual disability.

Thirty-three patients consented to participate in this study, but one was excluded because of an organic disease (subdural hygroma), and another declined to undergo MRI because of possible pregnancy. A controlled, randomized study was conducted with two groups. Using a central registration system, participants were randomly assigned to either a CRT group ($n = 16$) that was treated immediately or a waitlist control group ($n = 15$) that continued treatment as usual (TAU) for 12 weeks before beginning CRT. All participants were followed up for 12 weeks, underwent T1-weighted MRI, and underwent clinical and neuropsychological assessments before and after intervention, which was performed by personnel blinded to the group assignments.

Treatments

All participants were prescribed antipsychotics and received standard outpatient treatment. Participants in the CRT group completed computerized Jcores training, which exercises a broad range of cognitive functions, including attention, psychomotor speed, learning, verbal fluency, memory, and executive function. Each domain of the Jcores includes three to seven game types, and each game has five difficulty levels. Participants were asked to select specific cognitive domains and to adjust the task difficulty according to their abilities. For 12 weeks, the CRT group completed twice-weekly, hour-long computerized training sessions and weekly, hour-long group sessions, the purposes of which were to help establish associations between the computerized CRT and daily life or work performance as well as to aid in setting and tracking each participant's individualized community life and/or work goals [7]. This study's VCAT-J training procedures were identical to those of our previous study [11]. Psychiatrists or psychologists with computer-assisted CRT [6] study experience monitored all VCAT-J sessions.

TAU group participants primarily received medication and medical care from psychiatrists. Participants in the TAU group were also referred for social welfare and received assistance from a medical social worker as needed.

Clinical assessments

Symptom severity was assessed using the Positive and Negative Syndrome Scale [19]. Neurocognitive function was assessed using the BACS-J, which has been validated as a reliable and practical evaluation of neurocognitive function in patients with schizophrenia [20]. The BACS-J tests verbal memory, working memory, motor speed, verbal fluency, attention and information processing speed, and executive function. Composite BACS-J scores were calculated by averaging z-scores from the six subcomponents, which were in turn calculated from the means and standard deviations extracted from a dataset of 64 healthy control Japanese individuals [21], age-matched to this study's participants.

Functions related to daily life and community interactions were assessed using the Life Assessment Scale for the Mentally Ill [22], which measures a patient's social skills in five categories of daily life: 1) daily living, 2) interpersonal relations, 3) work skills, 4) endurance and stability, and 5) self-recognition. Each category has several items that are rated on a five-point scale (0 = "no problem," 4 = "serious problem"). In this study, we used scores from the interpersonal relations and work skills categories.

All neuropsychological assessments were evaluated by psychiatrists or psychologists uninvolved in CRT or regular outpatient treatment.

MRI data acquisition

All MRI examinations were performed using a 3.0-T clinical scanner (Magnetom Verio; Siemens, Erlangen, Germany) with a 32-channel phased-array brain coil. High-resolution, three-dimensional T1-weighted images were acquired using a magnetization-prepared rapid gradient-echo sequence (repetition time = 1800 ms, echo time = 2.4 ms, flip angle = 10°, field of view = 256 mm; 208 sagittal plane sections; acquisition matrix = 256 × 256; acquired resolution = 1 × 1 × 1 mm^3).

Image processing

Image preprocessing and statistical analyses were performed with the SPM12 software (Wellcome Trust Centre for Neuroimaging, London, UK; http://www.fil.ion.ucl.ac.uk/spm), and voxel-based morphometry was performed using the Computational Anatomy Toolbox for SPM (CAT12; Jena University Hospital Departments of Psychiatry and Neurology, Jena, Germany; http://dbm.neuro.uni-jena.de/cat/) running on MATLAB R2014a (MathWorks, Natick, MA). We used the default preprocessing approach to analyze longitudinal data in CAT12. T1-weighted images were subjected to intra-subject re-alignment, bias correction, tissue segmentation into GM, white matter, and cerebrospinal fluid; and registration using linear (affine registration) and nonlinear transformations through Diffeomorphic Anatomical Registration Through Exponentiated Lie Algebra [23] within a unified model [24]. GM segments were subsequently analyzed by multiplying them by the nonlinear components derived from the normalization matrix to preserve actual local GM values (modulated GM volumes). Finally, the modulated and normalized GM segments (voxel size = 1.5 × 1.5 × 1.5 mm^3) were smoothed using a Gaussian kernel of 8-mm full-width at half-maximum.

Statistical analysis

We performed between-group comparisons of baseline demographic and clinical characteristics using two-sample student's t and chi-square tests. Post-intervention changes in psychiatric symptoms, neurocognitive function, and social function were examined using analyses of variance (ANOVAs). We defined statistical significance as $P < 0.05$.

We performed an voxel-based analysis to investigate the relationship between post-CRT rehabilitation and GM volume changes, organizing a two-time (baseline versus 12-week follow-up) × two-group (CRT group versus TAU group) flexible factorial design in SPM12. We thus had four conditions: the CRT group at baseline, CRT group at follow-up, TAU group at baseline, and TAU group at follow-up. To test our hypothesis that rehabilitation would increase regional brain volumes, we investigated the interaction effect of increased post-rehabilitation volume by comparing volume increases in the CRT group to those in the TAU group. We used global scaling by total intracranial volume (TIV) to correct for different brain sizes. To avoid possible edge effects between different tissue types, we excluded all voxels outside the GM with absolute threshold masking. The mean TIV was 1619 cm^3, and all images were globally scaled to a value of 50, creating an overall scaling of 50/1619. To obtain an absolute threshold of 0.2, we multiplied 0.2 by 50/1619. As this was a hypothesis-led analysis, we applied a liberal significance threshold of $P < 0.001$ with a 35-voxel whole-brain extent. Volumes of interest (VOIs) were determined from clusters where significant interactions were found. Regional volumes were calculated by averaging the values for all voxels within the VOIs. VOI volume changes over the intervention were compared between groups using repeated-measures ANOVAs.

We used Spearman's correlation analysis to examine how VOI volume changes were related to various metrics in which the CRT group exhibited significantly greater improvements than the TAU group. Statistical analyses were performed using SPSS for Windows v. 21.0 (IBM, Armonk, NY).

Results and statistical analyses

Demographic and clinical data

Table 1 summarizes subject demographic and clinical characteristics. The CRT and TAU groups did not significantly differ in terms of demographics or baseline psychiatric symptoms, social function, or neurocognitive function.

Table 1 Demographic data and baseline clinical characteristics

	CRT group (n = 16)		TAU group (n = 15)			
	Mean	SD	Mean	SD	t or χ^2	P
Sex (male/female)	10/6		9/6		$\chi^2 = 0.02$	0.59
Age (years)	36.1	7.7	37.4	11.0	$t = -0.39$	0.70
Handedness (right/left)	16/0		13/2		$\chi^2 = 2.28$	0.23
Years of education	14.3	2.4	13.0	2.0	$t = 1.69$	0.10
Years from onset of schizophrenia	12.1	7.8	13.9	13.2	$t = -0.47$	0.65
Number of hospitalizations	1.0	1.2	2.1	1.9	$t = -2.00$	0.056
JART	102.6	11.8	97.8	12.2	$t = 1.10$	0.28
Drugs						
Mean dosage of antipsychotics[a]	440.3	265.1	680.3	530.9	$t = -1.61$	0.12
Mean dosage of anticholinergics[b]	0.75	1.65	1.30	1.51	$t = -0.97$	0.34
PANSS						
Positive symptoms	14.8	4.9	14.3	4.2	$t = 0.26$	0.80
Negative symptoms	20.7	4.4	20.6	7.2	$t = 0.04$	0.97
General psychopathology	39.6	7.8	41.5	10.5	$t = -0.57$	0.57
LASMI						
Interpersonal relations	11.1	3.9	11.5	7.9	$t = -2.13$	0.83
Work skills	10.6	3.4	12.6	5.7	$t = -1.22$	0.23
BACS (z-score)						
Verbal memory	−1.8	1.0	−2.0	1.1	$t = 0.56$	0.58
Working memory	−1.3	1.2	−1.3	1.2	$t = -0.18$	0.86
Motor speed	−2.4	1.4	−2.8	1.6	$t = 0.76$	0.45
Verbal fluency	−1.4	0.8	−0.9	0.8	$t = -1.68$	0.10
Attention and speed of information processing	−1.6	0.8	−2.1	0.9	$t = 1.45$	0.16
Executive functions	−0.4	2.3	−1.1	1.6	$t = 0.97$	0.34
Composite score	−1.5	0.9	−1.7	0.9	$t = 0.63$	0.53

Abbreviations: *BACS* Brief Assessment of Cognition in Schizophrenia, *CRT* cognitive remediation therapy, *JART* National Adult Reading Test, Japanese Version, *LASMI* Life Assessment Scale for the Mentally Ill, *PANSS* Positive and Negative Syndrome Scale, *SD* standard deviation, *TAU* treatment as usual
[a]Chlorpromazine-equivalent dose (mg/day)
[b]Biperiden-equivalent dose (mg/day)

Changes in psychometric scores

As shown in Table 2, the CRT group exhibited significantly greater improvements in verbal fluency (F = 7.12, $P = 0.012$) and BACS-J composite scores (F = 4.21, $P = 0.049$) than the TAU group. No evidence of significant differences between groups were found regarding psychiatric symptoms or social function.

Increased regional GM volumes following rehabilitation

Voxel-based analysis revealed that the CRT group exhibited significantly greater increases in right hippocampal GM volume than the TAU group ([x, y, z] = [35, − 21, − 21], cluster voxel size = 35, $T = 3.70$; Fig. 1). A repeated measures ANOVA revealed a significant group effect on right hippocampal and total intracranial raw volume changes (group-by-volume interaction, $F_{(1, 29)} = 16.1$; $P < 0.001$, Fig. 2).

Relationship between volume and psychometric scores

Next, we tested the relationship between hippocampal volume changes and changes in verbal fluency and BACS-J composite scores. We found that right hippocampal and total intracranial raw volume changes were positively correlated with verbal fluency improvements in both groups ($r = 0.53$, $P = 0.001$; Fig. 3), but no significant correlation was found with BACS-J composite score changes in either group.

Discussion

This is the first study to show hippocampal volume increases in patients with schizophrenia following targeted CRT intervention. We found that 12 weeks of computer-assisted CRT produced significantly greater increases in right hippocampal GM volume than were accomplished with conventional TAU. One

Table 2 ANOVAs of post-intervention clinical variable changes

	CRT group (*n* = 16)		TAU group (*n* = 15)			
	Mean	SD	Mean	SD	F	P
PANSS						
Positive symptoms	−0.88	2.16	0.33	3.09	1.61	0.21
Negative symptoms	−2.63	2.03	−0.67	5.04	2.06	0.16
General psychopathology	−2.38	4.13	0.40	8.17	1.45	0.24
LASMI						
Interpersonal relations	−1.75	2.18	−0.33	5.02	1.06	0.31
Work skills	−0.69	1.85	−0.33	1.29	0.38	0.54
BACS (z-score)						
Verbal memory	1.02	0.85	0.55	0.81	2.40	0.13
Working memory	0.24	0.66	−0.13	0.98	1.56	0.22
Motor speed	0.38	1.18	0.08	1.41	0.41	0.53
Verbal fluency	0.56	0.82	– 008	0.47	7.12	0.012
Attention and speed of information processing	0.25	0.52	0.04	0.50	1.33	0.26
Executive functions	0.48	1.85	0.42	1.37	0.01	0.92
Composite score	0.49	0.42	0.15	0.50	4.21	0.049

Abbreviations: *ANOVA* analysis of variance, *BACS* Brief Assessment of Cognition in Schizophrenia, *CRT* cognitive remediation therapy, *JART* National Adult Reading Test, Japanese Version, *LASMI* Life Assessment Scale for the Mentally Ill, *PANSS* Positive and Negative Syndrome Scale, *SD* standard deviation, *TAU* treatment as usual

potential mechanism underlying this increase could be enhanced levels of brain-derived neurotrophic factor (BDNF), as Vinogradov et al. [25] reported that individuals with schizophrenia who engaged in a 10-week computerized cognitive training program showed significantly greater increases in serum BDNF than were observed in control subjects. BDNF plays a critical role in maintaining adult hippocampal volumes [26] by increasing axonal branching, dendrite complexity [27], spine density [28], and the number of neurons with hippocampal projections [26]. However, as we did not measure BDNF levels in the current study, we cannot confirm whether the observed increase in hippocampal GM volume is attributable to enhanced BDNF. Further studies on this question are needed.

We also found a significant association between changes in verbal fluency scores and right hippocampal volumes. Verbal fluency—thought to reflect semantic processing—

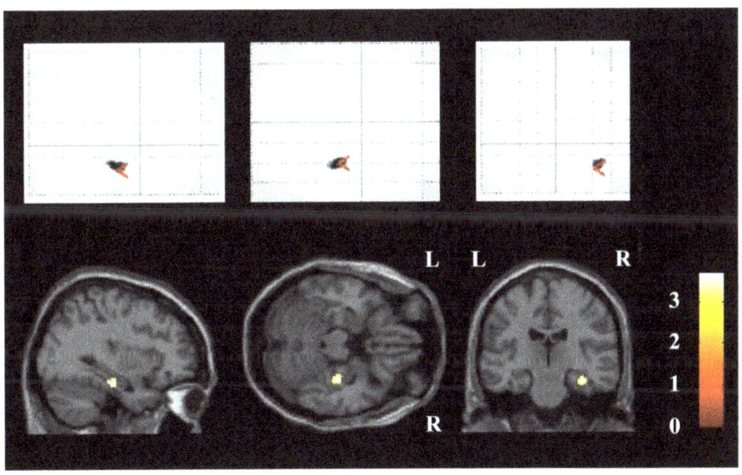

Fig. 1 Regional GM increases among participants receiving CRT versus TAU. Increases in GM volume in the CRT and TAU groups, as assessed using voxel-based analysis. We detected areas where the CRT group's GM volume growth was significantly greater than that of the TAU group (uncorrected $P < .005$ in 200 or more contiguous voxels). Statistical parametric mapping projections were then superimposed onto representative transaxial ($z = -21$), sagittal ($x = 35$), and coronal ($y = -21$) magnetic resonance images. Abbreviations: CRT, cognitive remediation therapy; GM, gray matter; L, left; R, right; TAU, treatment as usual

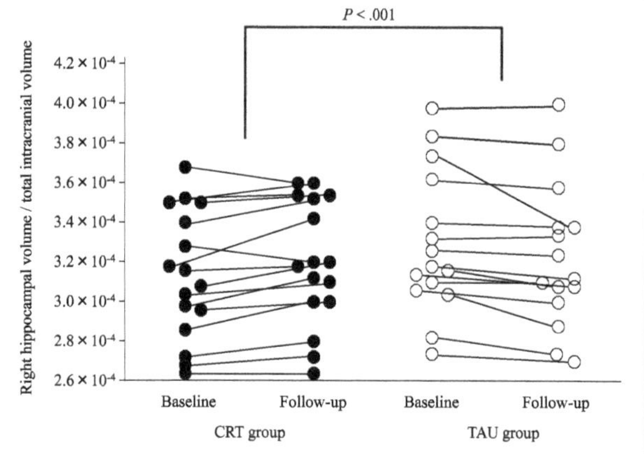

Fig. 2 Changes in right hippocampal volume as a proportion of total intracranial volume. Scatterplots showing right hippocampal volume changes in the CRT and TAU groups. VOI clusters were placed where a voxel-based analysis indicated that the CRT group exhibited significantly greater volume increases than the TAU group. Abbreviations: CRT, cognitive remediation therapy; TAU, treatment as usual; VOI, volume of interest

is the ability to recall words from long-term memory in accordance with certain conditions [29]. The Jcores includes several tasks that require semantic processing and information categorization, such as combining letters to form as many words as possible and forming a word beginning with another word's last character. Therefore, the Jcores is thought to be effective in improving verbal fluency in terms of semantic processing. The medial temporal lobe is necessary for retrieving semantically associated words, and is thus required for categorical fluency tasks. Indeed, functional neuroimaging studies in healthy individuals have reported hippocampal activation during verbal fluency tasks [30]. If CRT encourages neural activation and facilitates changes in hippocampal morphology, increased GM volume in this region might explain the observed improvements in verbal fluency.

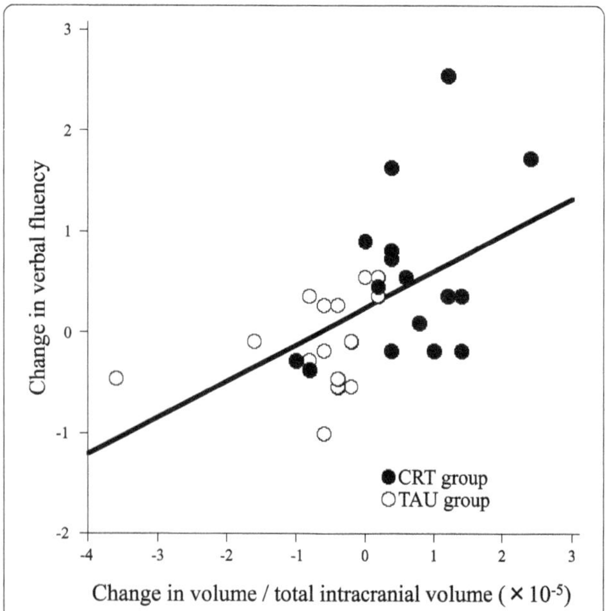

Fig. 3 Association between changes in verbal fluency and right hippocampal volume in both groups. We observed a significant, positive correlation in the relationship between changes in verbal fluency and in raw right hippocampal volume as a proportion of total intracranial volume in the CRT and TAU groups ($r = 0.53$, $P = 0.001$, $y = 0.25 + [3.6 \times 10^4]\,x$). CRT, cognitive remediation therapy; TAU, treatment as usual

In this study, hippocampal volume only increased on the right side. Interestingly, similar rightward lateralization patterns have also been reported in studies with healthy individuals. Kuhn et al. [16] investigated the effects of 2 months of video game training and found that the gaming group exhibited significantly greater GM increases than the control group. Similarly, Koch et al. [15] found that 14 weeks of extensive learning in medical students significantly increased right hippocampal GM volume. These results and ours suggest that hippocampus-dependent activity and/or learning affects hippocampal neuroplasticity on the right more than the left side of the brain. Future studies should investigate the laterality of activity-dependent hippocampal structure changes.

The ability of 12 weeks of CRT to increase hippocampal volume has notable implications for the neurodegenerative hypothesis of schizophrenia. Progressive brain-wide GM loss, including in the hippocampus, has been repeatedly reported in patients with schizophrenia [3]. Birchwood et al. [31] proposed that the majority of the biological, psychological, and social changes that occur in patients with schizophrenia take place in the first 5 years of disease onset; however, our participants had a mean illness duration of 12.1 years (standard deviation = 7.8 years), suggesting that clinically stable, chronically ill patients with schizophrenia also retain hippocampal plasticity. This study contributes to the development of therapeutic strategies and the understanding of the pathophysiology which underlies schizophrenia. We therefore believe that CRT for patients with schizophrenia should receive more attention as its further development will promote functional recovery.

Our study has some limitations that should be addressed. First, there exists the issue of the sample size being small. We referred to the sample size of a previous study [12], but through analysis using G*Power 3 [32], the optimal sample size would be 53 or larger (effect size $f = 0.25$, α error probability = 0.05 and power [1-β error probability] = 0.95). The sample size in the present study did not have sufficient power for detailed analyses, and in this respect, careful judgment is required in the interpretation of the results. We believe that additional testing with larger sample sizes is required to obtain conclusive results. Second, in this study, the intervention period was 12 weeks, and it remains necessary to verify the long-term effects of the intervention with a longer follow-up in future study. Third, ANOVA was used to compare changes in all psychometric items between groups after 12 weeks of intervention, without adjustment for the years of education and number of hospitalizations, which showed trend significance at baseline ($p = 0.10$ and 0.056, respectively). Therefore, these two psychometric items may have affected the results. Fourth, we did not control for any potential antipsychotic drug effects. The synergistic effect of neurocognitive remediation combined with antipsychotic drugs is unknown [11], and some antipsychotics may affect cerebral parenchymal volume [33]. Thus, future studies should regulate medications as much as possible. Fifth, we could not find an association between increased volumes in the right hippocampus and improved composite BACS-J scores following CRT. As this result might be due to the small sample size of this investigation, further studies with larger samples are necessary for any definitive conclusions. Sixth, we did not evaluate changes in hippocampal neural activity following CRT. We intend to use imaging technologies, including functional MRI, to address this question in the future.

Conclusion

In summary, we found that computer-assisted CRT can promote right hippocampal GM growth in patients with schizophrenia. We also found that right hippocampal volume changes were positively correlated with alterations in verbal fluency scores. These findings enhance our understanding of hippocampal neuroplasticity and encourage the development of CRT interventions to improve cognitive and daily functions in patients with schizophrenia.

Abbreviations

BACS-J: Brief Assessment of Cognition in Schizophrenia; BDNF: brain-derived neurotrophic factor; CRT: cognitive remediation therapy; GM: gray matter; JART: National Adult Reading Test, Japanese Version; Jcores: Japanese Cognitive Rehabilitation Program for Schizophrenia; LASMI: Life Assessment Scale for the Mentally Ill; MRI: magnetic resonance imaging; PANSS: Positive and Negative Syndrome Scale; SD: standard deviation; TAU: treatment as usual; TIV: total intracranial volume; VCAT-J: Vocational Cognitive Ability Training by Jcores; VOI: volume of interest

Acknowledgments

We thank Shunichi Furukawa, MD from the Department of Psychiatry at Tokyo Metropolitan Police Hospital in Tokyo, Japan; Sayaka Sato, PhD from the Department of Psychiatric Rehabilitation, National Center of Neurology and Psychiatry at the National Institute of Mental Health in Tokyo, Japan; Norifumi Hatsuse, PhD from the Department of Psychiatry at Teikyo University School of Medicine in Tokyo, Japan; Kazuhiko Iwata, MPH at the Center for Clinical Research and Development Initiative, Osaka Psychiatric Medical Center in Osaka, Japan; Mieko Kimura, PhD, independent; and Nobuhiro Tsukie, PhD at the Cyber Creative Institute; for their help in developing VCAT-J. We also express our appreciation to the staff of the MRI facility at the Nara Medical University Department of Radiology in Japan for subject care and data acquisition during the MRI procedures.

Funding

This work was supported by the Japan Society for the Promotion of Science Grants-in-Aid for Scientific Research Program [grant numbers JP25861024, JP16K19779, and JP16H05377].

Authors' contributions

TM1 contributed to the management of the project and wrote the manuscript. YM managed the literature review and analysis. EI and TK coordinated the research design and managed the study. HK supervised the development of the Jcores software. KM and FY supervised the MRI analysis and evaluated the acquired images. TT, TM2, and KK oversaw the MRI scanning. All authors contributed to and have approved the final manuscript.

Consent for publication

Not applicable.

Competing interests

The authors declare that they have no competing interests.
TM1 and TM2. TM1 would correspond to the author furthest up on the author list.

Author details

[1]Department of Psychiatry, Nara Medical University School of Medicine, 840 Shijo-cho, Kashihara, Nara 634-8522, Japan. [2]Department of Psychiatry, Teikyo University School of Medicine, 2-11-1 Kaga, Itabashi ku, Tokyo 173-8605, Japan. [3]School of Computer Science, Tokyo University of Technology, 1404-1 Katakuramachi, Hachioji City, Tokyo 192-0982, Japan. [4]Department of Radiology, Nagoya University Hospital, 65 Tsurumai-cho, Showa-ku, Nagoya, Aichi 466-8550, Japan. [5]Department of Radiology, Nara Medical University School of Medicine, 840 Shijo-cho, Kashihara, Nara 634-8522, Japan.

References

1. Strauss JS, Carpenter WT Jr. The prognosis of schizophrenia: rationale for a multidimensional concept. Schizophr Bull 1978;4:56–67.
2. Sponheim SR, Jung RE, Seidman LJ, Mesholam-Gately RI, Manoach DS, O'Leary DS, Ho BC, Andreasen NC, Lauriello J, Schulz SC. Cognitive deficits in recent-onset and chronic schizophrenia. J Psychiatr Res. 2010;44:421–8.
3. Vita A, De Peri L, Deste G, Sacchetti E. Progressive loss of cortical grey matter in schizophrenia: a meta-analysis and meta-regression of longitudinal MRI studies. Transl Psychiatry. 2012;2:e190.
4. Harvey PD, Keefe RS. Studies of cognitive change in patients with schizophrenia following novel antipsychotic treatment. Am J Psychiatry. 2001;158:176–84.
5. Keefe RS, Sweeney JA, Gu H, Hamer RM, Perkins DO, McEvoy JP, Lieberman JA. Effects of olanzapine, quetiapine, and risperidone on neurocognitive function in early psychosis: a randomized, double-blind 52-week comparison. Am J Psychiatry. 2007;164:1061–71.
6. Sato S, Iwata K, Furukawa SI, Matsuda Y, Hatsuse N, Ikebuchi E. The effects of the combination of cognitive training and supported employment on improving clinical and working outcomes for people with schizophrenia in Japan. Clin Pract Epidemiol Ment Health. 2013;10:18–27.
7. McGurk SR, Mueser KT, Xie H, Welsh J, Kaiser S, Drake RE, Becker DR, Bailey E, Fraser G, Wolfe R, et al. Cognitive enhancement treatment for people with mental illness who do not respond to supported employment: a randomized controlled trial. Am J Psychiatry. 2015;172:852–61.
8. Medalia A, Choi J. Cognitive remediation in schizophrenia. Neuropsychol Rev. 2009;19:353–64.
9. McGurk SR, Twamley EW, Sitzer DI, McHugo GJ, Mueser KT. A meta-analysis of cognitive remediation in schizophrenia. Am J Psychiatry. 2007;164:1791–802.
10. Chan JY, Hirai HW, Tsoi KK. Can computer-assisted cognitive remediation improve employment and productivity outcomes of patients with severe mental illness? A meta-analysis of prospective controlled trials. J Psychiatr Res. 2015;68:293–300.

11. Matsuda Y, Morimoto T, Furukawa S, Sato S, Hatsuse N, Iwata K, Kimura M, Kishimoto T, Ikebuchi E. Feasibility and effectiveness of a cognitive remediation programme with original computerised cognitive training and group intervention for schizophrenia: a multicentre randomised trial. Neuropsychol Rehabil. 2016;6:1–11.
12. Penadés R, Pujol N, Catalán R, Massana G, Rametti G, García-Rizo C, Bargalló N, Gastó C, Bernardo M, Junqué C. Brain effects of cognitive remediation therapy in schizophrenia: a structural and functional neuroimaging study. Biol Psychiatry. 2013;73:1015–23.
13. Eack SM, Hogarty GE, Cho RY, Prasad KM, Greenwald DP, Hogarty SS, Keshavan MS. Neuroprotective effects of cognitive enhancement therapy against grey matter loss in early schizophrenia: results from a 2-year randomized controlled trial. Arch Gen Psychiatry. 2010;67:674–82.
14. Pohlack ST, Meyer P, Cacciaglia R, Liebscher C, Ridder S, Flor H. Bigger is better! Hippocampal volume and declarative memory performance in healthy young men. Brain Struct Funct. 2014;219:255–67.
15. Koch K, Reess TJ, Rus OG, Zimmer C. Extensive learning is associated with grey matter changes in the right hippocampus. NeuroImage. 2016;125:627–32.
16. Kühn S, Gleich T, Lorenz RC, Lindenberger U, Gallinat J. Playing super Mario induces structural brain plasticity: grey matter changes resulting from training with a commercial video game. Mol Psychiatry. 2013;19:265–71.
17. Pereira AC, Huddleston DE, Brickman AM, Sosunov AA, Hen R, McKhann GM, Sloan R, Gage FH, Brown TR, Small SA. An in vivo correlate of exercise-induced neurogenesis in the adult dentate gyrus. Proc Natl Acad Sci U S A. 2007;104:5638–43.
18. Maass A, Düzel S, Goerke M, Becke A, Sobieray U, Neumann K, Lövdén M, Lindenberger U, Bäckman L, Braun-Dullaeus R, et al. Vascular hippocampal plasticity after aerobic exercise in older adults. Mol Psychiatry. 2015;20:585–93.
19. Kay SR, Fiszbein A, Opfer LA. The positive and negative syndrome scale (PANSS) for schizophrenia. Schizophr Bull. 1987;13:261–76.
20. Kaneda Y, Sumiyoshi T, Keefe R, Ishimoto Y, Numata S, Ohmori T. Brief assessment of cognition in schizophrenia: validation of the Japanese version. Psychiatry Clin Neurosci. 2007;61:602–9.
21. Kaneda Y, Sumiyoshi T, Nakagome K, Ikezawa S, Ohmori T, Noboru Y. Evaluation of cognitive functions in a normal population in Japan using the brief assessment of cognition in schizophrenia Japanese version (BACS-J) [in Japanese]. Seishin Igaku. 2013;55:167–75.
22. Iwasaki S, Miyauchi M, Oshima I, Murata N, Nonaka T, Kato H, Ueno Y, Fujii K. Development of the life assessment scale for the mentally ill: a reliability assessment [in Japanese]. Seishin Igaku. 1994;36:1139–51.
23. Ashburner J. A fast diffeomorphic image registration algorithm. NeuroImage. 2007;38:95–113.
24. Ashburner J, Friston KJ. Unified segmentation. NeuroImage. 2005;26:839–51.
25. Vinogradov S, Fisher M, Holland C, Shelly W, Wolkowitz O, Mellon SH. Is serum brain-derived neurotrophic factor a biomarker for cognitive enhancement in schizophrenia? Biol Psychiatry. 2009;66:549–53.
26. von Bohlen HO. Involvement of BDNF in age-dependent alterations in the hippocampus. Front Aging Neurosci. 2010;2:36.
27. Tolwani RJ, Buckmaster PS, Varma S, Cosgaya JM, Wu Y, Suri C, Shooter EM. BDNF overexpression increases dendrite complexity in hippocampal dentate gyrus. Neuroscience. 2002;114:795–805.
28. Alonso M, Medina JH, Pozzo-Miller L. ERK1/2 activation is necessary for BDNF to increase dendritic spine density in hippocampal CA1 pyramidal neurons. Learn Mem. 2004;11:172–8.
29. Miyajima M, Omiya H, Yamashita K, Miyata T, Yambe K, Matsui M, Denda K. The effects of cognitive remediation therapy using the frontal/executive program for autism spectrum disorder. Int J Psychiatry Med. 2016;51:223–35.
30. Pihlajamaki M, Tanila H, Hanninen T, Kononen M, Laakso MP, Partanen K, Soininen H, Aronen HJ. Verbal fluency activates the left medial temporal lobe: a functional magnetic resonance imaging study. Ann Neurol. 2000;47:470–6.
31. Birchwood M, Patrick M, Jackson H. Early intervention in schizophrenia. Br J Psychiatry. 1997;170:2–5.
32. Faul F, Erdfelder E, Lang AG, Buchner A. G*power 3: a flexible statistical power analysis program for the social, behavioral, and biomedical sciences. Behav Res Methods. 2007;114:175–91.
33. Okugawa G, Nobuhara K, Takase K, Saito Y, Yoshimura M, Kinoshita T. Olanzapine increases grey and white matter volumes in the caudate nucleus of patients with schizophrenia. Neuropsychobiology. 2007;55:43–6.

5

Possible multiple system atrophy with predominant parkinsonism in a patient with chronic schizophrenia

Hiroshi Komatsu[1*], Masaaki Kato[2], Teiko Kinpara[3], Takashi Ono[1] and Yoshihisa Kakuto[1]

Abstract

Background: Multiple system atrophy (MSA) is an adult-onset, rare, and progressive neurodegenerative disorder characterized by a varying combination of autonomic failure, cerebellar ataxia, and parkinsonism. MSA is categorized as MSA-P with predominant parkinsonism, and as MSA-C with predominant cerebellar features. The prevalence of MSA has been reported to be between 1.86 and 4.9 cases per 100,000 individuals. In contrast, approximately 1% of the population is affected by schizophrenia during their lifetime; therefore, MSA-P comorbidity is very rare in schizophrenic patients. However, when the exacerbation or progression of parkinsonism occurs in patients with schizophrenia treated with antipsychotics, it is necessary to consider rare neurodegenerative disorders, including MSA-P, in the differential diagnosis of parkinsonism.

Case presentation: A 60-year-old female patient with chronic schizophrenia developed possible MSA-P. She had been treated mainly with typical antipsychotics, and presented with urinary incontinence, nocturnal polyuria, and dysarthria around 2011. In 2014, she developed worsening parkinsonian symptoms and autonomic dysfunction. Although her antipsychotic medication was switched to an atypical antipsychotic and the dose reduced, her parkinsonism was not improved. In 2015, modified electroconvulsive therapy produced slight improvements in the symptoms; however, she shortly returned to her symptomatic state. A combination of cardiac ^{123}I-meta-iodobenzylguanidine scintigraphy and ^{123}I-FP-CIT single-photon emission computed tomography imaging, in addition to brain magnetic resonance imaging findings, helped to discriminate MSA-P from other sources of parkinsonism. L-dopa had been prescribed, but she responded poorly and died in the spring of 2016.

Conclusions: This case report highlights the importance of considering MSA-P in the differential diagnosis for parkinsonism in a patient being treated with antipsychotics for chronic schizophrenia. MSA-P should be considered in patients presenting with worsening and progressing parkinsonism, especially when accompanied by autonomic dysfunction or cerebellar ataxia. Although a definite diagnosis of MSA-P requires autopsy confirmation, a combination of brain magnetic resonance imaging and nuclear medicine scans may help to differentiate suspected MSA-P from the other parkinsonian syndromes. This case also demonstrates that MSA with parkinsonism that is poorly responsive to L-dopa may improve shortly after modified electroconvulsive therapy without worsening psychiatric symptoms.

Keywords: Multiple system atrophy, Schizophrenia, Antipsychotics, Parkinsonism, Autonomic dysfunction, Cardiac 123I-meta-iodobenzylguanidine scintigraphy, 123I-FP-CIT single-photon emission computed tomography image, Magnetic resonance imaging, Modified electroconvulsive therapy

* Correspondence: hkomatsu1019@gmail.com
[1]Department of Psychiatry, Miyagi Psychiatric Center, Mubanchi, Tekurada, Natori 981-1231, Japan
Full list of author information is available at the end of the article

Background

Multiple system atrophy (MSA) is an adult-onset, sporadic, and rare progressive neurodegenerative disorder characterized mainly by parkinsonism that responds poorly to levodopa, cerebellar symptoms, and autonomic failure.

MSA is categorized as MSA-P when parkinsonism is predominant, and as MSA-C when associated with dominant cerebellar features. MSA-P or MSA-C is categorized by the dominant symptoms at the time of evaluation and can change by the time of diagnosis. Moreover, the diagnostic criteria for definite, probable, and possible MSA were determined at the Second Consensus Conference on the Diagnosis of MSA, held in 2007 [1].

The incidence of the disease has been estimated to be 0.6 and 0.7 cases per 100,000 persons, while the prevalence is between 1.86 and 4.9 cases per 100,000 persons [2–8]. In Asian populations, the majority of MSA cases are of the MSA-C type, whereas MSA-P type predominates in the European population [9, 10].

Schizophrenia is a chronic and serious mental disorder characterized by positive symptoms (i.e., delusions and hallucination) and/or negative symptoms (i.e., blunted affect, loss of motivation, and poverty of speech) and/or cognitive dysfunction (i.e., impairment in several cognitive domains, including working memory, attention, verbal memory and executive functions) [11]. Approximately 1% of the population is affected by schizophrenia during an individual's lifetime, in which socio-occupational functioning is significantly impaired [12]. Antipsychotic medications are effective for relieving both positive and negative symptoms, but can cause extrapyramidal symptoms (EPS) (i.e., parkinsonian symptoms, dystonia, akathisia, and tardive dyskinesia) as a side effect. It is important to note that EPS tend to be more associated with typical antipsychotics than atypical antipsychotics [13].

Herein, we report a case involving a 60-year-old female patient with schizophrenia being treated with long-term antipsychotic medication, who developed possible MSA-P. We adhered to the CARE guidelines/methodology, which was created by an international group of experts that helps authors reduce bias and increase the accuracy, transparency, and usefulness of case reports (http://www.care-statement.org/).

Case presentation

The patient was the first-born of 4 children, with no family history of psychiatric illness and no developmental delay. In 1972, she first presented hallucination-delusions at 16 years of age and was diagnosed with schizophrenia in another hospital. After being hospitalized two times there, she visited the Miyagi Prefecture Center (MPC, Japan) at 25 years of age in 1981. An acute change in her emotions, behavior, and thoughts occurred a few days before the first consultation at the MPC.

At the first examination, she was very talkative and presented severely disorganized thoughts and behavior, as well as inappropriately expressed emotions. She was readmitted to the hospital for treatment of psychotic episodes. After discharge, she was continuously treated as an outpatient; however, symptoms including avolition, asociality, moderately disorganized thinking, and emotional vulnerability to psychological stress in daily life persisted. She married at 28 years of age in 1984, and gave birth to a boy the following year. She was maintained in a generally stable mental state with the support of a community health nurse and her family. Long-acting injectable (LAI) fluphenazine enanthate was introduced in 1993 to overcome poor adherence when she was 37 years of age. At approximately the same time, she was treated for diabetes. In 1994, at 38 years of age, an overnight stay with her sister-in-law resulted in rehospitalization for a worsening of disorganized thought, anxiety, and impatience. After being admitted for a few weeks, she regularly visited our hospital as an outpatient. In 2004, she transiently presented with dizziness from standing up too quickly at around 48 years of age. In 2011, she began complaining of urinary incontinence, nocturnal polyuria, and dysarthria at approximately 55 years of age; however, it was unlikely that such symptoms were side effects of her antipsychotics or diabetic autonomic neuropathy. When she was 56 years of age, she gradually developed pain in the right knee and was diagnosed with osteoarthritis of the right knee. In the following year, she underwent artificial joint replacement surgery for her right knee in the Department of Orthopaedic Surgery, Tohoku Rosai Hospital. Bilateral hand muscle weakness, predominantly in the right hand, and dysarthria were observed while she was hospitalized in 2013. Although she underwent brain magnetic resonance imaging (MRI), findings revealed no remarkable abnormalities (Fig. 1). She used a pick-up walker at home after the knee surgery; however, at the end of the same year, she fell at home and was diagnosed with a right femoral neck fracture. She was treated operatively for the fracture in the same orthopedic surgery department as before. After 4 months as an inpatient, she was discharged to her home, and resumed outpatient treatment at the MPC in 2014. She presented with depressed mood, decreased appetite, and body weight loss after discharge, and was prescribed sertraline for symptoms of depression. In 2014, at 58 years of age, she underwent video fluoroscopic examination of her swallowing, demonstrating increased dysphagia, bradykinesia, and upper-limb muscle rigidity, predominantly in the right limb. Drug-induced parkinsonism was suspected based on the results of the examination, which indicated no organic abnormality. LAI fluphenazine enanthate was

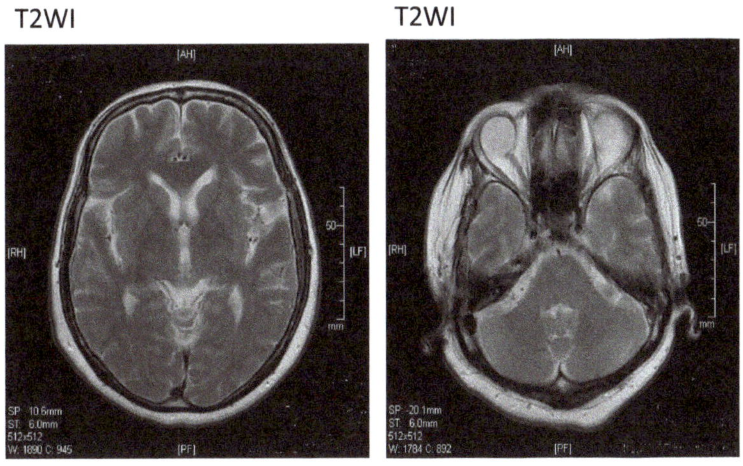

Fig. 1 Brain magnetic resonance images of the patient at 57 years of age (2013). T2-weighted images (T2WI) demonstrated no remarkable abnormalities, including fresh cerebral infarction, bleeding, space-occupying lesions, and prominent atrophic changes in brain regions including the bilateral putamen. Moreover, there was no high-intensity signal of the lateral rim of the putamen

discontinued, and she was switched from oral haloperidol to aripiprazole. She was readmitted to our hospital at 58 years of age upon appearance of emotional instability, hallucinations, and negativism following the drug switch. Moreover, she also presented with worsening of urinary incontinence and retention, which required urethral catheterization. The volume of post-catheterization urinary output was greater than 600 mL. Dosage adjustment of the antipsychotics, including tests with aripiprazole, zotepine, blonanserin, and perospirone, failed to improve the parkinsonism, mutism, and negativism (e.g., food and drug rejection); consequently, modified electroconvulsive therapy (mECT) was administered for 20 treatments. mECT produced slight improvements in the symptoms, and it became possible for her to ingest a small amount of food and speak a little (2015). However, she returned to her symptomatic state after a short period of time. She then underwent careful examination for persistent parkinsonism and autonomic dysfunction (including urinary retention, urinary incontinence, and constipation) in the Department of Neurology, Kohnan Hospital (2015). Brain MRI revealed a T2-hyperintense lateral rim and hypointense putamen that had progressed over the year (Fig. 2). Cardiac ^{123}I-meta-iodobenzylguanidine (MIBG) scintigraphy demonstrated normal myocardial MIBG uptake (Fig. 3). In ^{123}I-FP-CIT (DaTscan) single-photon emission computed tomography (SPECT) imaging, decreased uptake of ^{123}I-FP-CIT was observed in the bilateral striatum, but predominantly in the left dorsolateral striatum (Fig. 4). MSA-P was thus suspected from the clinical features (including parkinsonism, urinary dysfunction, and constipation), neuroimaging, and nuclear medicine findings. L-dopa was prescribed and the dose was increased to 700 mg/day; however, her response was poor, and she died of aspiration pneumonia in 2016 at 60 years of age.

Discussion

MSA is a rare neurodegenerative disorder in general, and MSA-P is significantly less common than MSA-C in the Japanese population [9, 10]. In fact, to our knowledge, this is the first report to describe a 60-year-old

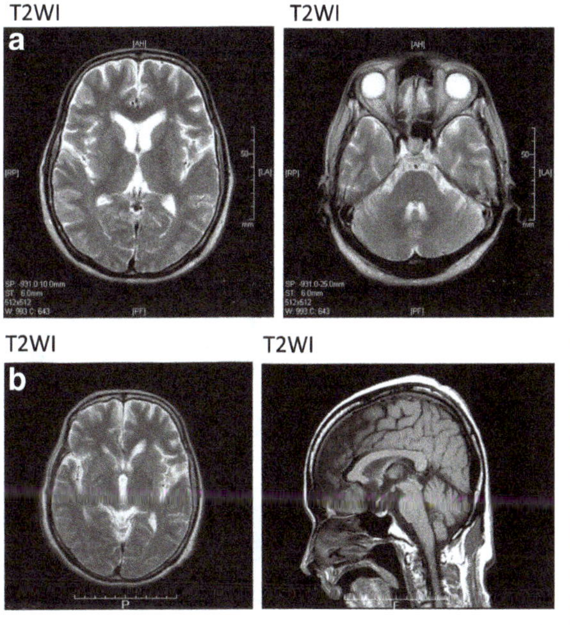

Fig. 2 Brain magnetic resonance images of the patient at 58 years of age (spring 2015) (**a**) and 59 years of age (winter 2015) (**b**). **a** Putaminal atrophic change and low- and high-intensity signals of the lateral rim of the putamen were observed predominantly in the left putamen in the T2-weighted image (T2WI). However, T2WI did not show the hot-cross bun sign, which may reflect pontine atrophy. **b** As in the previous year, magnetic resonance imaging findings revealed putaminal atrophic change and both low- and high-intensity signals of the lateral rim of the bilateral putamen, again predominantly in the left putamen. There were slight atrophic changes in the cerebellum and brain stem

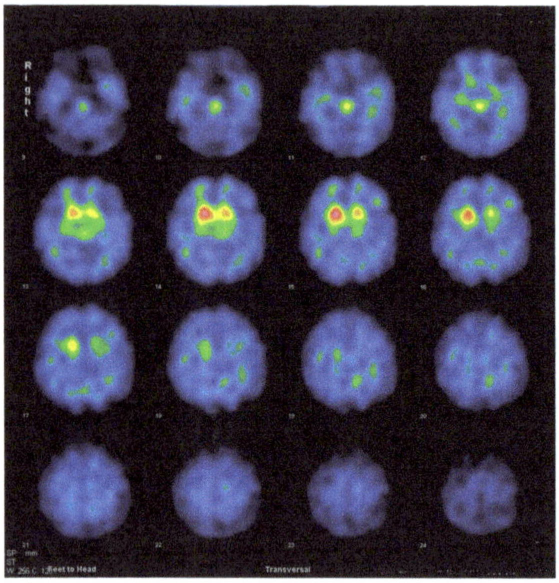

Fig. 3 ^{123}I-FP-CIT (DaTscan) SPECT image results in 2015. DaTscan data demonstrate reduced bilateral striatal ioflupane (^{123}I) uptake predominantly in the dorsolateral striatum. There were asymmetrical changes, with a greater decrease in ^{123}I uptake in the left dorsolateral striatum

female patient with chronic schizophrenia with possible MSA-P.

In 1900, Joseph Jules Dejerine and André Thomas first reported two cases presenting cerebellar ataxia and pathological lesions in the cerebellum and brainstem, which they described as olivopontocerebellar atrophy [14]. Subsequently, Shy and Drager described two patients with parkinsonism and autonomic symptoms including orthostatic hypotension in 1960 [15]. Van der Eecken et al. reported cases with parkinsonism and striatonigral degeneration at autopsy in the same year [16]. In 1969, Graham and Oppenheimer first introduced the term 'MSA' to represent all three diagnoses.

Papp et al. demonstrated the presence of argyrophilic glial cytoplasmic inclusions in the central nervous system of patients diagnosed with MSA in 1989 [17]; these inclusions were later reported to be positive for α-synuclein in 1998, and recent studies provide evidence for classifying MSA as an α-synucleinopathy, together with Parkinson's disease and dementia with Lewy bodies [18, 19].

The first consensus conference reported by Gilman et al. categorized MSA into MSA-P and MSA-C [20]. Moreover, the conference defined diagnostic criteria to define three levels of certainty: possible, probable, and definite. The second consensus conference, held in 2007, revised the diagnostic criteria such that the criteria for probable MSA were simplified, requiring at least one feature suggesting autonomic dysfunction; also, additional features for the diagnosis of possible MSA, and features supporting MSA (red flags) were introduced (Table 1) [1].

Patients with MSA-P exhibit early development of autonomic dysfunction and more rapid progression than those with Parkinson's disease. Low et al. reported that the mean remaining lifespan ranged from 6.2 to 10 years after symptoms first appear [21–25]. The most common causes of death have been reported to be nocturnal sudden death and aspiration pneumonia [26].

Autonomic features are a key characteristics in patients with MSA [8]. The urogenital and cardiovascular systems are most frequently affected. Criteria for diagnosis of probable MSA according to Gilman et al. (Table 1) include

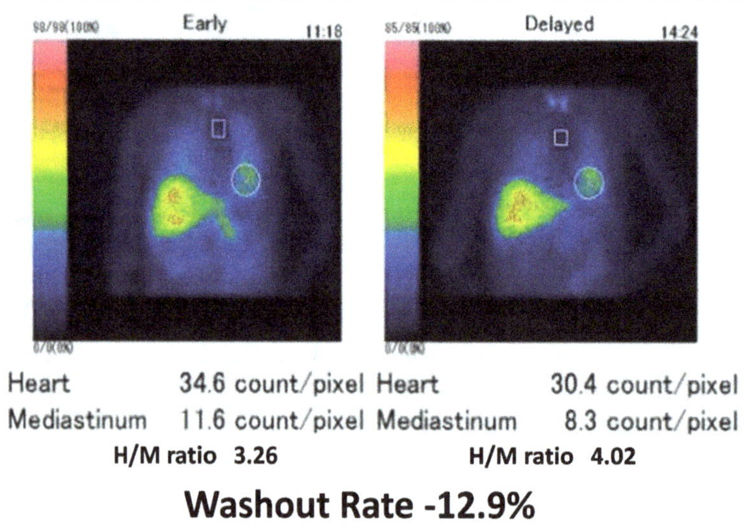

Fig. 4 Cardiac ^{123}I-meta-iodobenzylguanidine (MIBG) scintigraphy results in 2015. The values of the heart to mediastinum (H/M) ratio in the early and delayed phases were 3.26 and 4.02 (normal range is > 2.20), respectively. The washout rate was – 12.9% (normal range is < 22%). ^{123}I-MIBG scintigraphy showed normal cardiac MIBG uptake

Table 1 Diagnostic Criteria for definite, probable, and possible multiple system atrophy (MSA) [1]

Definite MSA

- Neuropathological demonstration of α-synclein-positive glial cytoplasmic inclusions with neurodegenerative changes in striatonigral or olivopontocerebellar structures
- A sporadic and progressive adult onset (>30 y) disease characterized by the symptoms below

Probable MSA

- Autonomic dysfunction including urinary dysfunction (inability to control the release of urine from the bladder, with erectile dysfunction in males) or orthostatic hypotension (decrease of blood pressure within 3 min by at least 30 mm Hg systolic or 15 mm Hg diastolic
- Plus parkinsonism (bradykinesia with rigidity, tremor, or postural instability), which responds poorly to L-dopa, or cerebellar symptoms (gait ataxia with dysathria, limb ataxia, or cerebellar oculomotor dysfunction)

Possible MSA

- Parkinsonism (bradykinesia with rigidity, tremor, or postural instability) or same cerebellar symptoms as Probable MSA
- Plus at least one feature suggesting autonomic dysfunction (otherwise unexplained urinary urgency, frequency or incomplete bladder emptying, erectile dysfunction in males, or orthostatic hypotension not meeting criteria of Probable MSA) and at least one of the additional features below

Additional features of Possible MSA

MSA-P or MSA-C

- Babinski sign with hyperreflexia
- Stridor

Possible MSA-P

- Rapidly progressive parkinsonism
- Poor response to L-dopa
- Postural instability within 3 y of motor onset
- Gait ataxia, cerebellar dysarthria, or cerebellar oculomotor dysfunction
- Dysphasia within 5 y of motor onset
- Atrophy in MRI of putamen, middle cerebellar penducle, pons, or cerebellum
- Hypometabolism in putamen, brainstem, or cerebellum on FDG-PET

Possible MSA-C

- Parkinsonism (bradykinesia and rigidity)
- Atrophy in MRI of putamen, middle cerebellar penducle, or pons
- Hypometabolism in putamen on FDG-PET
- Presynaptic nigrostriatal dopaminergic denervation in SPECT or PET imaging

Features supporting (red flag) and not supporting a diagnosis of MSA

Supporting features

- Orofacial dystonia

Table 1 Diagnostic Criteria for definite, probable, and possible multiple system atrophy (MSA) [1] *(Continued)*

- Disproportionate antecollis
- Severe dysphoria
- Contractures of hands or feet
- Inspiration signs
- Camptocormia (severe anterior flexion of the spine) and/or Pisa syndrome (severe lateral flexion of the spine)
- Severe dysarthria
- New or increased snoring
- Cold hands and feet
- Pathologic laughter or crying
- Jerky, myoclonic postural/action tremor

Nonsupporting features

- Classic pill-rolling rest tremor
- Clinically significant neuropathy
- Hallucination not induced by drugs
- Onset after age 75 y
- Family history of ataxia or parkinsonism
- Dementia (for DSM-IV)
- White matter lesions supporting multiple sclerosis

MSA Multiple system atrophy
MSA-P Multiple system atrophy with predominant parkinsonism
MSA-C Multiple system atrophy with predominant cerebellar features
MRI Magnetic resonance imaging
FDG [18F]fluorodeoxyglucose
PET Positron emission tomography
SPECT Single photon emission computed tomography
DSM-IV Diagnostic and Statistical Manual of Mental Disorders, Fourth Edition

autonomic dysfunction including urinary incontinence (inability to the release of urine from the bladder or orthostatic hypotension (decrease of blood pressure within 3 min of standing by at least 30 mmHg systolic or 15 mmHg diastolic). Orthostatic hypotension has been reported to be apparent in 43 to 81% of patients with MSA [24, 27–30].

Olfactory function has been reported to be preserved or mildly impaired in MSA, in contrast to a marked impairment in Parkinson's disease [31–37]. Olfactory function is evaluated with odor discrimination, threshold detection, or identification. Combination of assessment of olfactory function and other biomarkers including Cardiac MIBG Scintigraphy can be useful to discriminate Parkinson's disease from atypical parkinsonian disorders [33, 38, 39].

Cerebellar ataxia in MSA demonstrates a poor response to medical treatment; however, in approximately 30 to 40% of patients with MSA, parkinsonism may be at least transiently responsive to L-dopa therapy in the early stages of the disease [40, 41]. However, patients with MSA are typically less responsive to L-dopa therapy than those with Parkinson's disease.

Brain MRI may be a useful tool to distinguish MSA from other parkinsonian syndromes. Brain MRI in patients with MSA frequently reveal atrophic changes in the cerebellum, pons, and putamen. While middle cerebellar peduncle and cerebellar atrophy is more common in MSA-C than in MSA-P, putaminal atrophy is more pronounced in patients with MSA-P, which is consistent with the clinical symptoms [42]. Low intensity in the dorsolateral putamen and a slit-like, highly intense signal in the lateral margin of the putamen are commonly observed in T2-weighted MRI (T2WI) of MSA-P [42, 43]. In contrast, in addition to atrophic changes in the inferior or middle cerebellar peduncle, hot-cross bun sign, which may reflect pontine atrophy, is more commonly found in T2WI of MSA-C [8].

Nuclear medicine scans have been reported to be useful in the differential diagnosis of parkinsonism. In contrast to patients with Parkinson's disease and dementia with Lewy bodies, patients with MSA often exhibit normal or only mildly reduced cardiac MIBG uptake in both the early and delayed image phases in MIBG-uptake cardiac scintigraphy [44, 45]. Reduced striatal ^{123}I-FP-CIT uptake is observed in ^{123}I-FP-CIT (DaTscan) SPECT imaging of Parkinson's disease and other atypical parkinsonian diseases such as MSA [46]. Moreover, there are also a relatively limited number of studies reporting reduced DaTscan caused by excessive post-synaptic dopamine D2 blockade due to antipsychotic medication activity or even by the disease itself [47–53].

Clinical features and brain MRI findings together may help to differentiate MSA-P from progressive supranuclear palsy (PSP) and corticobasal degeneration (CBD). Patients with PSP develop vertical supranuclear eye movement disturbances, and exhibit atrophy of the mesencephalic tegmentum, superior colliculus, and superior cerebellar peduncle on brain MRI [54, 55]. However, patients with CBD typically exhibit pronounced frontoparietal asymmetrical atrophy that is particularly distinctive near the central sulcus in brain MRI [55].

To our knowledge, there have been no consistent reports to date demonstrating the effect of antipsychotic treatment on putaminal structure. Recent large-scale, multisite, subcortical brain volumetric studies revealed larger putaminal volume in schizophrenia compared with healthy subjects [56, 57]. Therefore, brain MRI findings, including putaminal atrophy, do not appear to be attributed to antipsychotic medications and schizophrenia itself.

Our patient developed autonomic dysfunction, including urinary incontinence and nocturnal polyuria, at around 55 years of age (2011). By 58 years of age (2014), she exhibited progression of her autonomic dysfunction (i.e., otherwise unexplained urinary incontinence and retention) and parkinsonian symptoms (i.e., postural instability, bradykinesia, and limb muscle rigidity). Consistent with previous reports, she exhibited no clinical symptoms suggesting olfactory dysfunction, although no objective test could be performed (e.g., odor discrimination test, odor identification test, etc.) because she was not able to follow instructions in the inspection test given her worsening psychiatric symptoms. Her parkinsonism did not improve after altering her dose and type of antipsychotics, and brain MRI findings revealed a T2-hyperintense lateral rim and hypointense putamen (Fig. 2). Although her cardiac MIBG scintigraphy results were normal, she exhibited decreased uptake of ^{123}I-FP-CIT in the bilateral striatum, although predominantly in the left dorsolateral striatum. Finally, her parkinsonian symptoms responded poorly to L-dopa therapy (700 mg/day). This combination of clinical features, and neuroimaging and nuclear medicine results, led us to diagnose possible MSA-P.

Notably, her parkinsonism symptoms slightly improved after a number of mECT treatments; this is consistent with previous reports describing the efficacy of mECT against parkinsonism [58, 59].

Psychiatric symptoms, including emotional incontinence, depression, and anxiety, can appear in patients with MSA: 39 to 62% of patients with MSA have been reported to experience mild to severe depression. A few case reports of MSA patients developing psychosis have also been published [60–67]. Papapetropoulos et al. reported that 9.5% of patients with MSA-P experienced hallucinations [65]. There is recent, increasing evidence from brain imaging, genetic association studies, and postmortem brain studies that oligodendrocyte dysfunction is implicated in the pathogenesis of both schizophrenia and major depressive disorder [68–70]. In patients with MSA, variable degrees of olivopontocerebellar atrophy and striatonigral degeneration are typically found at postmortem confirmation, which broadly reflect the cerebellar ataxia and parkinsonism [8]. In 1989, Papp et al. demonstrated the presence of argyrophilic oligodendroglial cytoplasmic inclusions in the central nervous system of patients diagnosed with MSA [17]; these inclusions were later reported to be positive for α-synuclein in 1998. The density of α-synuclein-positive oligodendroglial cytoplasmic inclusion broadly reflects the distribution of neurogenerative changes in patients with MSA [8]. Moreover, dopamine and norepinephrine were found to be profoundly depleted in various brain regions of patients with MSA, especially in the corpus striatum, nucleus accumbens, substantia nigra, locus coeruleus, hypothalamus, and septal nuclei [71]. These findings indicate that depression and psychosis in patients with MSA may be attributed to oligodendrocyte dysfunction and catecholaminergic disturbance(s).

Our patient presented with depressive symptoms and worsening of psychosis with progress of MSA. Although it was difficult to distinguish worsening of schizophrenia from depression and psychosis development by progression of MSA, these affective and psychotic symptoms may be caused partly by oligodendrocyte dysfunction and catecholaminergic disturbance(s) accompanied by progression of MSA. The exact neuropathology of schizophrenia and depression remain unclear. Therefore, it may be worthwhile to investigate the biological mechanisms underlying psychosis and depression in patients with MSA to elucidate a patho-etiology for these diseases.

Finally, there are some limitations to our study that should be addressed. First, definite MSA requires postmortem (autopsy) confirmation of α-synuclein-positive inclusions in oligodendrocytes. However, we could not confirm a diagnosis of definite MSA due to the lack of qualified pathologists/medical doctors able to perform autopsy in our hospital. Second, we could not confirm whether significant orthostatic hypotension met the diagnostic criteria for MSA in the head-up tilted position, despite the patient's complaints of transient dizziness from standing up. Third, we could not perform any objective urological evaluation (e.g., urodynamic testing, or post void residual volume) because of her worsening psychiatric symptoms, although frequent urinary incontinence and severe urinary retention requiring urethral catheterization suggested the presence of underactive detrusor.

Conclusions

To our knowledge, this is the first report to describe a 60-year-old female patient with chronic schizophrenia found to have developed possible MSA-P. Although MSA-P comorbidity in patients with schizophrenia may be very rare, MSA-P should be considered when such patients present with worsening and progression of parkinsonism, especially when accompanied by autonomic dysfunction or cerebellar ataxia. In this case, the combination of SPECT imaging and brain MRI, as well as her clinical features, helped us to discriminate MSA-P from the other parkinsonian syndromes in our differential diagnosis.

Abbreviations

CBD: Corticobasal degeneration; EPS: Extrapyramidal symptoms; LAI: Long-acting injectable; mECT: Modified electroconvulsive therapy; MIBG: 123I-meta-iodobenzylguanidine; MPC: Miyagi Prefecture Center; MRI: Magnetic resonance imaging; MSA: Multiple system atrophy; MSA-C: Multiple system atrophy with predominant cerebellar features; MSA-P: Multiple system atrophy with predominant parkinsonism; PSP: Progressive supranuclear palsy; SPECT: Single-photon emission computed tomography; T2WI: T2-weighted magnetic resonance images

Acknowledgements

The authors are very thankful to the patient and her family. We also would like to thank Editage (www.editage.jp) for English language editing. No specific funding was obtained for reporting this case.

Authors' contributions

HK and MK contributed to the treatment of the clinical case. HK drafted and wrote the paper. TK and MK performed neurological examinations and critically revised the manuscript. TK, MK, TO, and YK reviewed and edited the manuscript. All authors read and approved the final version of the manuscript.

Consent for publication

Written informed consent was obtained from the husband of the patient for publication of this case report and any accompanying images. A copy of the written consent is available for review by the Editor of this *Journal*.

Competing interests

The authors declare that they have no competing interests.

Author details

[1]Department of Psychiatry, Miyagi Psychiatric Center, Mubanchi, Tekurada, Natori 981-1231, Japan. [2]Department of Neurology, Minami Tohoku Hospital, Iwanuma 989-2483, Japan. [3]Department of Neurology, Kohnan Hospital, Sendai 982-8523, Japan.

References

1. Gilman S, Wenning GK, Low PA, Brooks DJ, Mathias CJ, Trojanowski JQ, et al. Second consensus statement on the diagnosis of multiple system atrophy. Neurology. 2008;71:670–6.
2. Bower JH, Maraganore DM, McDonnell SK, Rocca WA. Incidence of progressive supranuclear palsy and multiple system atrophy in Olmsted County, Minnesota, 1976 to 1990. Neurology. 1997;49:1284–8.
3. Schrag A, Ben-Shlomo Y, Quinn NP. Prevalence of progressive supranuclear palsy and multiple system atrophy: a cross-sectional study. Lancet. 1999;354:1771–5.
4. Wenning GK, Colosimo C, Geser F, Poewe W. Multiple system atrophy. Lancet Neurol. 2004;3:93–103.
5. Vanacore N. Epidemiological evidence on multiple system atrophy. J Neural Transm (Vienna). 2005;112:1605–12.
6. Bjornsdottir A, Gudmundsson G, Blondal H, Olafsson E. Incidence and prevalence of multiple system atrophy: a nationwide study in Iceland. J Neurol Neurosurg Psychiatry. 2013;84:136–40.
7. Ciolli L, Krismer F, Nicoletti F, Wenning GK. An update on the cerebellar subtype of multiple system atrophy. Cerebellum Ataxias. 2014;1:14.
8. Fanciulli A, Wenning GK. Multiple-system atrophy. N Engl J Med. 2015;372:249–63.
9. Watanabe H, Saito Y, Terao S, Ando T, Kachi T, Mukai E, et al. Progression and prognosis in multiple system atrophy: an analysis of 230 Japanese patients. Brain. 2002;125:1070–83.
10. Yabe I, Soma H, Takei A, Fujiki N, Yanagihara T, Sasaki H. MSA-C is the predominant clinical phenotype of MSA in Japan: analysis of 142 patients with probable MSA. J Neurol Sci. 2006;249:115–21.
11. Owen MJ, Sawa A, Mortensen PB. Schizophrenia. Lancet. 2016;388:86–97.
12. Mueser KT, McGurk SR. Schizophrenia. Lancet. 2004;363(9426):2063–72.
13. Leucht S, Cipriani A, Spineli L, Mavridis D, Orey D, Richter F, et al. Comparative efficacy and tolerability of 15 antipsychotic drugs in schizophrenia: a multiple-treatments meta-analysis. Lancet. 2013;382(9896):951–62.
14. Dejerine J, Thomas A. L' atrophie olivo-ponto-cérébelleuse. Nouvelle iconographie de la Salpêtrière. 1900;13:330–70.
15. Shy GM, Drager GA. A neurological syndrome associated with orthostatic hypotension: a clinical-pathologic study. Arch Neurol. 1960;2:511–27.
16. Van Eecken HAR. Van Bogaert, L Striatopallidal-nigral degeneration. J Neuropath Exp Neurol. 1960;19:159–66.
17. Papp MI, Kahn JE, Lantos PL. Glial cytoplasmic inclusions in the CNS of patients with multiple system atrophy (striatonigral degeneration, olivopontocerebellar atrophy and shy-Drager syndrome). J Neurol Sci. 1989;94:79–100.
18. Wakabayashi K, Yoshimoto M, Tsuji S, Takahashi H. Alpha-synuclein immunoreactivity in glial cytoplasmic inclusions in multiple system atrophy. Neurosci Lett. 1998;249:180–2.
19. Goedert M, Jakes R, Spillantini MG. The Synucleinopathies: twenty years on. J Parkinsons Dis. 2017;7(Suppl 1):S53–71.
20. Gilman S, Low PA, Quinn N, Albanese A, Ben-Shlomo Y, Fowler CJ, et al. Consensus statement on the diagnosis of multiple system atrophy. J Auton Nerv Syst. 1998;74:189–92.
21. Low PA, Reich SG, Jankovic J, Shults CW, Stern MB, Novak P, et al. Natural history of multiple system atrophy in the USA: a prospective cohort study. Lancet Neurol. 2015;14:710–9.

22. Kim HJ, Jeon BS, Lee JY, Yun JY. Survival of Korean patients with multiple system atrophy. Mov Disord. 2011;26:909–12.
23. Ben-Shlomo Y, Wenning GK, Tison F, Quinn NP. Survival of patients with pathologically proven multiple system atrophy: a meta-analysis. Neurology. 1997;48:384–93.
24. Wenning GK, Geser F, Krismer F, Seppi K, Duerr S, Boesch S, et al. The natural history of multiple system atrophy: a prospective European cohort study. Lancet Neurol. 2013;12:264–74.
25. Schrag A, Wenning GK, Quinn N, Ben-Shlomo Y. Survival in multiple system atrophy. Mov Disord. 2008;23:294–6.
26. Shimohata TOT, Nakayama H, Tomita M, Shinoda H, Nishizawa M. Frequency of nocturnal sudden death in patients with multiple system atrophy. J Neurol. 2008;255:1483–5.
27. Fereshtehnejad SM, Lökk J. Orthostatic hypotension in patients with Parkinson's disease and atypical parkinsonism. Parkinsons Dis. 2014;2014:475854.
28. Pavy-Le Traon A, Piedvache A, Perez-Lloret S, Calandra-Buonaura G, Cochen-De Cock V, Colosimo C, et al. New insights into orthostatic hypotension in multiple system atrophy: a European multicentre cohort study. J Neurol Neurosurg Psychiatry. 2016;87:554–61.
29. Sun Z, Jia D, Shi Y, Hou X, Yang X, Guo J, et al. Prediction of orthostatic hypotension in multiple system atrophy and Parkinson disease. Sci Rep. 2016;12:21649.
30. Sakakibara R, Hattori T, Uchiyama T, Kita T, Asahina M, Suzuki A, et al. Urinary dysfunction and orthostatic hypotension in multiple system atrophy: which is the more common and earlier manifestation? J Neurol Neurosurg Psychiatry. 2000;68:65–9.
31. Wenning GK, Shephard B, Hawkes C, Petruckevitch A, Lees A, Quinn N. Olfactory function in atypical parkinsonian syndromes. Acta Neurol Scand. 1995;91:247–50.
32. Haehner A, Hummel T, Reichmann H. Olfactory dysfunction as a diagnostic marker for Parkinson's disease. Expert Rev Neurother. 2009;9:1773–9.
33. Kikuchi A, Baba T, Hasegawa T, Sugeno N, Konno M, Takeda A. Differentiating Parkinson's disease from multiple system atrophy by [123I] meta-iodobenzylguanidine myocardial scintigraphy and olfactory test. Parkinsonism Relat Disord. 2011;17:698–700.
34. Garland EM, Raj SR, Peltier AC, Robertson D, Biaggioni I. A cross-sectional study contrasting olfactory function in autonomic disorders. Neurology. 2011;76:456–60.
35. Suzuki M, Hashimoto M, Yoshioka M, Murakami M, Kawasaki K, Urashima M. The odor stick identification test for Japanese differentiates Parkinson's disease from multiple system atrophy and progressive supra nuclear palsy. BMC Neurol. 2011;11:157.
36. Doty RL. Olfactory dysfunction in Parkinson disease. Nat Rev Neurol. 2012;8: 329–39.
37. Krismer F, Pinter B, Mueller C, Mahlknecht P, Nocker M, Reiter E, et al. Sniffing the diagnosis: olfactory testing in neurodegenerative parkinsonism. Parkinsonism Relat Disord. 2017;35:36–41.
38. Goldstein DS, Holmes C, Bentho O, Sato T, Moak J, Sharabi Y, et al. Biomarkers to detect central dopamine deficiency and distinguish Parkinson disease from multiple system atrophy. Parkinsonism Relat Disord. 2008;14:600–7.
39. Fujita H, Suzuki K, Numao A, Watanabe Y, Uchiyama T, Miyamoto T, et al. Usefulness of cardiac MIBG scintigraphy, olfactory testing and substantia Nigra Hyperechogenicity as additional diagnostic markers for distinguishing between Parkinson's disease and atypical parkinsonian syndromes. PLoS One. 2016;11:e0165869.
40. Constantinescu R, Richard I, Kurlan R. Levodopa responsiveness in disorders with parkinsonism: a review of the literature. Mov Disord. 2007;22:2141–8.
41. Wenning GK, Tison F, Ben Shlomo Y, Daniel SE, Quinn NP. Multiple system atrophy: a review of 203 pathologically proven cases. Mov Disord. 1997;12:133–47.
42. Feng JY, Huang B, Yang WQ, Zhang YH, Wang LM, Wang LJ, et al. The putaminal abnormalities on 3.0T magnetic resonance imaging: can they separate parkinsonism-predominant multiple system atrophy from Parkinson's disease? Acta Radiol. 2015;56:322–8.
43. Massey LA, Micallef C, Paviour DC, O'Sullivan SS, Ling H, Williams DR, et al. Conventional magnetic resonance imaging in confirmed progressive supranuclear palsy and multiple system atrophy. Mov Disord. 2012;27:1754–62.
44. Taki J, Yoshita M, Yamada M, Tonami N. Significance of 123I-MIBG scintigraphy as a pathophysiological indicator in the assessment of Parkinson's disease and related disorders: it can be a specific marker for Lewy body disease. Ann Nucl Med. 2004;18:453–61.
45. Raffel DM, Koeppe RA, Little R, Wang CN, Liu S, Junck L, et al. PET measurement of cardiac and nigrostriatal denervation in parkinsonian syndromes. J Nucl Med. 2006;47:1769–77.
46. Jin S, Oh M, Oh SJ, Lee SJ, Chung SJ, Lee CS, et al. Differential diagnosis of parkinsonism using dual-phase F-18 FP-CIT PET imaging. Nucl Med Mol Imaging. 2013;47:44–51.
47. Mateos JJ, Lomeña F, Parellada E, Font M, Fernandez E, Pavia J, et al. Decreased striatal dopamine transporter binding assessed with [123I] FP-CIT in first-episode schizophrenic patients with and without short-term antipsychotic-induced parkinsonism. Psychopharmacology. 2005;181:401–6.
48. Mateos JJ, Lomeña F, Parellada E, Font M, Fernández E, Pavia J, et al. Striatal dopamine transporter density decrease in first episode schizophrenic patients treated with risperidone. Rev Esp Med Nucl. 2006;25:159–65.
49. Mateos JJ, Lomeña F, Parellada E, Mireia F, Fernandez-Egea E, Pavia J, et al. Lower striatal dopamine transporter binding in neuroleptic-naive schizophrenic patients is not related to antipsychotic treatment but it suggests an illness trait. Psychopharmacology. 2007;191:805–11.
50. Tinazzi M, Ottaviani S, Isaias IU, Pasquin I, Steinmayr M, Vampini C, et al. [123I]FP-CIT SPET imaging in drug-induced parkinsonism. Mov Disord. 2008; 23:1825–9.
51. Tinazzi M, Antonini A, Bovi T, Pasquin I, Steinmayr M, Moretto G, et al. Clinical and [123I]FP-CIT SPET imaging follow-up in patients with drug-induced parkinsonism. J Neurol. 2009;256:910–5.
52. Tinazzi M, Cipriani A, Matinella A, Cannas A, Solla P, Nicoletti A, et al. [^{123}I]FP-CIT single photon emission computed tomography findings in drug-induced parkinsonism. Schizophr Res. 2012;139:40–5.
53. Tinazzi M, Morgante F, Matinella A, Bovi T, Cannas A, Solla P, et al. Imaging of the dopamine transporter predicts pattern of disease progression and response to levodopa in patients with schizophrenia and parkinsonism: a 2-year follow-up multicenter study. Schizophr Res. 2014;152:344–9.
54. Kurata T, Kametaka S, Ohta Y, Morimoto N, Deguchi S, Deguchi K, et al. PSP as distinguished from CBD, MSA-P and PD by clinical and imaging differences at an early stage. Intern Med. 2011;50:2775–81.
55. Boxer AL, Geschwind MD, Belfor N, Gorno-Tempini ML, Schauer GF, Miller BL, et al. Patterns of brain atrophy that differentiate corticobasal degeneration syndrome from progressive supranuclear palsy. Arch Neurol. 2006;63:81–6.
56. Okada N, Fukunaga M, Yamashita F, Koshiyama D, Yamamori H, Ohi K, et al. Abnormal asymmetries in subcortical brain volume in schizophrenia. Mol Psychiatry. 2016;21:1460–6.
57. Van Erp TG, Hibar DP, Rasmussen JM, Glahn DC, Pearlson GD, Andreassen OA, et al. Subcortical brain volume abnormalities in 2028 individuals with schizophrenia and 2540 healthy controls via the ENIGMA consortium. Mol Psychiatry. 2016;21:547–53.
58. Hooten WM, Melin G, Richardson JW. Response of the parkinsonian symptoms of multiple system atrophy to ECT. Am J Psychiatry. 1998;155:1628.
59. Roane DM, Rogers JD, Helew L, Zarate J. Electroconvulsive therapy for elderly patients with multiple system atrophy: a case series. Am J Geriatr Psychiatry. 2000;8:171–4.
60. Parsa MA, Simon M, Dubrow C, Ramirez LF, Meltzer HY. Psychiatric manifestations of olivo-ponto-cerebellar atrophy and treatment with clozapine. Int J Psychiatry Med. 1993;23:149–56.
61. Ehrt U, Brieger P, Broich K, Marneros A. Psychotic symptoms as initial manifestation of a multiple system atrophy. Fortschr Neurol Psychiatr. 1999; 67:104–7.
62. Benrud-Larson LM, Sandroni P, Schrag A, Low PA. Depressive symptoms and life satisfaction in patients with multiple system atrophy. Mov Disord. 2005;20:951–7.
63. Duggal HS. Cognitive affective psychosis syndrome in a patient with sporadic olivopontocerebellar atrophy. J Neuropsychiatry Clin Neurosci. 2005;17:260–2.
64. Malone D, Dennis MS. Multiple system atrophy and hallucinations–a short report. Int J Geriatr Psychiatry. 2005;20:699–700.
65. Papapetropoulos S, Tuchman A, Laufer D, Mash DC. Hallucinations in multiple system atrophy. Parkinsonism Relat Disord. 2007;13:193–4.
66. Schrag A, Sheikh S, Quinn NP, Lees AJ, Selai C, Mathias C, et al. A comparison of depression, anxiety, and health status in patients with progressive supranuclear palsy and multiple system atrophy. Mov Disord. 2010;25:1077–81.

67. Zhang LY, Cao B, Zou YT, Wei QQ, Ou RW, Zhao B, et al. Depression and anxiety in multiple system atrophy. Acta Neurol Scand. 2017;137:33–7.
68. Tkachev D, Mimmack ML, Ryan MM, Wayland M, Freeman T, Jones PB, et al. Oligodendrocyte dysfunction in schizophrenia and bipolar disorder. Lancet. 2003;362:798–805.
69. Takahashi N, Sakurai T, Davis KL, Buxbaum JD. Linking oligodendrocyte and myelin dysfunction to neurocircuitry abnormalities in schizophrenia. Prog Neurobiol. 2011;93:13–24.
70. Miyata S, Hattori T, Shimizu S, Ito A, Tohyama M. Disturbance of oligodendrocyte function plays a key role in the pathogenesis of schizophrenia and major depressive disorder. Biomed Res Int. 2015;2015:492367.
71. Spokes EG, Bannister R, Oppenheimer DR. Multiple system atrophy with autonomic failure: clinical, histological and neurochemical observations on four cases. J Neurol Sci. 1979;43:59–82.

6

Assessment of sexual dysfunction and associated factors among patients with schizophrenia in Ethiopia, 2017

Tolesa Fanta[1*], Kibrom Haile[1], Dessie Abebaw[1], Dawit Assefa[2] and Getahun Hibdye[3]

Abstract

Background: Sexual dysfunction is remarkably prevalent amongst psychiatric patients than general population. This might be due to either the nature of the illness itself or the unwanted effect of the medication they are taking for the illness which limits the capability of forming interpersonal and sexual relationships. This issue is rarely raised in developing countries, and the aim of this study was to assess magnitude and factors contributing to sexual dysfunction among patients with Schizophrenia.

Method: Hospital based cross sectional study was conducted at Amanuel Mental Specialized Hospital from January to June 2017. The sample required for this study was determined by using single population proportion formula and the final sample size was 423; and systematic random sampling was used to select participants. We used Change in Sexual Functioning Questionnaire to measure sexual dysfunction. The collected data was cleaned, interred in to Epi data and transferred to SPSS version 20 for farther analysis. The OR with 95% CI was used to measure association and *P*-value < 0.05 was used as statistically significant.

Result: A total of 422 patients with Schizophrenia were involved in the study. The prevalence of General Sexual dysfunction was 82.7%; and in male and female patients the prevalence was 84.5 and 78.6% respectively. Marital status (Unmarried, Divorced and widowed, history of relapse and poor quality of life were associated significantly to global sexual dysfunction.

Conclusion: The magnitude of Sexual dysfunction was found to be high among patients with schizophrenia and it is associated with different factors like unmarried, divorced, widowed, relapse and poor quality of life. Treating physicians should be conscious to sexual dysfunction during evaluation and treatment of patients with Schizophrenia. Special attention should be given to single, divorced, widowed patients and patients with history of relapse to improve quality of life of this patients.

Keywords: Sexual dysfunction, Schizophrenia, Amanuel hospital

Background

Sexual life is a natural and complex component of human behaviors that is determined by many physiological and psychological factors. Sexual dysfunction is a public health issue which affects an estimate of 43% women and 31% men in US [1]. The commonest dysfunction among women is sexual desire dysfunction complained by around 30 % of women. The commonest dysfunctions among men are erectile dysfunction and premature ejaculation. Any problem in main area of sexual behavior; interest, arousal, orgasm/ejaculation and like can arise as the result of either pathophysiological or psychological mechanisms [2].

Sexual dysfunction is extremely prevailing in psychiatric patients than general population. This is related to either the nature of the illness itself (negative symptoms like avolition, anhedonia and blunted affect) or the unwanted effect of the medication they are taking for the illness (effect on prolactin secretion and obesity) which

* Correspondence: tole.fanta@gmail.com
[1]Amanuel Mental Specialized Hospital Research and Training Department, Addis Ababa, Ethiopia

limits the capability of forming interpersonal and sexual relationships [1].

The peak age of onset of schizophrenia in both sexes is during the reproductive period. Consequently impaired sexual functioning among persons with schizophrenia can affect their ability to have a family, and, thus, to fulfill traditional social expectations [3]. The role of antipsychotic drugs in sexual functioning of people with schizophrenia is becoming a recent concern of researchers since this side-effect may decrease adherence to treatment, especially among males, because they are more concerned about sexual functioning than females) [4].

Sexual dysfunction has many impacts on patients with Schizophrenia. It has direct or indirect association with quality of life, adherence, difficulty to form and maintain family, and lastly may develop depression and suicidality [3, 5, 6].

Despite the importance and high prevalence of the problem, this patients do not inform the problem either due to feeling of discomfiture or for the reason that they do not view it as a treatable problem [6]. In other hand psychiatrists and other specialists significantly undervalue or even neglect the existence of the problem probably due to embarrassment of talking about sexual problems with patients, lack of time and viewing difficulties in this area as minor compared to psychotic symptoms. In spite of these realities there are limited or no researches conducted in this country regarding sexual dysfunction and its influence on patients with Schizophrenia. Therefore, this study aims to evaluate the prevalence of sexual dysfunction among patients with schizophrenia and see if there is any association between socio-demographic factors, different clinical factors like medication related factors, co-morbid physical or psychiatric conditions, and substance use and sexual dysfunction among patients with Schizophrenia.

Methods

Study design and study period

Institutional based cross sectional study was conducted from January to June 2017.

Study area

The study was conducted at Amanuel Mental Specialized Hospital (ASMH) located in the country's capital, Addis Ababa. Amanuel mental specialized hospital is the only mental specialized hospital where patients mainly afflicted with severe mental illness, including schizophrenia, are treated. The hospital gives service for patients from all over the country. It has a case load of more than 10,000 patients per month and schizophrenia is the number one diagnosis, diagnosed in more than 60% of the patients visiting the hospital.

Population

All patients with Schizophrenia who are on follow up at AMSH are the source populations and people with Schizophrenia in the age group 18 & above who were on treatment at AMSH during the study period were study population.

Eligibility criteria

All patients with Schizophrenia in age group 18 and above were included in the study and the patients in exacerbation phase were excluded from the study.

Sample size

The minimum number of sample required for this study wasdetermined by using single population proportion formula and the final sample size for this study with 10% nonresponse rate was 423.

Sampling procedure

Systematic random sampling technique with interval of 11 was used to select the participants from 4885 patients with schizophrenia came for follow up during data collection period.

Study variables

The outcome variable for this study was Sexual Dysfunction. Socio-demographic factors, duration of the illness, duration on treatment, medication, dosage and frequency, comorbid known chronic medical illness, history of admission and relapse, adherence to drug, Quality of life, Suicide, Depression and history of substance use were explanatory variables for this study.

Instruments

The gold standard instrument which is Structured Clinical Interview for DSM- IV-TR axis I disorders (SCID) was used to confirm a diagnosis of Schizophrenia. Sexual dysfunction was measured by using Changes in Sexual Functioning Questionnaires (CSFQ-14). It has separate forms for female (CSFQ –F-C) and for Male (CSFQ-M-C) Clinical Version. It contains14 items and is used to assess the presence/absence of sexual dysfunction in study participants. All the 14 items should be answered on a five Likert scale to assess global sexual dysfunction. The score < =47 for male and < =41 for female indicates the presence of global sexual dysfunction. The tool can also measure the sexual dysfunction components: Pleasure (Item 1), Desire/frequency (Item 2 and 3), Desire/interest (Item 4, 5 and 6), Arousal/erection (Item 7, 8 and 9) and Orgasm/ejaculation (Item 11, 12 and 13) It has Cronbach's α of 0.91 and 0.93 for male and female scales, respectively [7, 8]. WHOQOL-BREF was used to measure quality of life. This instrument is cross culturally validated and currently in use in

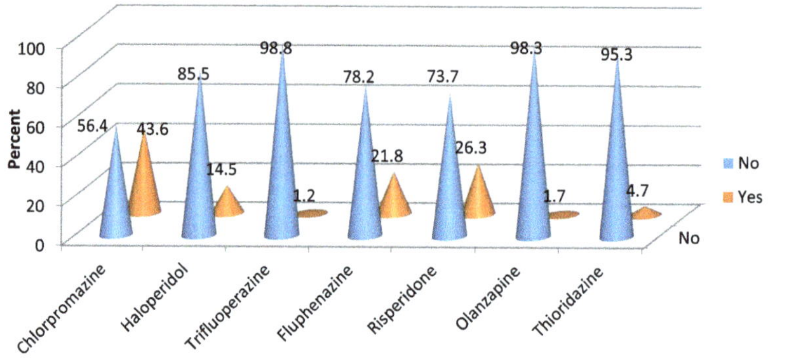

Fig. 1 Antipsychotic Medications prescribed for the participants

different languages [9]. PHQ-9 was used to measure depression in patients with schizophrenia. This instrument has sensitivity of 86% and specificity of 67%in diagnosing depression [10]. Eight –item Morisky medication adherence Scale was used to measure medication adherence. It is valid and reliable with Cronbach's α of 83%; and, sensitivity and specificity of 93 and 53% respectively [11]. The English version of the instruments was translated to local language and back retranslated to English by language professionals and psychiatrists.

Data quality control

17 masters level mental health students were hired for data collection and two masters level mental health professionals were hired to supervise the data collectors. The data collectors were given a two days training on questionnaire and way of assessment. Pre-test was conducted 15 days before the start of actual data collection to know the time needed to complete one questionnaire and to know whether the questionnaire used is understandable to the study participants or not. The data collected during the pre-test was not included in the final analysis.

Data processing and analysis

Data was coded and entered to Epi data and transferred to Statistical Package for Social Sciences version 20 (SPSS-20) for further analysis. Descriptive statistical analysis was used to estimate the frequencies and percentages of the variables. Bivariate and multivariate logistic regression analysis was used to see the association between outcome and explanatory variables. The strength of the association was measured by odds ratio with 95% CI and *P*-value less than 0.05 was considered as statistically significant.

Ethical consideration

Ethical clearance was obtained from Amanuel Mental Specialized Hospital Ethical Review Committee. The Four Item Abbreviated Mental Test (AMT4) was used to measure the capacity of the patient to give consent. Then the purpose, importance and confidentiality of the information gathered was explained to each of the competent participant before the start of interview. Participants were also informed that they will never get any benefit because of participation in the study and no harm on them if they would not agree to participate or withdraw from participation during the data collection

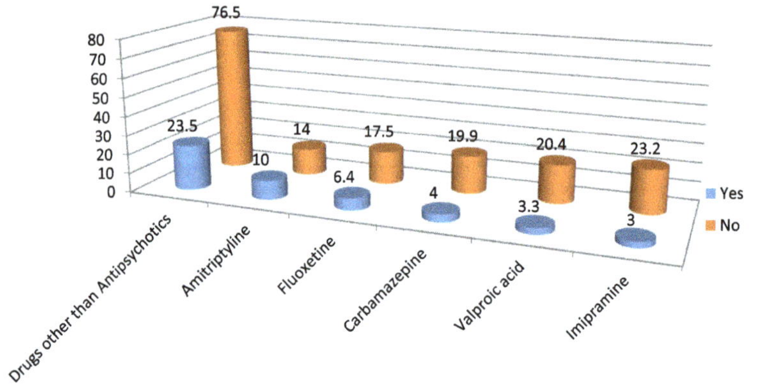

Fig. 2 Medications prescribed for comorbid psychiatric problems

Table 1 Distribution of participants by socio-demographic factors and clinical factors

No.	Variables	Variables category	Frequency (422)	Percentage (100%)
1	Age	18–24	35	8.3
		25–34	174	41.2
		35–44	150	35.5
		> = 45	63	14.9
2	Sex	Female	132	31.3
		Male	290	68.7
3	Marital Status	Married	154	36.5
		Single	224	53.1
		Divorced and Widowed	44	10.4
4	Ethnicity	Oromo	140	33.2
		Amhara	126	29.9
		Gurage	98	23.2
		Others*	58	13.7
5	Religion	Orthodox	228	54
		Protestant	79	18.7
		Muslim	115	27.3
6	Educational Status	No formal education	31	7.3
		Primary school	137	32.5
		High School	164	38.9
		Diploma	46	10.9
		Degree and above	44	10.4
7	Occupation	Private	135	32
		Governmental	42	11.1
		Unemployed	142	33.6
		Others(House wife, Daily labourers)	98	23.2
8	Residence	Urban	353	83.6
		Rural	69	16.4
9	Frequency of Chlorpromazine per day	Once/day	149	81.0
		> = 2	35	19
10	Frequency of Haloperidol per day	Once/day	46	75.4
		> = 2	15	24.6
11	Frequency of Trifluoperazine per day	Once/day	3	60
		> = 2/day	2	40
12	Frequency of Fluphenazineper day	Once/month	91	90.9
		> = 2/month	1	1.1
13	Frequency of Resperidone per day	Once/day	71	64.5
		> = 2/day	39	35.5
14	Frequency of Olanzapine per day	Once/day	5	62.5
		> = 2/day	2	37.5
15	Frequency of Thioridazine per day	Once/day	20	100
		> = 2/day	0	0
16	Duration of the illness	<=5 years	174	41.2
		6-10 years	119	28.2
		> = 11 years	129	30.6

Table 1 Distribution of participants by socio-demographic factors and clinical factors *(Continued)*

No.	Variables	Variables category	Frequency (422)	Percentage (100%)
17	Duration on treatment	<=5 years	207	49.1
		6-10 years	103	24.4
		> = 11 years	112	26.5
18	Admission	No	254	60.2
		Yes	168	39.8
19	Number of admission	<=1	96	57.1
		> = 2	72	42.9
20	Relapse	No	226	53.6
		Yes	196	46.4
21	Number of relapse	<=1	96	49
		> = 2	100	51
22	Depression	No	346	82
		Yes	76	18
23	Non-Adherence	No	203	48.1
		Yes	219	51.9
24	Poor Quality of life	No	217	51.4
		Yes	205	48.6
		Yes	0	0
25	Suicidal Ideation	No	373	88.4
		Yes	49	11.6
26	Suicidal Attempt	No	406	96.2
		Yes	16	3.8

process. Finally, their willingness to be involved in the study was asked and written consent was obtained.

At the time of data collection the investigator, supervisor and data collectors followed 'code of ethics' and obeyed the rules & regulations of the hospital. Participant's privacy was kept strictly at the time of data collection.

Result

A total of 422 patients with schizophrenia participated on the study with response rate of 99.76%. Among the participants 290(68.7%) were male and 132(31.3%) were female in gender. The mean age of the participants is 35.46 with ± 9.25 standard deviation. Majority of the participants 353(83.6%) were from urban area. The most frequently prescribed antipsychotic drug is chlorpromazine 184(43.6%) followed by Resperidone 111 (26.3%) (Fig. 1). Amitriptyline is the most frequently prescribed drug among the medications ordered for other comorbid psychiatric conditions 42(41.6%) followed by Fluoxetine 27(26.7%) (Fig. 2). Most of the participants take their medications once in twenty four hours (Table 1). Among

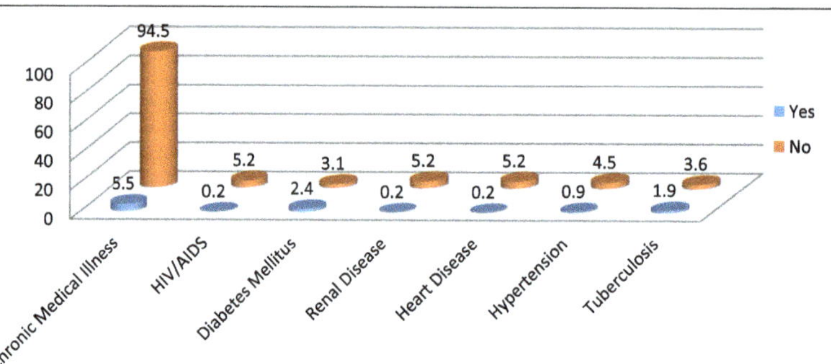

Fig. 3 Magnitude of Chronic Medical Illness among Patients with Schizophrenia

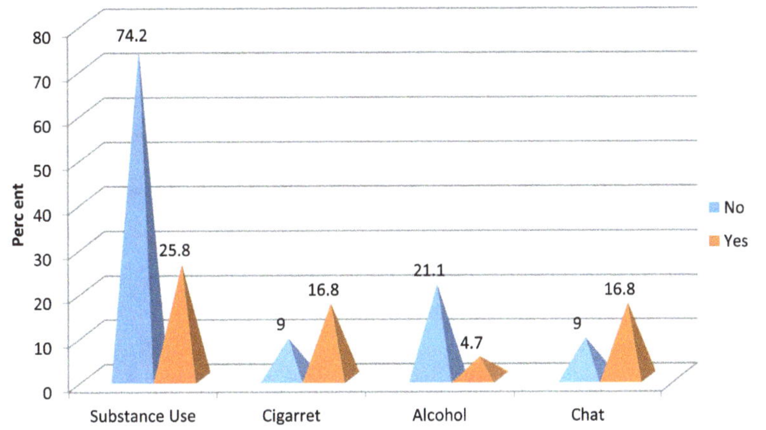

Fig. 4 Magnitude of Substance Use among Patients with Schizophrenia

the study participants, 23(5.5%) were found to have at least one comorbid other medical illness. The most frequently occurring chronic medical illness in patients with Schizophrenia is Diabetes Mellitus 10(2.4%) followed by Tuber Closes (TB) 8(1.9%) (Fig. 3). Among the substance users 71(16.8%) use cigarette and khat users were 71(16.8%) (Khat and Cigarette are equally consumed) (Fig. 4). The median score of duration of the illness is 7 years with inter quartile range of 6, and the median score of duration on treatment is 6 years with inter quartile range of 10. The median score for frequency of admission is 1 with inter quartile range of 1, and the median score for frequency of relapse is 2 with inter quartile range of 2. The mean score of Quality of Life of the participants is 60.59 with standard deviation of ± 9.43 (Table 1).

Prevalence of sexual dysfunction among patients with schizophrenia

The prevalence of General sexual dysfunction among the study participants was 349(82.7%) with 95% confidence interval of (78.9, 86.3). The overall sexual dysfunction among male participants was 246(84.5%) with 95% confidence interval of (80.3, 88.7) and it was 103(78.6%) with 95% confidence interval of (71, 84.7) in female Schizophrenic patients (Fig. 5). Erectile dysfunction 277(95.2%) is highly prevalent followed by pleasure dysfunction 274(94.2%) in male participants (Fig. 6). In female participants who had sexual dysfunction the most prevalent sexual dysfunction was pleasure dysfunction 125(94.7%) followed by arousal/excitement dysfunction 123(93.2%) (Fig. 7).

Bivariate and multivariate analysis

After bivariate logistic regression analysis, five variables (Marital status, Resperidone use, Relapse, Depression and Quality of life) met the requirement to proceed to multivariate logistic regression analysis. After multivariate analysis, marital status, history of relapse, and quality of life were found to be significantly associated with global sexual dysfunction. Compared to the married ones, being single, [aOR 4.19, 95% CI (2.30, 7.64)], and being divorced [aOR 2.86,

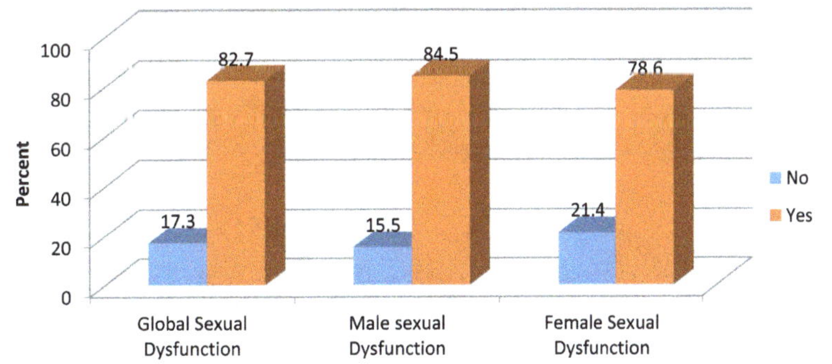

Fig. 5 Global sexual Dysfunction and sexual Dysfunction across Male and Female participants

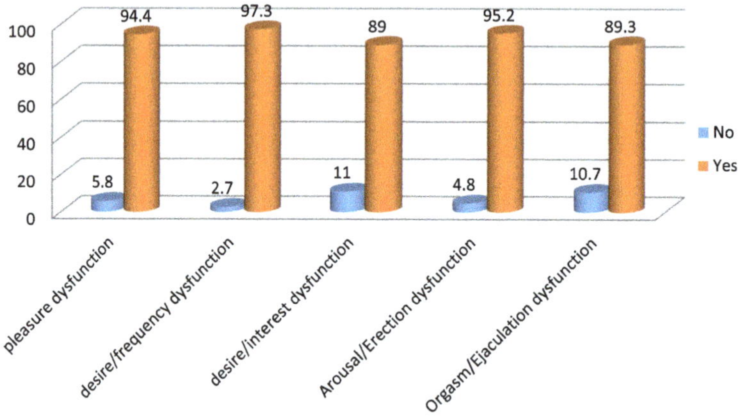

Fig. 6 Components of Sexual Dysfunction among male participants

95% CI (1.03, 7.90)] were significantly associated with General sexual dysfunction. History of relapse, [aOR 2.21, 95% CI (1.25, 3.91)], and poor quality of life, [aOR 5.57, 95% CI (2.79, 11.09)] were also significantly associated with General sexual dysfunction at p-value< 0.05 (Table 2).

Discussion

This study found that magnitude of General sexual dysfunction, and sexual dysfunction across male and female patients with Schizophrenia is extremely high and needs immediate intervention. The prevalence of general sexual dysfunction among patients with Schizophrenia in this study is supported by the comparative study conducted in Egypt on paranoid and non-paranoid schizophrenic patients in which Prevalence of general sexual dysfunction was 80% in patients with paranoid schizophrenia and 86.7% in patients with non-paranoid Schizophrenia [7]. The magnitude of general sexual dysfunction in this study is very high when compared to the study conducted in Britain and Iran which was 45 and 31.1% respectively [12, 13]. The reason for this significant difference may be explained by socio-cultural difference and difference in measurement instrument to assess sexual dysfunction. In case of the study conducted in Britain, they used Sexual Functioning Questionnaire (SFQ) to assess sexual dysfunction, and the study conducted in Iran used Arizona Sexual Experience Scale (ASEX) [12, 13].

Prevalence of sexual dysfunction among male Schizophrenic patients in our study which is 84.5% in lines with the study conducted by Macdonald in which the magnitude of sexual dysfunction in male Schizophrenic patients is 82% [14]. Magnitude of sexual dysfunction among female schizophrenic patients in this study which is 78.6% is lower than that of Macdonald in which prevalence of sexual dysfunction among female schizophrenic patients is 92%, and is higher than that of USA and Turkey in which prevalence of female sexual dysfunction is 59 and 68% respectively [14–16]. The reason for the discrepancy is probably due to difference in culture and living style which may differ in different countries and population. Difference in measurement tool to assess sexual dysfunction in this particular population is

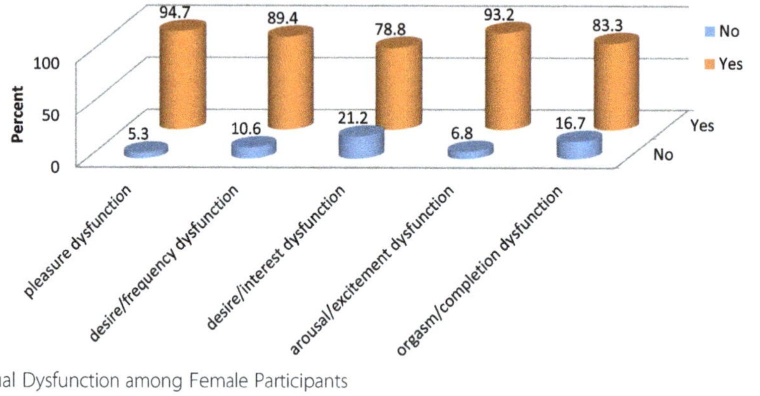

Fig. 7 Components of Sexual Dysfunction among Female Participants

Table 2 Factors Associated With Sexual Dysfunction Among Patients With Schizophrenia At Amanuel Mental Specialized Hospital/2017

Explanatory variables	Variables category	Sexual Dysfunction		Bivariate and Multivariate Analysis		*P*-Value
		Absent	Present	Bivariate Analysis COR (95% CI)	Multivariate Analysis aOR (95% CI)	
Marital Status	Married	44	110	1:00	1:00	
	Single	23	201	3.49(2.01,6.10)	4.19(2.30,7.64)	0.000
	Divorced and Widowed	6	38	2.53(1.00,6.6.42)	2.86(1.03,7.90)	0.043
Resperidone	No	62	249	1.00	1.00	
	Yes	11	100	2.264(1.15,4.48)	1.69(0.82,3.51)	
Relapse	No	30	196			
	Yes	43	153	1.84(1.10,3.06)	2.21(1.25,3.91)	0.007
Depression	No	67	279	1.00	1.00	
	Yes	6	70	2.80(1.17,6.72)	1.49(0.58,3.83)	
Quality of life	Good	60	157	1.00	1.00	
	Poor	13	192	5.64(2.99,10.66)	5.57(2.79,11.09)	0.000

also possible reason for observed difference. In case of USA they used the Global Impression of Sexual Function (GISF) and in Turkey they used Arizona Sexual Experience Scale (ASEX) to assess sexual dysfunction [15, 16]. Another possible reason for the difference might be criterion used to include the participants in the study. The study conducted in USA included patients who were on conventional antipsychotics and Resperidone where as in our study all schizophrenic patients on any antipsychotic medication were included in the study [16]. Sample size difference across the studies is also possible reason for the discrepancy. Among the factors hypothesized to be contributing factors to sexual dysfunction, unmarried participants were four times more likely to develop sexual dysfunction compared to married participants and Divorced and widowed participants were three times more likely to develop sexual dysfunction compared to married participants. This finding is supported by the study conducted in Nigeria [17]. The possible reason for the association is that the infrequent sexual activity in single and divorced/widowed individuals probably decreases frequency of sexual desire. Having history of relapse exposes two times more to sexual dysfunction compared to the patients without history of relapse. This may be explained by, the more the relapse is frequent the more the illness becomes deteriorated with predomination of negative symptoms of Schizophrenia which potentially affect sexual performance. The need for higher doses of antipsychotics in case of frequent relapse is also another possible reason for this significant association. In this study sexual dysfunction is found to be highly associated with poor quality of life. This result is supported by the study conducted by Olfson and Kandrakonda S [18, 19]. This may be due to the fact that an inproper sexual functioning may affect maintaining a satisfying intimate relationship which is the major component of Quality of life.

Conclusion

Prevalence of Sexual dysfunction is found to be high among patients with Schizophrenia and it needs special attention. The current prevalence of general sexual dysfunction among Schizophrenic patients in our study is high. Regarding sexual dysfunction across sex, male and female sexual dysfunction was also high. Among the hypothesized factors to be risk factors for sexual dysfunction, marital status (single, divorced, widowed), history of relapse and poor quality of life were significantly associated with sexual dysfunction.

Recommendation

To Amanuel Mental Specialized Hospital.

All Psychiatrists and mental health specialists have to be conscious to sexual dysfunction which is highly prevalent among the patients they are treating, and all patients who are on follow up at this hospital for the case of Schizophrenia should be screened for sexual dysfunction. The overall treatment and care delivered by the hospital should focus on improving quality of life by diagnosing and managing sexual dysfunction properly, rather than focusing only on decreasing the symptom of the illness. Special consideration should be given to a patients with history of relapse, single, widowed and divorced.

Abbreviations
AMSH: Amanuel Mental Specialized Hospital; CSFQ: Changes in Sexual Functioning Questionnaires; PHQ-9: Patients Health Questionnaire nine; SD: Sexual Dysfunction; SMI: Severe Mental Illness; SPSS: Statistical Package of Social Science; USA: United States of America; WHOQOL: World Health Organization Quality of Life

Acknowledgements
We are grateful to the data collectors and supervisors for their unreserved effort. Our gratitude also goes to Amanuel Mental Specialized Hospital for funding this study. Finally we are grateful to the study participants for their patience.

Funding
Funding for this study was provided by Amanuel Mental Specialized Hospital.

Authors' contributions
TF involved in designing and coordinating overall progress of the study; KH, DA[1], GH and DA[2] equally contributed in the design of the study, performed the statistical analyses and critically revised the manuscript. All authors read and approved the final manuscript.

Competing interests
The authors declare that they have no competing interests.

Author details
[1]Amanuel Mental Specialized Hospital Research and Training Department, Addis Ababa, Ethiopia. [2]Amanuel Mental Specialized Hospital, Addis Ababa, Ethiopia. [3]Amanuel Mental Specialized Hospital Clinical Service Department, Addis Ababa, Ethiopia.

References
1. Zemishlany Z, Weizman A. The impact of mental illness on sexual dysfunction. InSexual Dysfunction 2008 Apr 8 (Vol. 29, pp. 89–106). Karger Publishers.
2. Baggaley M. Sexual dysfunction in schizophrenia: focus on recent evidence. Hum Psychopharmacol Clin Exp. 2008 Apr 1;23(3):201–9.
3. Kelly DL, Conley RR. Sexuality and schizophrenia: a review. Schizophr Bull. 2004 Jan 1;30(4):767–79.
4. Hanssens L, L'Italien G, Loze JY, Marcus RN, Pans M, Kerselaers W. The effect of antipsychotic medication on sexual function and serum prolactin levels in community-treated schizophrenic patients: results from the schizophrenia trial of aripiprazole (STAR) study (NCT00237913). BMC psychiatry. 2008 Dec 22;8(1):1.
5. Kikuchi T, Iwamoto K, Sasada K, Aleksic B, Yoshida K, Ozaki N. Sexual dysfunction and hyperprolactinemia in Japanese schizophrenic patients taking antipsychotics. Prog Neuro-Psychopharmacol Biol Psychiatry. 2012 Apr 27;37(1):26–32.
6. Hashem A.H., Abd El-Gawad T., Ezzat M., Assal A., Goueily T. *and* El Rakhawy M. A comparative study of sexual function in paranoid versus non-paranoid schizophrenic patients and its relation to serum prolactin Level.Current psychiatry. Vol 13. No. 2. July 2006.
7. Maria Paz Garcia-Portilla, MD, PhD et al. Psychometric properties of the Spanish version of the changes in sexual functioning questionnaire short-form (CSFQ-14) in patients with severe mental disorders. International Society for Sexual Medicine J Sex Med 2011;8:1371–1382..
8. Liu-Seifert H, Kinon BJ, Tennant CJ, Sniadecki J, Volavka J. Sexual dysfunction in patients with schizophrenia treated with conventional antipsychotics or risperidone. Neuropsychiatr Dis Treat. 2009 Apr 8;5:47–54.
9. Oyekanmi AK, Adelufosi AO, Abayomi O, Adebowale TO. Demographic and clinical correlates of sexual dysfunction among Nigerian male outpatients on conventional antipsychotic medications. BMC research notes. 2012 Jun 7;5(1):1.
10. Olfson M, Uttaro T, Carson WH, Tafesse E. Male sexual dysfunction and quality of life in schizophrenia. J Clin psychiatry. 2005 Mar;66(3):331–8.
11. Kandrakonda S, Jally MR, Kesava Reddy SR, Miryala G. Prevalence of sexual dysfunction in patients with mental illness receiving psychotropic medication. AP J Psychol Med. 2014;15(2):235–9.
12. CLAYTON ELMaAH. Reliability and construct validity of the changes in sexual functioning questionnaire short-form (CSFQ-14):. Journal of Sex & Marital Therapy,. 2006;32:43–52. Departments of Psychiatric Medicine & Health Evaluation Sciences, University of Virginia, Charlottesville, Virginia, USA.
13. WHO. WHOQOL, user manual, division of mental health and prevention of substance abuse. Geneva, Switzerland.. 1998.
14. Gelaye B, et al. Validity of the patient health Questionnaire-9 for depression screening and diagnosis in East Africa. Psychiatry Res. 2013 December 15; 210(2) https://doi.org/10.1016/j.psychres.2013.07.015.
15. Morisky E, Ang A, Wood M. Predictive validity of a medication adherence measure in an outpatient setting. J Clin Hypertens (Greenwich). 2008;10: 348–54.
16. Smith S, O'KEANE VE, Murray R. Sexual dysfunction in patients taking conventional antipsychotic medication. Br J Psychiatry. 2002 Jul 1;181(1):49–55.
17. Ahmadzadeh G, Shahin A. Sexual dysfunctions in the patients hospitalized in psychiatric wards compared to other specialized wards in Isfahan, Iran, in 2012. Advanced biomedical research. 2015;4–225.
18. Macdonald S, Halliday J, MacEwan T, Sharkey V, Farrington S, Wall S, McCreadie RG. Nithsdale schizophrenia surveys 24: sexual dysfunction. Br J Psychiatry. 2003 Jan 2;182(1):50–6.
19. Hocaoglu C, Celik FH, Kandemir G, Guveli H, Bahceci B. Sexual dysfunction in outpatients with schizophrenia in Turkey: a cross-sectional study. Shanghai Arch Psychiatry. 2014 Dec 1;26(6):347–56.

7

High-density lipoprotein-cholesterol and antipsychotic medication in overweight inpatients with schizophrenia

Shin Ono[1,2], Takuro Sugai[2,3], Yutaro Suzuki[2,3], Manabu Yamazaki[4], Kazutaka Shimoda[2,5], Takao Mori[4], Yuji Ozeki[2,5], Hiroshi Matsuda[4], Norio Sugawara[2,6], Norio Yasui-Furukori[2,6], Kurefu Okamoto[4], Toyoaki Sagae[7] and Toshiyuki Someya[2,3*]

Abstract

Background: Patients with schizophrenia have an increased prevalence of metabolic disturbances compared with the general population. However, the mechanisms underlying the metabolic side effects of antipsychotics are unknown. The aim of the present study was to compare the levels of high-density lipoprotein (HDL)-cholesterol in Japanese schizophrenia patients medicated with olanzapine, risperidone, or aripiprazole monotherapy.

Methods: This study was a post-hoc analysis of a nationwide survey, which included 433 Japanese outpatients with schizophrenia and 674 inpatients. A brief questionnaire was compiled that covered demographic data, systolic blood pressure, diastolic blood pressure, and HDL-cholesterol after reviewing the relevant literature and guidelines. To compare demographic and clinical characteristics, analysis of variance was performed for continuous variables and the chi-square test was performed for categorical variables. For comparisons of HDL-cholesterol levels among the three antipsychotic groups, analysis of covariance was carried out with age, diastolic blood pressure, chlorpromazine-equivalent dosage, and waist circumference as confounding variables after stratification by body mass index (BMI) for each outpatient group and inpatient group.

Results: The mean age was 57.9 ± 14.0 years and the mean BMI was 23.4 ± 4.5 kg/m^2. HDL-cholesterol levels when stratified by BMI differed significantly ($p = 0.019$) between the three antipsychotic groups after age, diastolic blood pressure, chlorpromazine-equivalent dosage, and waist circumference in inpatients. A significant difference in HDL-cholesterol levels was only found in the overweight inpatient group, and no significant differences in HDL-cholesterol levels were found among the three antipsychotics for outpatients of all BMI stratifications or inpatients that were underweight or of normal weight. For post-hoc analysis of HDL-cholesterol levels in overweight inpatients, HDL-cholesterol was significantly lower in the olanzapine group than in the aripiprazole group ($p = 0.023$).

Conclusions: This study reveals a difference in HDL-cholesterol levels in overweight Japanese inpatients with schizophrenia resulting from the use of different antipsychotics. In the post-hoc analysis of HDL-cholesterol levels in overweight inpatients, HDL-cholesterol was significantly lower in the olanzapine group than in the aripiprazole group. Further studies incorporating more detailed evaluations, including diet and physical activity, are needed to clarify the differences in HDL-cholesterol according to antipsychotic use.

Keywords: Schizophrenia, Antipsychotics, High-density lipoprotein-cholesterol, Metabolic syndrome

* Correspondence: psy@med.niigata-u.ac.jp
[2]Japanese Society of Clinical Neuropsychopharmacology, Tokyo, Japan
[3]Department of Psychiatry, Niigata University Graduate School of Medical and Dental Sciences, Niigata, Japan
Full list of author information is available at the end of the article

Background

Patients with schizophrenia suffer from increased morbidity and mortality compared with the general population and have a life expectancy that is approximately 20% shorter [1]. Patients with schizophrenia also have an increased prevalence of cardiometabolic risk factors such as obesity, diabetes type 2, hypertension, hyperglycemia, and dyslipidemia compared with the normal population [2–4]. Low high-density lipoprotein (HDL)-cholesterol level, a cardiometabolic risk factor, is strongly and inversely associated with the risk of coronary heart disease [5]. Some studies attributed metabolic disturbance in schizophrenia to poor patient lifestyle choices such as sedentary lifestyle, smoking, poor diet, prolonged stress, as well as use of antipsychotic drugs, and genetic susceptibility [6].

Metabolic disorders associated with atypical antipsychotic drugs include abnormalities of glucose metabolism such as insulin resistance, hyperglycemia, dyslipidemia and weight gain [7–11]. In a meta-analysis study of second-generation antipsychotics, olanzapine increased cholesterol levels to a level higher than that induced by aripiprazole, risperidone, or ziprasidone [12]. However, the underlying causal mechanisms of metabolic side effects with antipsychotics are unknown. Apart from the effects of antipsychotics related to lipid abnormalities, patients with schizophrenia who are antipsychotic drug-naïve, or drug-free, also have low levels of HDL-cholesterol and are at high risk for metabolic syndrome [13].

Many confounding factors affect HDL-cholesterol levels. It is well known that HDL-cholesterol levels are decreased in overweight subjects [14, 15], and there is a negative association with body mass index (BMI) and HDL-cholesterol [16]. Additionally, smoking decreased HDL-cholesterol [17] while exercise increased HDL-cholesterol [18, 19]. As these various factors (e.g. diet, exercise, smoking, obesity, antipsychotics, and schizophrenia) influence HDL-cholesterol, it seems prudent to investigate HDL-cholesterol in schizophrenia in relation to BMI.

The prevalence of metabolic syndrome in schizophrenia patients treated with antipsychotics is higher than in the general population. In a previous nationwide survey on the prevalence of metabolic syndrome in the Japanese population, the prevalence in outpatients was approximately 3-fold higher than that in inpatients [20]. Japan has more psychiatric hospitals than other Organization for Economic Cooperation and Development (OECD) countries [21]. The average length of stay in psychiatric beds was 301.0 days according to surveys by the Ministry of Health, Labour and Welfare in Japan [22], and the length of stay in psychiatric beds in Japan was considered longer than that in other countries. The system for psychiatric treatment in Japan is different from other countries in terms of longer stay in psychiatric beds and higher number of psychiatric beds. Of note, there is a relatively uniform diet or exercise regime in a hospitalized environment compared with the outpatient environment in Japan. Drug adherence is also maintained in hospitals. Therefore, differences in medical care environments, such as hospitalization and outpatient treatment, should be taken into account when evaluating HDL-cholesterol in schizophrenic patients, especially in Japan.

The aim of the present study was to compare HDL-cholesterol levels between Japanese schizophrenia patients medicated with olanzapine, risperidone, or aripiprazole monotherapy as a post-hoc analysis of a previous nationwide survey.

Methods

Subjects

This study was a post-hoc analysis of a previous survey [20]. Of the 23,116 subjects in the original survey, only those receiving monotherapy with olanzapine, risperidone, or aripiprazole were included in the present study. The original sample included 7655 outpatients and 15,461 inpatients diagnosed with schizophrenia who had been taking the same antipsychotics. All of the subjects were diagnosed with schizophrenia based on International Statistical Classification of Diseases and Related Health Problems version 10 (ICD-10) or the Diagnostic and Statistical Manual of Mental Disorders, fourth edition, text revision (DSM-IV-TR) [23, 24]. The study protocol and informed consent procedure were approved by the Ethics Committee of the Japan Psychiatric Hospitals Association. The investigation was carried out in accordance with the Declaration of Helsinki. Each participant gave written informed consent prior to all study procedures.

The number of Japanese patients with schizophrenia was 795,000, and the majority of these patients were treated in hospitals in the Japan Psychiatric Hospitals Association in an investigation conducted by the Ministry of Health, Labour and Welfare in 2008. For the aim of assisting patients with schizophrenia, a joint project with the cooperation of the Japanese Society of Clinical Neuropsychopharmacology and the Japan Psychiatric Hospitals Association was started in Japan in 2012.

A questionnaire survey was conducted between January 2012 and July 2014. Responses were obtained from 7655 outpatients and 15,461 inpatients in 520 facilities for outpatients and 247 facilities for inpatients belonging to the Japan Psychiatric Hospitals Association. We excluded patients aged under 20 years; patients whose sex, BMI, and HDL-cholesterol data were not recorded; and patients medicated with polypharmacy of antipsychotics or monotherapy with drugs other than olanzapine, risperidone, or aripiprazole. The final study population comprised 1107 individuals.

Assessments

A brief questionnaire was compiled to cover demographic data (age and sex), systolic blood pressure, diastolic blood pressure, and HDL-cholesterol after reviewing the relevant literature and guidelines. Body weight, height, and waist circumference were measured, and BMI was calculated by weight (kg)/height squared (m^2). Blood pressure was measured twice with patients in a seated position after at least 5 min of rest, using a standard mercury sphygmomanometer. HDL-cholesterol was measured by standard analytical techniques.

Statistical analyses

Demographic and clinical variables are presented as the mean ± standard deviation (SD) or proportion. To compare demographic and clinical characteristics between the three antipsychotic groups, analysis of variance was performed for continuous variables and the chi-square test was performed for categorical variables. The threshold for significance was set at $p < 0.05$. SPSS Statistics 24 for Mac OS (IBM Japan, Tokyo, Japan) was used for statistical analyses. For comparisons of HDL-cholesterol levels among the three antipsychotic groups, analysis of covariance was carried out with age, diastolic blood pressure, chlorpromazine-equivalent dosage, and waist circumference as confounding variables after stratification by BMI (BMI < 18.5, underweight; 18.5 ≤ BMI < 25, normal weight; BMI ≥ 25, overweight) for each outpatient group and inpatient group. Post-hoc analyses were performed using the Bonferroni method.

Results

There were 433 outpatients and 674 inpatients with schizophrenia in this study. All were Japanese with a mean age of 57.9 ± 14.0 years and a mean BMI of 23.4 ± 4.5 kg/m^2. Table 1 summarizes the demographic and clinical characteristics of the entire study population ($n = 1107$). No significant intergroup differences were observed for sex, BMI, waist circumference, systolic blood pressure, or HDL-cholesterol. Significant differences were observed for age ($p < 0.001$), diastolic blood pressure ($p = 0.025$), and chlorpromazine-equivalent dosage of current atypical antipsychotics ($p < 0.001$). The HDL-cholesterol levels for overweight inpatients differed significantly among the three antipsychotic groups ($p = 0.019$) after adjustment for age, diastolic blood pressure, chlorpromazine-equivalent dosage, and waist circumference. For post-hoc analysis of HDL-cholesterol levels in overweight inpatients among the three antipsychotic groups, HDL-cholesterol was significantly lower in the olanzapine group than in the aripiprazole group ($p = 0.023$), and HDL-cholesterol levels were similar between the olanzapine and risperidone groups ($p = 0.160$). HDL-cholesterol levels in underweight and normal weight patients did not differ significantly (Table 2). No significant differences in HDL-cholesterol levels were found among the three antipsychotics for outpatients of all BMI stratifications (Table 3).

Discussion

This study reveals that overweight inpatients with schizophrenia treated with antipsychotics had significant differences in HDL-cholesterol after adjustment for age, diastolic blood pressure, chlorpromazine-equivalent dosage, and waist circumference. However, there was no difference in HDL-cholesterol among the antipsychotic treatments in the overall patient group, outpatients of all BMI stratifications or inpatients of normal weight and underweight. We believe this survey is the first large-scale questionnaire survey in Japan to show a difference in HDL-cholesterol levels between antipsychotic drugs by BMI stratification.

Regarding the effects of antipsychotics on cholesterol, antipsychotic treatments have been reported to be associated with increased total and low-density lipoprotein (LDL)-cholesterol as well as decreased HDL-cholesterol [10, 25]. In a previous 52-week comparison study of olanzapine and aripiprazole, olanzapine was associated with significantly greater weight gain than aripiprazole throughout the study [26]. The change in HDL-cholesterol from baseline was significantly lower in the olanzapine group than in the aripiprazole group at the 52-week end-point where weight gain related to the two drugs was highest [26]. Although this prospective study by Chrzanowski and colleagues [26] was methodologically different to our cross-sectional study, our results also show that HDL-cholesterol is lower in overweight inpatients in the olanzapine group than those in the aripiprazole group. A 1-year observation study on first-episode drug-naïve patients revealed significant differences in HDL-cholesterol decreases between groups of patients who gained > 20% or < 20% of their baseline BMI at 1 year, and no significant difference in HDL-cholesterol between olanzapine- and risperidone-treated patients [27]. This finding is in accord with the lack of difference observed between olanzapine and risperidone in overweight inpatients in the present study.

In a randomized comparative study of aripiprazole and olanzapine, no group differences were observed in the proportions of patients with potentially clinically significant fasting HDL cholesterol levels, because the weight gain at the study end-point was significantly greater with olanzapine than with aripiprazole [28]. The discrepancy with the present results may arise because there was no correction of HDL-cholesterol by baseline BMI, waist circumference, or weight change in their study. In a comparison between olanzapine and risperidone, the patients included across the all groups were, on average, overweight with a mean BMI of > 25 kg/m^2 and

Table 1 Comparisons of demographic and clinical characteristics of patients in the three antipsychotic groups

		Olanzapine (*N* = 356)	Risperidone (*N* = 529)	Aripiprazole (*N* = 222)	*p*-value
Age	years	56.4 ± 14.0	60.2 ± 13.2	54.8 ± 15.2	< 0.001
Females (males)		158 (198)	243 (286)	115 (107)	0.201
Outpatients (inpatients)		138 (218)	194 (335)	101 (121)	0.077
BMI	kg/m^2	23.2 ± 4.1	23.5 ± 4.5	23.5 ± 5.1	0.516
Waist circumference	cm	84.0 ± 11.5	84.8 ± 11.7	83.4 ± 14.1	0.297
Systolic blood pressure	mmHg	124.5 ± 18.9	122.7 ± 17.3	123.9 ± 19.1	0.355
Diastolic blood pressure	mmHg	77.2 ± 12.3	75.0 ± 12.5	74.9 ± 13.0	0.025
HDL-cholesterol	mg/dL	54.3 ± 18.6	55.4 ± 17.9	57.5 ± 17.9	0.126
CP-equivalent dosage of current AAP	mg	516.1 ± 261.7	420.8 ± 273.4	402.1 ± 231.7	< 0.001
Concomitant drugs					
Antidepressant		1	0	0	
Mood stabilizer		6	11	3	
Benzodiazepines		7	13	2	
Anticholinergic drug		0	9	0	

Data are shown as the mean ± SD or number of subjects
Age, BMI, waist circumference, systolic blood pressure, diastolic blood pressure, HDL-cholesterol, and CP-equivalent dosage of current AAP were compared among the three antipsychotics groups. The chi-square test was performed to analyze sex and outpatients (inpatients)
BMI body mass index, *HDL* high-density lipoprotein, *CP* chlorpromazine, *AAP* atypical antipsychotic

olanzapine-treated patients had significantly lower HDL-cholesterol levels than risperidone-treated patients [29]. Because the authors could not analyze inpatients and outpatients separately, their findings may not be consistent with the results of the current study.

In a study on the acute metabolic effects of olanzapine in healthy volunteers, there was a significant decrease in HDL-cholesterol, in the absence of changes in total cholesterol and LDL-cholesterol [30]. The decrease in HDL-cholesterol within a short time period suggested a direct effect of antipsychotics on HDL-cholesterol. Birkenaes and colleagues reported that even after correction for BMI, low HDL-cholesterol was observed in patients treated with olanzapine and clozapine [31]. Similarly, Kang and colleagues showed significant differences in the prevalence of low HDL-cholesterol after adjustment for BMI among atypical antipsychotic groups [32]. There may also be differences between antipsychotics regarding the direct effects on HDL-cholesterol.

In the present study, differences in HDL-cholesterol among patients treated with antipsychotics were not detected in outpatients. Although no direct comparisons of inpatients with outpatients were made in this study, a previous study reported that hypocholesterolemia was higher in inpatients than in outpatients or the general population [33, 34]. There was a possibility that drug adherence was decreased in outpatients compared with inpatients, and thus the effects of antipsychotic drugs on HDL-cholesterol may have been decreased in outpatients. In hospitalized patients, their diet is controlled, and the proportion of obese patients is lower compared with outpatients. Therefore, in the hospitalization environment, where drug adherence and diet are controlled, it may be possible to detect differences between the effects of different antipsychotics, unlike in outpatient environments. It was also reported that the most likely improvement in the lipid profile induced by physical activity was an increase in HDL-cholesterol [35]. Because the physical activity of outpatients is likely to be higher than that of inpatients, the effects of antipsychotics on HDL-cholesterol may be masked by the influence of physical activity, which may improve HDL-cholesterol

Table 2 Comparisons of HDL-cholesterol levels in the three antipsychotic groups with stratification by BMI for inpatients

			Olanzapine	Risperidone	Aripiprazole	*p*-value	Post-hoc (*p*-value)
HDL-cholesterol	BMI < 18.5	mg/dL	62.0 ± 20.5 (34)	58.6 ± 15.8 (55)	62.6 ± 21.6 (28)	0.490	
	18.5 ≤ BMI < 25	mg/dL	54.1 ± 21.5 (137)	55.0 ± 16.2 (196)	58.2 ± 15.8 (68)	0.282	
	BMI ≥ 25	mg/dL	43.8 ± 12.3 (47)	49.7 ± 15.0 (84)	54.7 ± 16.8 (25)	0.019	Olanzapine < Aripiprazole (0.023)

Data are shown as the mean ± SD (number of subjects)
Analyses of covariance among the three antipsychotics were performed for HDL-cholesterol with age, diastolic blood pressure, chlorpromazine-equivalent dosage and waist circumference as confounding variables
Post-hoc analyses were performed by the Bonferroni method
HDL high-density lipoprotein, *BMI* body mass index

Table 3 Comparisons of HDL-cholesterol levels in the three antipsychotic groups with stratification by BMI for outpatients

			Olanzapine	Risperidone	Aripiprazole	*p*-value
HDL-cholesterol	BMI < 18.5	mg/dL	72.1 ± 18.7 (8)	81.3 ± 30.4 (4)	62.5 ± 3.4 (4)	0.959
	18.5 ≤ BMI < 25	mg/dL	57.6 ± 13.4 (69)	61.4 ± 23.0 (96)	60.7 ± 17.7 (45)	0.442
	BMI ≥ 25	mg/dL	53.0 ± 15.6 (61)	52.7 ± 15.8 (94)	51.9 ± 18.4 (52)	0.819

Data are shown as the mean ± SD (number of subjects)
Analyses of covariance among the three antipsychotics were performed for HDL-cholesterol with age, diastolic blood pressure, chlorpromazine-equivalent dosage and waist circumference as confounding variables
Post-hoc analyses were performed by the Bonferroni method
HDL high-density lipoprotein, *BMI* body mass index

levels. Antipsychotics or physical activity may directly influence the decrease in HDL-cholesterol levels, and the differences seen between these antipsychotics may be caused by factors other than being overweight.

In the study of BMI status of hospitalized Japanese schizophrenia patients, underweight as well as obesity was a characteristic in schizophrenia inpatients compared with the general population [36]. Regarding the characteristics of underweight, a previous study showed that the prevalence of hypotriglyceridemia was significantly higher in the underweight group than in the normal weight group and overweight/obese schizophrenia inpatients [33]. In this study, we did not conduct a direct comparison of HDL-cholesterol levels between overweight, normal weight, and underweight groups. We also did not assess triglyceride levels in this study. Therefore, further studies including metabolic parameters such as triglycerides are necessary for the assessment of underweight patients with schizophrenia.

For overall patients, the olanzapine group had a statistically significant higher chlorpromazine-equivalent dosage compared with the two other groups in this study. The HDL-cholesterol levels for overweight inpatients differed significantly among the three antipsychotic groups after adjustment for chlorpromazine-equivalent dosage. Regarding the risk of metabolic syndrome in psychiatry inpatients, metabolic syndrome was associated with chlorpromazine-equivalent total daily doses, and specifically with clozapine, olanzapine, and quetiapine [37]. There was no consensus as to whether there was a dose-dependence on weight gain or metabolic effects [38].

This study reveals a difference in HDL-cholesterol in overweight Japanese inpatients with schizophrenia resulting from the use of different antipsychotics. Further studies incorporating more detailed evaluations including diet and physical activity, are needed to clarify the differences in HDL-cholesterol according to antipsychotic use.

Limitations

The present study had several limitations. First, the cross-sectional and antipsychotic treatments were not performed randomly, and thus bias in the antipsychotic prescriptions was not controlled. Second, the present analysis was a post-hoc analysis of a study that was not designed or powered to demonstrate differences between treatments, and thus the possibility of type II errors may remain. Third, comparisons with unmedicated schizophrenia patients or healthy controls could not be performed in this study. Fourth, we did not assess psychiatric symptoms or severity using the Brief Psychiatric Rating Scale, Positive and Negative Symptom Scale or Clinical Global Impressions in this study. Psychiatric symptoms might be related to body weight, physical activity, or antipsychotic drugs, so further study including the assessment of symptoms and severity is required.

Conclusions

This post-hoc study of a large questionnaire survey showed differences in HDL-cholesterol levels between different antipsychotic monotherapies in Japanese inpatients with schizophrenia. HDL-cholesterol was significantly lower in the olanzapine group than in the aripiprazole group in overweight inpatients. The difference was only revealed in overweight inpatients, and further study is needed to evaluate factors such as diet and physical activity to clarify the differences in HDL-cholesterol levels related to antipsychotic use.

Abbreviations

BMI: Body mass index; DSM-IV-TR: Diagnostic and Statistical Manual of Mental Disorders, fourth edition, text revision; HDL: High-density lipoprotein; ICD-10: International Statistical Classification of Diseases and Related Health Problems version 10; LDL: Low-density lipoprotein; OECD: Organization for Economic Cooperation and Development; SD: Standard deviations

Acknowledgements

We are grateful to the study participants and the facilities belonging to the Japan Psychiatric Hospitals Association that cooperated with this investigation. We would like to thank all of our coworkers for their contributions to the data collection and management. Wendy Brooks, PhD, from Edanz Group (https://www.edanzediting.com/) provided English language editing services for a draft of this manuscript.

Funding

This work was partially supported by Eisai Co. Ltd., Yoshitomi Pharmaceutical Industries, Dainippon Sumitomo Pharma Co. Ltd., Astellas Pharma Inc., Meiji Seika Pharma Co. Ltd., Eli Lilly Japan K.K., Otsuka Pharmaceutical Co. Ltd., GlaxoSmithKline K.K., Janssen Pharmaceutical K.K., MSD K.K., Shionogi & Co. Ltd., Asahi Kasei Pharma Corp., Novartis Pharma Co. Ltd., Takeda Pharmaceutical Co. Ltd., Ono Pharmaceutical Co. Ltd., and Tsumura & Co. The funders had no role in the study design, data collection and analysis, decision to publish, or preparation of the manuscript.

Authors' contributions

Conceptualization: SO, TSugai, YS, YO, NS, NYF, TSomeya. Data curation: SO, TSugai, YS, MY, KS, TM, YO, HM, NS, NYF, KO, TSagae. Formal analysis: SO, TSugai. Investigation: SO, TSugai, YS, MY, KS, TM, YO, HM, NS, NYF, KO, TSagae, TSomeya. Methodology: SO, TSugai, MY, TM, HM, KO, TSagae. Project administration: TSugai, YS, TSomeya. Supervision: TSugai, YS, TSomeya. Validation: SO, TSugai, YS, KS, YO, NS, NYF. Visualization: SO. Writing – original draft: SO, TSugai, YS, TSomeya. Writing – review & editing: SO, TSugai, YS, MY, KS, TM, YO, HM, NS, NYF, KO, TSagae, TSomeya. All authors read and approved the final manuscript.

Competing interests

Toshiyuki Someya has received research support or honoraria from Asahi Kasei Pharma Corp., Astellas Pharma Inc., Daiichi Sankyo Co. Ltd., Dainippon Sumitomo Pharma Co. Ltd., Eisai Co. Ltd., Eli Lilly Japan K.K., GlaxoSmithKline K.K., Janssen Pharmaceutical K.K., Meiji Seika Pharma Co. Ltd., Mitsubishi Tanabe Pharma Co. Ltd., Mochida Pharmaceutical Co. Ltd., MSD K.K., Otsuka Pharmaceutical Co. Ltd., Pfizer Japan Inc., Shionogi & Co. Ltd., Tsumura & Co., and Yoshitomi Pharmaceutical Industries. Yutaro Suzuki has received research support or honoraria from Janssen Pharmaceutical K.K., Mitsubishi Tanabe Pharma Co. Ltd., and Otsuka Pharmaceutical Co. Ltd. Kazutaka Shimoda has received research support or honoraria from Daiichi Sankyo Co. Ltd., Dainippon Sumitomo Pharma Co. Ltd., Eisai Co. Ltd., Eli Lilly Japan K.K., GlaxoSmithKline K.K., Meiji Seika Pharma Co. Ltd., Novartis Pharma K.K., Otsuka Pharmaceutical Co. Ltd., Pfizer Japan Inc., Shionogi & Co. Ltd., Takeda Pharmaceutical Co. Ltd., Tsumura & Co., Yoshitomi Pharmaceutical Industries Ltd., Asahi Kasei Pharma Corporation, Astellas Pharma Inc., Janssen Pharmaceutical K.K., Kowa Pharmaceutical Co. Ltd., Meiji Seika Pharma Co., Mitsubishi Tanabe Pharma Corporation Ltd., MSD K.K., Novartis Pharma K.K., and Ono Pharmaceutical Co. Ltd. Norio Yasui-Furukori has received research support or honoraria from Astellas Pharma Inc., Dainippon Sumitomo Pharma Co. Ltd., Eli Lilly Japan K.K., GlaxoSmithKline K.K., Janssen Pharmaceutical K.K., Meiji Seika Pharma Co., Mochida Pharmaceutical Co. Ltd., MSD K.K., Otsuka Pharmaceutical Co. Ltd., Pfizer Japan Inc., Takeda Pharmaceutical Co. Ltd., and Yoshitomi Pharmaceutical Industries. Norio Sugawara has received grant or research support from a Grant-in-Aid for Young Scientists (B), Ministry of Education, Culture, Sports, Science and Technology, Japan Grant B., a Karoji Memorial Fund for Medical Research Grant, and The Senshin Medical Research Foundation. Shin Ono has received grant or research support from the Hospitals Bureau Niigata Prefecture Government and a Grant-in-Aid for Scientific Research (C). There are no patents, products in development, or marketed products to declare. The other authors declare no potential conflicts of interest.

Author details

[1]Department of Community Psychiatric Medicine, Niigata University Graduate School of Medical and Dental Sciences, Niigata, Japan. [2]Japanese Society of Clinical Neuropsychopharmacology, Tokyo, Japan. [3]Department of Psychiatry, Niigata University Graduate School of Medical and Dental Sciences, Niigata, Japan. [4]Japan Psychiatric Hospital Association, Tokyo, Japan. [5]Department of Psychiatry, Dokkyo Medical University School of Medicine, Mibu, Japan. [6]Department of Neuropsychiatry, Hirosaki University School of Medicine, Hirosaki, Japan. [7]Department of Health and Nutrition, Yamagata Prefectural Yonezawa University of Nutrition Sciences Faculty of Health and Nutrition, Yonezawa, Japan.

References

1. Harris EC, Barraclough B. Excess mortality of mental disorder. Br J Psychiatry. 1998;173:11–53.
2. Dixon L, Weiden P, Delahanty J, Goldberg R, Postrado L, Lucksted A, et al. Prevalence and correlates of diabetes in national schizophrenia samples. Schizophr Bull. 2000;26:903–12.
3. McEvoy JP, Meyer JM, Goff DC, Nasrallah HA, Davis SM, Sullivan L, et al. Prevalence of the metabolic syndrome in patients with schizophrenia: baseline results from the Clinical Antipsychotic Trials of Intervention Effectiveness (CATIE) schizophrenia trial and comparison with national estimates from NHANES III. Schizophr Res. 2005;80:19–32.
4. Meyer JM, Stahl SM. The metabolic syndrome and schizophrenia. Acta Psychiatr Scand. 2009;119:4–14.
5. Chirovsky DR, Fedirko V, Cui Y, Sazonov V, Barter P. Prospective studies on the relationship between high-density lipoprotein cholesterol and cardiovascular risk: a systematic review. Eur J Cardiovasc Prev Rehabil. 2009;16:404–23.
6. De Hert M, Schreurs V, Vancampfort D, Van Winkel R. Metabolic syndrome in people with schizophrenia: a review. World Psychiatry. 2009;8:15–22.
7. Lieberman JA, Stroup TS, McEvoy JP, Swartz MS, Rosenheck RA, Perkins DO, et al. Effectiveness of antipsychotic drugs in patients with chronic schizophrenia. N Engl J Med. 2005;353:1209–23.
8. Melkersson K, Dahl ML. Adverse metabolic effects associated with atypical antipsychotics: literature review and clinical implications. Drugs. 2004;64:701–23.
9. Newcomer JW. Abnormalities of glucose metabolism associated with atypical antipsychotic drugs. J Clin Psychiatry. 2004;65:36–46.
10. Newcomer JW. Second-generation (atypical) antipsychotics and metabolic effects: a comprehensive literature review. CNS Drugs. 2005;19(Suppl 1):1–93.
11. Newcomer JW, Haupt DW. The metabolic effects of antipsychotic medications. Can J Psychiatr. 2006;51:480–91.
12. Rummel-Kluge C, Komossa K, Schwarz S, Hunger H, Schmid F, Lobos CA, et al. Head-to-head comparisons of metabolic side effects of second generation antipsychotics in the treatment of schizophrenia: a systematic review and meta-analysis. Schizophr Res. 2010;123:225–33.
13. Enez Darcin A, Yalcin Cavus S, Dilbaz N, Kaya H, Dogan E. Metabolic syndrome in drug-naïve and drug-free patients with schizophrenia and in their siblings. Schizophr Res. 2015;166:201–6.
14. Albrink MJ, Krauss RM, Lindgrem FT, von der Groeben J, Pan S, Wood PD. Intercorrelations among plasma high density lipoprotein, obesity and triglycerides in a normal population. Lipids. 1980;15(9):668–76.
15. Wilson DE, Lees RS. Metabolic relationships among the plasma lipoproteins. Reciprocal changes in the concentrations of very low and low density lipoproteins in man. J Clin Invest. 1972;51:1051–7.
16. Shamai L, Lurix E, Shen M, Novaro GM, Szomstein S, Rosenthal R, et al. Association of body mass index and lipid profiles: evaluation of a broad spectrum of body mass index patients including the morbidly obese. Obes Surg. 2011;21(1):42–7.
17. Phillips NR, Havel RJ, Kane JP. Levels and interrelationships of serum and lipoprotein cholesterol and triglycerides. Association with adiposity and the consumption of ethanol, tobacco, and beverages containing caffeine. Arteriosclerosis. 1981;1(1):13–24.
18. Wood PD, Haskell WL. The effect of exercise on plasma high density lipoproteins. Lipids. 1979;14(4):417–27.
19. Superko HR. Exercise and lipoprotein metabolism. J Cardiovasc Risk. 1995; 2(4):310–5.
20. Sugai T, Suzuki Y, Yamazaki M, Shimoda K, Mori T, Ozeki Y, et al. Difference in prevalence of metabolic syndrome between Japanese outpatients and inpatients with schizophrenia: a nationwide survey. Schizophr Res. 2016;171:68–73.
21. Organisation for Economic Cooperation and Development. OECD health statistics 2017.
22. Ministry of Health and Welfare. Summary of Static/Dynamic Surveys of Medical Institutions and Hospital Report 2010. Statistics and Information Department, Minister's Secretariat, Ministry of Health and Welfare, Tokyo.
23. American Psychiatric Association. Diagnostic and Statistical Manual of Mental Disorders. 4th ed. Washington, DC: American Psychiatric Press; 2000. Text Revision
24. World Health Organization. International statistical classification of diseases and related health problems 10th revision. 2004.
25. Newcomer JW. Antipsychotic medications: metabolic and cardiovascular risk. J Clin Psychiatry. 2007;68(Suppl 4):8–13.
26. Chrzanowski WK, Marcus RN, Torbeyns A, Nyilas M, McQuade RD. Effectiveness of long-term aripiprazole therapy in patients with acutely relapsing or chronic, stable schizophrenia: a 52-week, open-label comparison with olanzapine. Psychopharmacology. 2006;189:259–66.
27. Perez-Iglesias R, Mata I, Pelayo-Teran JM, Amado JA, Garcia-Unzueta MT, Berja A, et al. Glucose and lipid disturbances after 1 year of antipsychotic treatment in a drug-naïve population. Schizophr Res. 2009;107:115–21.
28. Fleischhacker WW, McQuade RD, Marcus RN, Archibald D, Swanink R, Carson WH. A double-blind, randomized comparative study of aripiprazole and

olanzapine in patients with schizophrenia. Biol Psychiatry. 2009;65:510–7.
29. Wirshing DA, Boyd JA, Meng LR, Ballon JS, Marder SR, Wirshing WC. The effects of novel antipsychotics on glucose and lipid levels. J Clin Psychiatry. 2002;63:856–65.
30. Albaugh VL, Singareddy R, Mauger D, Lynch CJ. A double blind, placebo-controlled, randomized crossover study of the acute metabolic effects of olanzapine in healthy volunteers. PLoS One. 2011;6:e22662.
31. Birkenaes AB, Birkeland KI, Engh JA, Faerden A, Jonsdottir H, Ringen PA, et al. Dyslipidemia independent of body mass in antipsychotic-treated patients under real-life conditions. J Clin Psychopharmacol. 2008;28:132–7.
32. Kang SH, Lee JI. Metabolic disturbances independent of body mass in patients with schizophrenia taking atypical antipsychotics. Psychiatry Investig. 2015;12:242–8.
33. Suzuki Y, Sugai T, Fukui N, Watanabe J, Ono S, Tsuneyama N, et al. High prevalence of underweight and undernutrition in Japanese inpatients with schizophrenia. Psychiatry Clin Neurosci. 2014;68(1):78–82.
34. Sugai T, Suzuki Y, Yamazaki M, Shimoda K, Mori T, Ozeki Y, et al. High prevalence of obesity, hypertension, hyperlipidemia, and diabetes mellitus in Japanese outpatients with schizophrenia: a nationwide survey. PLoS One. 2016;11:e0166429.
35. Mann S, Beedie C, Jimenez A. Differential effects of aerobic exercise, resistance training and combined exercise modalities on cholesterol and the lipid profile: review, synthesis and recommendations. Sports Med. 2014;44:211–21.
36. Inamura Y, Sagae T, Nakamachi K, Murayama N. Body mass index of inpatients with schizophrenia in Japan. Int J Psychiatry Med. 2012;44(2):171–81.
37. Centorrino F, Masters GA, Talamo A, Baldessarini RJ, Öngür D. Metabolic syndrome in psychiatrically hospitalized patients treated with antipsychotics and other psychotropics. Hum Psychopharmacol. 2012;27(5):521–6.
38. Simon V, van Winkel R, De Hert M. Are weight gain and metabolic side effects of atypical antipsychotics dose dependent? A literature review. J Clin Psychiatry. 2009;70(7):1041–50.

8

Health-related quality of life in prisoners with attention-deficit hyperactivity disorder and head injury

Susan Young[1,2*], Rafael A. González[3], Moshe Fridman[4], Paul Hodgkins[5], Keira Kim[6] and Gisli H. Gudjonsson[2,7]

Abstract

Background: Attention-deficit hyperactivity disorder (ADHD) and head injury (including traumatic brain injury (TBI)) manifest in high levels across prison samples and guidance from the National Institute for Health and Care Excellence notes that people with acquired brain injury may have increased prevalence of ADHD. We aimed to examine the association of ADHD with TBI and the impact of the association upon health-related quality of life (HRQoL) and service use among imprisoned adults.

Methods: An observational study was performed in 2011–2013, at Porterfield Prison, Inverness, United Kingdom (UK). The all male sample included 390 adult prison inmates with capacity to consent and no history of moderate or severe intellectual disability. Head injury was measured with a series of self-reported questions, addressing history of hits to the head: frequency, severity, loss of consciousness (LOC), and sequelae. Participants were interviewed using the Diagnostic Interview for ADHD in Adults 2.0. The Health Utilities Index Mark 3 was used to measure health status, and to calculate attribute specific HRQoL and Quality-Adjusted Life Year (QALY) scores.

Results: 72% of prisoners sampled reported at least one head injury in their lifetime. Among those, 70% of head injuries occurred before age 16 and 70% experienced LOC. Prisoners with ADHD were nearly twice more likely to have TBI. Prisoners with ADHD-only and ADHD with co-morbid TBI had significantly lower scores in several HRQoL attributes, compared with TBI only or the absence of either condition. Adjusted logistic regression models indicated an average reduction of 0.20 QALYs in inmates with ADHD-only and 0.30 QALY loss in those with ADHD with co-morbid TBI compared with inmates with neither condition.

Conclusions: There is a robust association between ADHD and TBI, and ADHD with co-morbid TBI confers significantly greater impairment in terms of HRQoL. Managing the short and long-term consequences of TBI is essential to improving care for prisoners and to addressing the criminogenic factors related to them.

Keywords: Attention deficit/hyperactivity disorder, Head injury, Traumatic brain injury, Prison population, Health-related quality of life, Co-morbidity

Background

Despite the high prevalence of both attention-deficit hyperactivity disorder (ADHD; 26%) [1] and head injury (including traumatic brain injury (TBI; 60%)) [2] in the prison populations, little is known about their association with each other and their impact on health-related quality of life (HRQoL) measures. The recently revised National Institute for Health and Care Excellence guideline on the recognition of ADHD (NICE guideline NG87) noted that people with acquired brain injury may have increased prevalence of ADHD compared with the general population [3]. Hence the present study is topical in investigating quality of life in offenders with ADHD and head injury.

ADHD is a childhood onset neurodevelopmental disorder, characterised by a persistent pattern of inattention and/or hyperactivity-impulsivity [4]. ADHD is associated with executive functioning deficits [5] and combined

* Correspondence: suzyyoung@aol.com
[1]Psychology Services Limited, PO Box 1735, Croydon CR97AE, UK
[2]Reykjavik University, Reykjavik, Iceland

with conduct problems is associated with an increased risk for adult criminality [6]. Compared with world-wide prevalence rates (2.5% adults [7], 5.3% children [8]), there is a five-fold increase of ADHD among youth prisoners (< 18 years) and a ten-fold increase of ADHD among adult prisoners (> 18 years) [1]. A systematic review and meta-analysis study indicated that among incarcerated adults with ADHD there is an increased rate of co-morbid psychiatric disorders (29% conduct disorder (CD), 74% substance use disorder, 66% mood disorder, 55% depressive disorder, 68% anxiety disorder, and 60% personality disorders) [9]. A study of 1.92 million individuals in Denmark demonstrated a significant increase in the mortality rate among people with ADHD compared to those without ADHD ($p < 0.0001$), with accidents being the leading cause of death [10].

Prevalence rates for head injury and TBI vary depending on the source of information, definition, the occurrence of loss of consciousness (LOC), and/or loss of memory. A meta-analysis indicated that 60% of the overall offender population is reported to have TBI with LOC [2], which is significantly higher than the general population estimates of 12% in adults [11] and 24% in adolescents [12]. A recent systematic review reported that between 16.5 to 72.1% of incarcerated youths have TBI [13]. Two studies indicated that prisoners commonly report a history of repeated head trauma incidents [14, 15]. A population study based on Swedish registry data reported that individuals with TBIs are at significant risk of violent crime [16]. Furthermore, prisoners with TBI were reported to be significantly younger at the time of their first offence, compared with prisoners without TBI [17].

The possible association between ADHD and head injuries is complex. Difficulties with the ability to self-regulate have been described as an executive function that is central to ADHD symptoms [18], which may be an antecedent for impulsive behaviour or aggression [19]. Therefore, having ADHD may increase the risk of head injuries [10, 20]. Additionally, there is some evidence to suggest that brain injuries in school-age children may lead to the development of ADHD later in childhood [20, 21]. Furthermore, ADHD and TBI share similar risk factors, such as low socioeconomic status and history of risk-taking behaviours [22, 23] and similar symptoms. TBI is usually accompanied by attention deficits, frontal-executive compromise, and self regulation difficulties [24]. Because TBI is often the outcome of certain risk taking behaviours, confounding effects from co-existing disorders such as ADHD and conduct problems may play an important role in associations.

In considering impairments and functional states that may be affected by disease, injury, and treatment, the Health Utilities Index Mark 3 (HUI3) is an effective tool to evaluate overall health status and quality of life outcomes [25, 26]. Results from HUI3 can be used to calculate attribute specific health-related quality of life (HRQoL) and quality-adjusted life years (QALY) scores, which represent the impact that health status has on quality of life and life span.

To the best of our knowledge this is the first study addressing the health status of adult prison inmates with ADHD and TBI using the HUI3. We hypothesize that: 1) there is a significant association between ADHD and TBI amongst prison inmates, and 2) prisoners with ADHD and co-morbid TBI have an increased likelihood of adverse health, intellectual ability, and quality of life outcomes, compared with those with ADHD only, TBI only, or neither.

Methods

Participants and sample selection

Following approval from the Scottish Prison Service Research Access and Ethics Committee and in accordance with the Declaration of Helsinki, prisoners were recruited by opportunity sampling from Porterfield Prison, Scotland, UK, over a period of 18 months in 2011–2013. Participants included 390 adult male prisoners who consented to participate. Those with moderate or severe learning difficulties, lack of fluency in the English language, and severe mental illness were excluded from participating.

Participants in the study were indirectly compensated. The study group deposited £20 per participant into a Prison Common Good Fund, which was managed by a group of prisoners. The fund was then used to purchase items for the common good of all prisoners to enhance prison life.

Prisoners who indicated interest attended an appointment with the researcher where they were given detailed (oral and written) information about the study and consent procedures. After obtaining consent, two psychology researcher assistants administered a comprehensive battery of measures, which took approximately 4 h to complete (usually split across 2 or 3 sessions). The researchers received comprehensive training to administer the Diagnostic Interview for ADHD in Adults 2.0 (DIVA-2) from the Maudsley Hospital Adult ADHD Service, which included observations and training on reaching diagnostic classification to ensure inter-rater reliability [27]. The researchers sat down with the participants throughout the sessions, administered the DIVA-2 and self-report questionnaires. Participants received assistance to do the latter, when required. Out of the 390 participants, 81 (20.8%) required assistance with reading the questionnaires. The request for assistance was most frequent among the 53 participants in the combined ADHD and co-morbid TBI group (41.5%), in contrast to 17.5% among the remaining 337 participants (Chi^2 (df 1) = 8.20. $p < 0.01$).

Measures

History of head injury

Head injury was measured via a self-reported questionnaire addressing history of hits to the head. The key question "Have you ever been hit in the head?" was followed by further questions detailing the injury and its consequences including: frequency, age of onset, occurrence of LOC, cause, related medical service use, and occurrence of related memory loss.

Definitions of TBI are often based on the occurrence of any LOC and on the extent of post-traumatic amnesia (PTA). Considering that head injury incidents were self-reported by prisoners, we aimed to make the identification of a likely TBI more robust. Recording the number of head injuries increased the threshold level and minimised false positives, and also helped to distinguish those most likely to have had any form of sequelae after their injuries.

Our strict definition of a likely TBI

We determined the lifetime prevalence of a likely TBI based upon the occurrence of the following:

1) At least one head injury **and**
2) Occurrence of LOC **and**
3) Any additional indicator of head injury severity (such as an LOC > 20 min, requiring surgery, and/or caused memory loss) **or**
4) Medical service utilisation related to the head injury (such as a visit to the doctor or Accident and Emergency (A&E) services).

Because head injury history was not entered into prisoners' medical records, we were unable to formally apply the commonly used Mayo Classification System (MCS) [28]. But, by restricting our likely TBI cases to include only those with LOC (whilst also including a parameter of severity); all of our defined cases could be interpreted to be mild or moderate-severe by the MCS.

Health utilities index mark 3 (HUI3)

The HUI3 is a multi-attribute health status classification system that enables researchers to map levels of: vision, hearing, speech, ambulation, dexterity, emotion, cognition, and pain; using decision tables and coding algorithms, which can be represented in terms of attribute specific HRQoL scores [26]. The HRQoL scoring system provides utility scores ranging from 0.00 (dead) to 1.00 (perfect health), and meets the criteria for calculating Quality-Adjusted Life Years (QALY) [26]. The HUI health-based classification systems have been validated worldwide. In their paper [26] Horseman and colleagues direct readers to "the HUI web page at http://www.healthutilities.com and review the annotated references of articles from hundreds of studies worldwide for evidence of HUI validity (face validity, content validity, construct validity, convergent validity, discriminative validity, predictive validity), reliability and responsiveness."

Prisoners' were asked to answer HUI3 questions based upon their health status in the 4 weeks prior to the interview. The HUI3 composite score was used to calculate QALYs and was extrapolated to one year to represent the study health evaluation time frame.

ADHD diagnosis and CD screening

All participants underwent a comprehensive evaluation for ADHD and were interviewed using the Diagnostic Interview for ADHD in Adults 2.0 (DIVA-2) [29]. The DIVA-2 is a validated semi-structured clinical interview of ADHD in adults based on DSM-IVR criteria [4]. It is a clinical diagnostic tool and the associated website provides information about its validity (see www.eunetworkadultadhd.com/validation-of-diva-2-0/). Questions addressed their current and childhood (ages 5 to 12) presentation of ADHD symptoms and scope of impairment.

All participants were screened for conduct disorder using the CD scale of the Barkley Adult ADHD Rating Scale-IV (BAARS-IV) [30], which corresponds with DSM-5 criteria. Endorsement of three or more criteria indicated likelihood of the disorder.

Service use

Medical service utilization was obtained through inspection of prison medical records. Researchers recorded service use over the three months prior to the interview date, such as: visits to medical doctor, visits to accidents and emergency room (A&E), admission to hospital and length of stay, and surgeries. The authors chose to include three months of service for practical reasons; and additionally felt this time period fairly represented the service use of all prisoners given the variance in prison stays.

Intelligence

IQ was estimated using the vocabulary subtest of the Wechsler Abbreviated Scale of Intelligence (WASI) [31]. The vocabulary subtest is reported to be a robust predictor of general IQ regardless of brain injury [32].

Analytical strategy

Frequencies were reported for all categorical variables, and means (with standard deviations) for continuous variables. Student t-tests were used to contrast age and age of first injury by groups. Logistic regression models were fitted using ADHD as the exposure for any head injury, TBI, causes and consequences of head injury, and service utilisation. Ordered logistic regression was used to analyze number of head injuries reported.

Odds ratios (OR) were reported as indicators of the magnitude of associations in binary (e.g. presence or absence of head injury) and on the ordered categorical outcome (head injuries reported) models. Logistic regression analyses were repeated exclusively on those who reported their first injury before age 16. This analysis allowed us to examine whether a TBI occurring before age 16 may be associated with ADHD. We used age 16 because it represented the threshold for legal adulthood in the UK.

Tobit regressions were used in favour of traditional ordinary least-squares (OLS) regression models to estimate the relationship between inmate groups of ADHD only, TBI only, ADHD with co-morbid TBI, and groups having neither (reference group); and HUI3 HRQoL and QALY scores. The *Tobit* model is designed to estimate linear relationships between variables when there are ceiling or flooring effects on the outcome [33]. In our case, we considered the upper limit of 1.0 of the outcome variable as censored. Post-estimation linear combinations of coefficients allowed contrasting the ADHD with co-morbid TBI group with either ADHD only or TBI only group. Differences in estimated IQ were examined via linear regression models.

All models were adjusted for age at time of survey and for the presence of CD whenever necessary. We established the significance level at $p \leq 0.05$ for all statistical tests. All analyses were performed using Stata version 13 (StataCorp) [34].

Results

Descriptive statistics

The all male sample was essentially Caucasian British (99.0%) with an average age of 30.3 years (sd 8.3). Mean ages for each of the groups were: 28.6 years (sd 7.9) for ADHD only, 32.3 years (sd 8.4) for TBI only, 27.9 years (sd 7.2) for ADHD with co-morbid TBI, and 30.2 years (sd 8.5) for neither ADHD nor TBI. Bonferroni post hoc analyses indicated a significantly younger age for the ADHD with co-morbid TBI group contrasted against the TBI only group.

Head injury and TBI: Prevalence, history, and sequelae

Two hundred eighty participants (71.8%) reported having experienced at least one head injury in their lifetime, and 169 (43.3%) were considered to have a likely TBI according to our strict definition (see Table 1). Among those with at least one head injury, the mean age of first injury was 12.5 years (sd 6.7); approximately 70% of which suffered their first injury before age 16 and reported having experienced LOC (see Table 2).

Among those who suffered at least one head injury; 79% required a visit to a medical doctor, 76% required a visit to accident and emergency (A&E) services, and 19.3% required surgery. Additionally, 23% reported experiencing either anterograde or retrograde memory loss. 44% of the head injuries were due to an accident, and 56% were the consequence of a violent assault (e.g. hit with bat) (see Table 2).

Head injury, TBI, and ADHD

24.6% of the prisoners met the criteria for a clinical diagnosis of ADHD. 79% of prisoners with ADHD and 69% of prisoners without ADHD reported at least one head injury ($p = 0.07$). Among prisoners reporting at least one head injury, prisoners with ADHD did not differ from those without ADHD in terms of cause, LOC, or sequelae (such as requiring emergency services, surgery, or experiencing memory loss) (see Table 2).

Using our strict definition of a likely TBI, there was a significant difference between prisoners with ADHD compared with those without ADHD. 55% of prisoners with ADHD had a likely TBI compared with 40% of those without ADHD ($p < 0.01$), with nearly twice the odds among those with ADHD to have experienced a TBI (see Table 1).

Among prisoners reporting head injuries, those with ADHD reported a significantly higher number of head injuries than those without ADHD (OR 2.19 (1.44, 3.31), $p < 0.001$). Notably, a significantly high proportion (82%) of those with ADHD and at least one head injury reported their first injury occurring before age 16 (OR 2.45 (1.26, 4.76), $p < 0.001$) (see Table 2).

Out of the total sample of 390, 153 (39.2%) met screening criteria for CD. There was a significant difference in CD screening diagnosis across the four groups: ADHD only; TBI only; ADHD/TBI; and remaining participants (Chi^2 (df 3) = 43.6 $p <$ 0.000). The rate was highest among the ADHD/TBI group (69.8%), followed by ADHD only (65.1%). The rate for TBI only was 29.3% and similar to the rate of 30.3% for none of the ADHD, TBI or combined conditions being met.

Analyses were repeated exclusively on those who reported their first injury before age 16. Although ADHD was associated with first injury occurring before age 16 it was no longer significant after adjustments were made for coexisting CD.

Health status, service use, and estimated IQ

Prisoners with ADHD only, TBI only, and ADHD with co-morbid TBI were compared against those with neither in specific HRQoL attribute and QALY loss, service use, and estimated intelligence (see Table 3).

Prisoners with ADHD-only had significantly poorer utility scores on emotion ($p < 0.05$) and cognition ($p < 0.01$) attributes. Those with ADHD with co-morbid TBI had the most impaired specific health attributes with significantly poorer scores on vision ($p < 0.001$), ambulation ($p < 0.05$), emotion ($p < 0.001$), cognition ($p < 0.01$) and pain ($p < 0.05$) attributes. Prisoners without ADHD or likely TBI had an

Table 1 Head Injury, TBI, and IQ Among Inmates without ADHD and with ADHD

	All Inmates *N* = 390 n (%)	without ADHD *n* = 294 n (%[a])	with ADHD *n* = 96 n (%[b])	OR (95% CI)	*p*
ADHD prevalence		294 (75.4[c])	96 (24.6[c])		
Head injury frequency					
None	110 (28.2)	90 (30.6)	20 (20.8)		
1	64 (16.4)	57 (19.4)	7 (7.3)		
2 to 3	82 (21.0)	61 (20.8)	21 (21.9)		
4 to 6	63 (16.2)	39 (13.3)	24 (25.0)		
7 to 10	43 (11.0)	32 (10.9)	11 (11.5)		
11 or more	28 (7.2)	15 (5.1)	13 (13.5)	2.19 (1.44, 3.31)[d]	< 0.001
Any head injury	280 (71.8)	204 (69.4)	76 (79.2)	1.68 (0.97, 2.91)	*0.070*
Likely TBI	169 (43.3)	116 (39.5)	53 (55.2)	1.89 (1.19, 3.01)	*0.007*
IQ estimate, *mean [sd]*	*76.9 [14.4]*	*78.2 [13.9]*	*72.9 [15.3]*	t 3.10 (385)[e]	*0.002*

[a]Percentage of inmates without ADHD
[b]Percentage of inmates with ADHD
[c]Percentage of all inmates
[d]Derived from ordered *logit* model. Proportionality of odds was established using a chi-square test ($p = 0.08$)
[e]t distribution and degrees of freedom

average QALY of 0.72 (sd 0.26) and both the ADHD-only and ADHD with co-morbid TBI groups had significantly greater loss (− 0.2 and − 0.3, respectively) than those with neither.

Prisoners with ADHD with co-morbid TBI had a significantly higher number of visits to mental health nurses ($p < 0.01$) and addiction services ($p < 0.05$) compared with those with neither. Adjusted models for IQ demonstrate that prisoners with ADHD with co-morbid TBI had significantly lower intelligence scores compared to those with neither ($p < 0.01$) (Table 3). Because only the ADHD with co-morbid TBI group was significantly different from the referent in terms of IQ and service use, we made no further contrasts.

Discussion

In the present study we set out to examine the potential association of ADHD with TBI in a UK prison sample and the impact that each has on health-related quality of life. Our hypotheses were supported. Our results indicate that prisoners with a clinical diagnosis of ADHD were significantly associated with our strict definition of a likely TBI; 55% were almost twice more likely to have TBI. Furthermore, our results indicate a high frequency

Table 2 Head Injury History and Sequelae Among Inmates without ADHD and with ADHD

	Any head injury *n* = 280 n (%[a])	without ADHD *n* = 204 n (%[b])	with ADHD *n* = 76 n (%[c])	OR (95% CI)	*p*
First injury age[d], *mean yr [sd]*	*12.5 [6.7]*	*13.1 [7.1]*	*10.9 [4.9]*	t 2.45 (273)[e]	0.01
at < 16 yr	192 (69.8)	132 (65.4)	60 (82.2)	2.45 (1.26, 4.76)	0.008
at ≥16 yr	83 (30.2)	70 (34.7)	13 (17.8)	Referent	–
LOC	195 (69.6)	137 (67.2)	58 (76.3)	1.58 (0.86, 2.88)	0.14
LOC > 20 mins.	61 (21.8)	41 (20.1)	20 (26.3)	1.42 (0.77, 2.63)	0.26
Memory loss	65 (23.3)	43 (21.1)	22 (29.3)	1.55 (0.85, 2.83)	0.15
Caused by accident	121 (43.8)	93 (46.3)	28 (37.3)	1.45 (0.84, 2.49)	0.18
Caused by assault	155 (56.2)	108 (53.7)	47 (62.7)	Referent	–
Required doctor visit	220 (78.6)	155 (76.0)	65 (85.5)	1.87 (0.91, 3.82)	0.09
Required A&E visit	214 (76.4)	155 (76.0)	59 (77.6)	1.10 (0.59, 2.06)	0.77
Required surgery	54 (19.3)	38 (18.6)	16 (21.1)	1.16 (0.61, 2.24)	0.65

[a]Percentage of inmates with more than one head injury
[b]Percentage of inmates without ADHD
[c]Percentage of inmates with ADHD
[d]Age is based on data for 275 inmates, missing first injury age for 5 inmates
[e]t distribution and degrees of freedom

Table 3 Health Status, Service Use, and Estimated IQ of Prisoners with ADHD only, TBI only, and ADHD with co-morbid TBI Compared with Inmates with Neither

	ADHD only $n = 43$, 11.0%	TBI only $n = 116$, 29.7%	ADHD with co-morbid TBI $n = 53$, 13.6%
HUI3 HRQoL specific attribute scores[a]	beta coef. (se)	beta coef. (se)	beta coef. (se)
Vision	−0.04 (0.02)	−0.01 (0.01)	− 0.05 (0.02)**
Hearing	− 0.50 (0.30)	−0.09 (0.24)	− 0.57 (0.30)
Speech	−0.07 (0.07)	− 0.05 (0.05)	−0.10 (0.06)
Ambulation	−0.37 (0.40)	−0.48 (0.32)	− 0.81 (0.37)*
Dexterity	− 0.02 (0.16)	− 0.21 (0.12)	− 0.06 (0.15)
Emotion	−0.17 (0.07)*	− 0.03 (0.05)	−0.23 (0.06)***
Cognition	− 0.24 (0.07)**	− 0.06 (0.05)	−0.32 (0.07)***
Pain	− 0.09 (0.10)	−0.15 (0.07)*	− 0.23 (0.09)*
QALY derived by HUI3 composite score[a,b,c]	− 0.20 (0.06)**	− 0.05 (0.04)	−0.30 (0.05)***†
Service use (3 months)	OR (95%CI)	OR (95%CI)	OR (95%CI)
General Practitioner	1.09 (0.33, 5.60)	2.15 (0.75, 6.14)	1.09 (0.36, 3.32)
Physical Health Nurse	1.67 (0.45, 6.19)	0.94 (0.41, 2.13)	1.57 (0.48, 5.12)
Mental Health Nurse	1.59 (0.79, 3.22)	0.99 (0.59, 1.65)	3.08 (1.59, 5.98)**
Addiction Nurse	0.51 (0.23, 1.12)	1.13 (0.69, 1.85)	2.12 (1.10, 4.09)*
Estimated IQ, *mean (sd)*[a]	− 4.68 (2.48)	−1.62 (1.72)	−7.62 (2.34)**

Note: The referent is inmates with neither ADHD nor TBI, $n = 178$

[a]Models adjusted for age and CD

[b]HUI3 composite score was based on 362 inmates with complete HUI3 data (missing some specific attribute scores on 28 inmates)

[c]All *tobit* models account for censoring at the upper level of the outcome (QALY)

†Linear combination of coefficients for ADHD/TBI *v.* ADHD-only is not statistically significant; Linear combination of coefficients for ADHD/TBI *v.* TBI-only 0.25 (0.06), $p < 0.001$

*$p < 0.05$

**$p < 0.01$

***$p < 0.001$

of head injury at an early age; 82% of prisoners with ADHD with at least one head injury reported that their first injury occurred before age 16. In addition, the risk for adverse health, intellectual ability, and quality of life outcomes, appears greater among prisoners having ADHD with co-morbid TBI than for those with ADHD-only, TBI-only, or neither.

Our results are not consistent with another study addressing head injury among youth offenders [35]. There the authors reported that the proportion of youth offenders who were screened for ADHD and other neurodevelopmental disorders was not significantly higher amongst youth offenders with TBI, compared with those without TBI [35]. This apparent lack of an association between ADHD and TBI may be explained by having a small sample of juvenile offenders and/or by using different methods of assessing ADHD.

Our results are consistent, however, with findings from a recent prison study examining externalizing symptoms and injury severity [36]. Increased rates of externalizing behaviours were reported amongst young adult survivors of paediatric TBI; 25% of all young people with a history of paediatric TBI developed significant levels of externalizing behaviours [36]. Our analyses demonstrating that prisoners with ADHD suffer a high frequency of head injuries before the age of 16 may be explained by the possible coexistence of CD. This may suggest that traumatic events before adulthood may be driven by behavioural problems coexisting with ADHD.

Our results are also consistent with reports from large cohort studies at the population level. Researchers have found evidence of a prospective association between head injury before age 2 and a later diagnosis of ADHD [20]. Nonetheless, they did not find robust evidence of a causal link, as there was also a similar increase in the probability of ADHD diagnosis amongst children who had suffered non-head injuries. They concluded that any accident before age 2 could be a marker for a later diagnosis of ADHD [6], concurring with the view that ADHD is a risk factor for accidents and ensuing injuries. Early brain injury may interact with other predisposing factors generating a "double-burden" on psychiatric disease. Further population-based research should aim to elucidate and expand potential mechanisms.

Prisoners in our study without ADHD or likely TBI had an average QALY of 0.72, which was notably lower than estimates for the general population. Using the HUI-3 and EQ-5D, general population norms in the US and UK estimate an average age-relevant QALY of 0.93 and 0.909, respectively [25, 37]. We analysed the impact of ADHD and TBI on HRQoL and QALYs. We calculated that adult prisoners with ADHD and ADHD with co-morbid TBI have an adjusted average QALY loss of 0.20 and 0.30 compared with those with neither. Prisoners with TBI-only showed no reduction in QALYs. Although the linear combination of coefficients for ADHD-only versus ADHD with co-morbid TBI was not statistically significant, the 0.10 point difference indicated clinical relevance according to the 0.03 difference threshold advised by the HUI3 developers [26]. Furthermore, prisoners with ADHD with co-morbid TBI had a remarkable and significant difference from the TBI-only group, which shows the extent of health impairment that may be attributable to ADHD, and its potential additivity when combined with TBI.

Analyses of specific HRQoL attributes demonstrated the types and extent of impairments. Our finding that prisoners with ADHD had significant impairments related to emotion and cognition, were to be expected, and may likely reflect the influence of co-morbid anxiety or mood disorder [9]. Our finding that prisoners with ADHD with co-morbid TBI had additional significant impairments related to vision, ambulation, and pain was also not a surprise given these groups reported related service use. Prisoners with ADHD with co-morbid TBI had the most visits to specialist mental health and addiction services. ADHD is a known risk factor for developing substance dependence, and a meta-analytic prison rate co-morbidity of 74% was recently established [9].

The significantly poorer vision score among the ADHD with TBI group may relate to their reading difficulties. In the present study, out of the 53 participants in the ADHD/TBI group, 22 (41.5%) required assistance with reading the questionnaires in comparison with only 17.5% of the other participants. With respect to mobility, the finding that prisoners with ADHD/TBI have significantly poorer ambulation problems may reflect that prisoners with the combined condition suffer more injuries that hinder their mobility compared with other prisoners. For example, data obtained from the Danish registry has reported that the morbidity rate is nearly three times higher if you have ADHD, and that 77.8% of unnatural deaths are accounted for by accidental injury [10].

To the best of our knowledge, this is the first study addressing the health status of adult prison inmates with ADHD and TBI using the HUI3. A previous study of children with ADHD reported that higher symptom dimensions of inattention, hyperactivity and impulsivity correlated with poorer HRQoL, along with conduct problems, physical complaints, and somatic symptoms [38]. Additionally, a UK cross-sectional study reported that children and adolescents with ADHD had poorer scores in most health domains compared with samples of healthy children and children with diabetes [39], highlighting the negative impact of ADHD on health. The impact of ADHD on HRQoL scores may be dependent on symptom severity and the presence of co-morbid conditions [40]. Our findings therefore provide initial evidence of the effect that ADHD and TBI has on health-related quality of life outcomes of a fairly large number of prison inmates.

Limitations

A key strength of the study is its large sample size and a methodology in which every participant was clinically diagnosed using the DIVA-2. Nonetheless, there are several limitations.

The cross-sectional design of the study limits any causal interpretation of the association between TBI and ADHD, and other response variables.

Definitions of TBI often vary depending on the source of information, occurrence of LOC and/or loss of memory, and because of this, many results in studies of TBI cannot be generalized. For example: study participants had to rely on their own or a family member's recollection of their trauma events. Recall bias is unaccounted for and may have been a factor on all reported measures of head injury, health status, and service use.

Another limitation is that our findings may not be applicable and generalized beyond the prison population and will likely require replication using other clinical samples. Furthermore, our study results may not be applicable and generalized to female or ethnic minority groups of prisoners. Females often present as clinically distinct from males in correctional services, as they have been found to have the potential for greater impairment in ADHD symptomatology and substance dependence rates [41].

Finally, there is an absence of data in our study on co-morbid factors associated with ADHD and TBI, such as conduct disorder, anxiety, mood disorders, substance misuse, antisocial behaviours, and aggression [42–46], which may impact the findings regarding quality of life. Therefore, the associations found with regard to ADHD, TBI, and HUI3 may be caused by variables not investigated in the present study.

Conclusions

Both ADHD and TBI manifest in high proportions across prison samples. We provide evidence of a strong direct association between them, and evidence to suggest that prisoners with ADHD with co-morbid TBI present with significant impairment in several aspects of HRQoL. Prison inmates with ADHD and those with ADHD with co-morbid TBI had reduced 0.20 and 0.30 QALY respectively when compared with inmates with neither.

The comprehensive health screening tool (CHAT) is an effective screen for both ADHD and TBI in youth offender institutions [35]. The brief version of the Barkley

Adult ADHD Rating Scale (B-BAARS) is an effective screen for ADHD with excellent sensitivity and specificity in adult prison populations [27]. Routine administration in all secure establishments of validated screens could support identification of ADHD and head injury. Furthermore, managing the short and long-term consequences of TBI in prisoners may be important in supporting their rehabilitation and reducing reoffending.

Abbreviations

A&E: Accident and emergency services; ADHD: Attention-deficit hyperactivity disorder; BAARS-IV: Barkley Adult ADHD Rating Scale-IV; B-BAARS: Brief version of the Barkley Adult ADHD Rating Scale; CD: Conduct disorder; CHAT: Comprehensive health screening tool; DIVA-2: Diagnostic Interview for ADHD in Adults 2.0; DSM-5: Diagnostic and Statistical Manual of Mental Disorders, 5th edn; HRQoL: Health-related quality of life; HUI3: Health Utilities Index Mark 3; LOC: Loss of consciousness; MCS: Mayo Classification System; OLS: Ordinary least-squares; OR: Odds ratios; QALY: Quality of life adjusted years; TBI: Traumatic brain injury; WASI: Wechsler Abbreviated Scale of Intelligence

Acknowledgments

We are grateful to the Scottish Prison Service and staff at Porterfield Prison in Inverness for their support of the study. We thank Laura Mutch and Isabella Mallet-Lambert for data collection.

Funding

This study was funded by Shire Pharmaceutical Development Limited, but the funder had no role in the design of the study, data collection, analysis, interpretation of data, and writing the manuscript.

Authors' contributions

SY, RG, MF, PH, and GG led the planning and scientific input of the study. RG conducted the statistical analysis and wrote the first draft with input from SY and GG. KK critically edited the data tables and manuscript; and wrote the final draft. All authors have read and approved the final manuscript.

Consent for publication

Not applicable.

Competing interests

SY has received honoraria for consultancy, travel, educational talks and/or research from Janssen, Eli Lilly, HB Pharma, and/or Shire. MF consulted for Amgen, CSL Behring, Merck, Novo Nordisk, Shire, and Vertex. GG and RG have no conflicts of interest. PH was an employee of Shire working on ADHD projects from 2009 to 2013. The study was supported by Shire Pharmaceutical Development Limited through a restricted grant. Shire had no role in the design and conduct of the study (collection, management, analysis, and interpretation of the data) or on the preparation, review, or approval of the manuscript, and the decision to submit the manuscript for publication. The study was also supported by the National Institute for Health Research (NIHR) Imperial Biomedical Research Centre. The views expressed are those of the authors and not necessarily those of the NHS, the NIHR or the Department of Health. Aside from KK, none of the authors received funds for their involvement in this manuscript.

Author details

[1]Psychology Services Limited, PO Box 1735, Croydon CR97AE, UK. [2]Reykjavik University, Reykjavik, Iceland. [3]East London NHS Foundation Trust, East London, UK. [4]AMF Consulting Inc., Los Angeles, CA, USA. [5]Sage Therapeutics, Cambridge, MA, USA. [6]Independent Medical Writer, San Diego, CA, USA. [7]Institute of Psychiatry, Psychology and Neuroscience, King's College London, London, UK.

References

1. Young S, Moss D, Sedgwick O, Fridman M, Hodgkins P. A meta-analysis of the prevalence of attention deficit hyperactivity disorder in incarcerated populations. Psychol Med. 2014;45(02):247–58.
2. Shiroma EJ, Ferguson PL, Pickelsimer EE. Prevalence of traumatic brain injury in an offender population: a meta-analysis. J of Correctional Health Care. 2010;16(2):147–59.
3. National Institute for Health and Care Excellence. Attention deficit hyperactivity disorder: diagnosis and management. NICE guideline (NG87). London, Author 2018.
4. Diagnostic and statistical manual of mental disorders, 5th EDN Washington, D.C. American Psychiatric Association; 2013.
5. Velez-Pastrana MC, Gonzalez RA, Rodriguez Cardona J, Purcell Baerga P, Alicea Rodriguez A, Levin FR. Psychometric properties of the Barkley deficits in executive functioning scale: a Spanish-language version in a community sample of Puerto Rican adults. Psychol Assess. 2015;28(5):483–98.
6. Satterfield JH, Faller KJ, Crinella FM, Schell AM, Swanson JM, Homer LD. A 30-year prospective follow-up study of hyperactive boys with conduct problems: adult criminality. J Am Acad Child Adolesc Psychiatry. 2007;46(5):601–10.
7. Simon V, Czobor P, Balint S, Meszaros A, Bitter I. Prevalence and correlates of adult attention-deficit hyperactivity disorder: meta-analysis. Br J Psychiatry. 2009;194(3):204–11.
8. Polanczyk G, de Lima MS, Horta BL, Biederman J, Rohde LA. The worldwide prevalence of ADHD: a systematic review and metaregression analysis. Am J of Psychiatry. 2007;164(6):942–8.
9. Young S, Sedgwick O, Fridman M, Gudjonsson G, Hodgkins P, Lantigua M, Gonzalez RA. Co-morbid psychiatric disorders among incarcerated ADHD populations: a meta-analysis. Psychol Med. 2015;45(12):2499–510.
10. Dalsgaard S, Øtergaard SD, Leckman JF, Mortensen PB, Pedersen MG. Mortality in children, adolescents, and adults with attention deficit hyperactivity disorder: a nationwide cohort study. Lancet. 2015;385(9983): 2190–6.
11. Frost RB, Farrer TJ, Primosch M, Hedges DW. Prevalence of traumatic brain injury in the general adult population: a meta-analysis. Neuroepidemiology. 2013;40(3):154–9.
12. Ilie G, Boak A, Adlaf EM, Asbridge M, Cusimano MD. Prevalence and correlates of traumatic brain injuries among adolescents. JAMA. 2013;309(24):2550.
13. Hughes N, Williams WH, Chitsabesan P, Walesby RC, Mounce LT, Clasby B. The prevalence of traumatic brain injury among young offenders in custody: a systematic review. J Head Trauma Rehabil. 2015;30(2):94–105.
14. Davies RC, Williams WH, Hinder D, Burgess CN, Mounce LT. Self-reported traumatic brain injury and postconcussion symptoms in incarcerated youth. J Head Trauma Rehabil. 2012;27(3):E21–7.
15. Moore E, Indig D, Haysom L. Traumatic brain injury, mental health, substance use, and offending among incarcerated young people. J Head Trauma Rehabil. 2014;29(3):239–47.
16. Fazel S, Lichtenstein P, Grann M, Langstrom N. Risk of violent crime in individuals with epilepsy and traumatic brain injury: a 35-year Swedish population study. PLoS Med. 2011;8(12):e1001150.
17. Pitman I, Haddlesey C, Ramos SD, Oddy M, Fortescue D. The association between neuropsychological performance and self-reported traumatic brain injury in a sample of adult male prisoners in the UK. Neuropsychol Rehabil. 2015;25(5):763–79.
18. Barkley RA, Fischer M. Deficient emotional self-regulation is a core component of ADHD. J of ADHD and Related Disorders. 2010;1(2):5–37.
19. Gonzalez RA, Gudjonsson GH, Wells J, Young S. The role of emotional distress and ADHD on institutional behavioral disturbance and recidivism among offenders. J Atten Disord. 2013;20(4):368–78.
20. Keenan HT, Hall GC, Marshall SW. Early head injury and attention deficit hyperactivity disorder: retrospective cohort study. BMJ. 2008;337:a1984.

21. Levin H, Hanten G, Max J, Li X, Swank P, Ewing-Cobbs L, Dennis M, Menefee DS, Schachar R. Symptoms of attention-deficit/hyperactivity disorder following traumatic brain injury in children. J Dev Behav Pediatr. 2007;28(2):108–18.
22. Chang Z, Lichtenstein P, D'Onofrio BM, Sjolander A, Larsson H. Serious transport accidents in adults with attention-deficit/hyperactivity disorder and the effect of medication: a population-based study. JAMA Psychiatry. 2014;71(3):319–25.
23. Larsson H, Sariaslan A, Langstrom N, D'Onofrio B, Lichtenstein P. Family income in early childhood and subsequent attention deficit/hyperactivity disorder: a quasi-experimental study. J Child Psychol Psychiatry. 2014;55(5): 428–35.
24. Williams WH, McAuliffe KA, Cohen MH, Parsonage M, Ramsbotham J. General the Lord D.: traumatic brain injury and juvenile offending: complex causal links offer multiple targets to reduce crime. J Head Trauma Rehabil. 2015;30(2):69–74.
25. Health Utilities Inc. http://www.healthutilities.com/. Accessed 29 Oct 2017.
26. Horsman J, Furlong W, Feeny D, Torrance G. The health utilities index (HUI): concepts, measurement properties and applications. Health Qual Life Outcomes. 2003;1:54.
27. Young S, González RA, Mutch L, Mallet-Lambert I, O'Rourke L, Hickey N, Asherson P, Gudjonsson GH. Diagnostic accuracy of a brief screening tool for attention deficit hyperactivity disorder in UK prison inmates. Psychol Med. 2016;46(07):1449–58.
28. Malec JF, Brown AW, Leibson CL, Flaada JT, Mandrekar JN, Diehl NN, Perkins PK. The mayo classification system for traumatic brain injury severity. J Neurotrauma. 2007;24(9):1417–24.
29. Kooij JJS. Diagnostic Interview for ADHD in Adults 2.0 (DIVA 2.0). Adult ADHD: Diagnostic assessment and treatment. Amsterdam, ND: Pearson Assessment and Information BV; 2010.
30. Barkley RA. Barkley adult ADHD rating scale-IV (BAARS-IV). New York, NY: Guilford; 2011.
31. Wechsler D. Wechsler Abbreviated Scale of Intelligence. The psychological corporation. New York, NY: Harcourt Brace & Company; 1999.
32. Lezak MD, Howieson DB, Bigler ED, Tranel D. Neuropsychological assessment. 5th ed. New York: Oxford University Press; 2012.
33. Long JS. Regression models for categorical and limited dependent variables: SAGE Publications; 1997.
34. StataCorp. Stata Statistical Software: Release 13. College Station, TX: StataCorp LP; 2013.
35. Chitsabesan P, Lennox C, Williams H, Tariq O, Shaw J. Traumatic brain injury in juvenile offenders: findings from the comprehensive health assessment tool study and the development of a specialist linkworker service. J Head Trauma Rehabil. 2015;30(2):106–15.
36. Ryan NP, Hughes N, Godfrey C, Rosema S, Catroppa C, Anderson VA. Prevalence and predictors of externalizing behavior in young adult survivors of pediatric traumatic brain injury. J of Head Trauma Rehabilitation. 2015; 30(2):75–85.
37. Kind P, Hardman G, Macran SUK. Population norms for EQ-5D. University of York: Centre for Health Econ; 1999.
38. Riley AW, Spiel G, Coghill D, Dopfner M, Falissard B, Lorenzo MJ, Preuss U, Ralston SJ, Group A.S. Factors related to health-related quality of life (HRQoL) among children with ADHD in Europe at entry into treatment. Eur Child Adolesc Psychiatry. 2006;15(Suppl 1):I38–45.
39. Coghill D, Hodgkins P. Health-related quality of life of children with attention-deficit/hyperactivity disorder versus children with diabetes and healthy controls. Eur Child Adolesc Psychiatry. 2015;
40. Klassen AF, Miller A, Fine S. Health-related quality of life in children and adolescents who have a diagnosis of attention-deficit/hyperactivity disorder. Pediatrics. 2004;114(5):e541–7.
41. Gonzalez RA, Velez-Pastrana MC, Ruiz Varcarcel JJ, Levin FR, Albizu-Garcia CE. Childhood ADHD symptoms are associated with lifetime and current illicit substance-use disorders and in-site health risk behaviors in a representative sample of Latino prison inmates. J Atten Disord. 2015;19(4):301–12.
42. Comai S, Bertazzo A, Vachon J, Daigle M, Toupin J, Cote G, Turecki G, Gobbi G. Tryptophan via serotonin/kynurenine pathways abnormalities in a large cohort of aggressive inmates: markers for aggression. Prog Neuro-Psychopharmacol Biol Psychiatry. 2016;70:8–16.
43. Rosler M, Retz W, Retz-Junginger P, Hengesch G, Schneider M, Supprian T, Schwitzgebel P, Pinhard K, Dovi-Akue N, Wender P, et al. Prevalence of attention deficit–/hyperactivity disorder (ADHD) and comorbid disorders in young male prison inmates. Eur Arch Psychiatry Clin Neurosci. 2004;254(6):365–71.
44. Retz W, Retz-Junginger P, Hengesch G, Schneider M, Thome J, Pajonk FG, Salahi-Disfan A, Rees O, Wender PH, Rosler M. Psychometric and psychopathological characterization of young male prison inmates with and without attention deficit/hyperactivity disorder. Eur Arch Psychiatry Clin Neurosci. 2004;254(4):201–8.
45. Sobanski E, Bruggemann D, Alm B, Kern S, Deschner M, Schubert T, Philipsen A, Rietschel M. Psychiatric comorbidity and functional impairment in a clinically referred sample of adults with attention-deficit/hyperactivity disorder (ADHD). Eur Arch Psychiatry Clin Neurosci. 2007;257(7):371–7.
46. Timonen M, Miettunen J, Hakko H, Zitting P, Veijola J, von Wendt L, Rasanen P. The association of preceding traumatic brain injury with mental disorders, alcoholism and criminality: the northern Finland 1966 birth cohort study. Psychiatry Res. 2002;113(3):217–26.

9

Olfactory impairment in first-episode schizophrenia: a case-control study, and sex dimorphism in the relationship between olfactory impairment and psychotic symptoms

Xiacan Chen[1†], Jiajun Xu[2*†], Bin Li[2], Wanjun Guo[2], Jun Zhang[2] and Junmei Hu[1*]

Abstract

Background: A body of studies has focused on the olfactory impairment among people with schizophrenia. The effect of sex on this relationship has attracted the attention of researchers. These issues have not been studied much in Chinese schizophrenia patients.

Methods: We conducted a case-control study of 110 first-episode antipsychotic medicine naïve schizophrenia patients aged 18–35 years and 110 controls, matched by age and sex. Odour threshold, discrimination and identification were assessed by the "Sniffin' Sticks" test. Psychotic symptoms were assessed by the Positive and Negative Syndrome Scale (PANSS).

Results: The odour threshold, discrimination and identification scores of patients with schizophrenia were significantly lower than those of the healthy control group. The difference in identification score had statistical significance between male and female patients with schizophrenia ($t = -2.45$, $P < 0.05$). Controlling for confounding factor, in male schizophrenia participants, the negative subscale score was significantly and inversely correlated with the discrimination ($\gamma = -0.37$, $p < 0.008$), identification ($\gamma = -0.45$, $p < 0.008$) and TDI ($\gamma = -0.50$, $p < 0.008$) scores; the general psychopathology subscale score was inversely and significantly correlated with the identification ($\gamma = -0.47$, $p < 0.008$) and TDI ($\gamma = -0.41$, $p < 0.008$) scores. For female schizophrenia patients, positive and general psychopathology subscale scores had a significant inverse correlation with the identification score (positive: $\gamma = -0.47$, $p < 0.008$; general psychopathology: $\gamma = -0.42$, $p < 0.008$).

Conclusions: Controlling for confounder, negative symptoms were related to impaired odour discrimination and identification in male schizophrenia patients, while positive symptoms were correlated with impaired odour identification in female schizophrenia patients. This sex dimorphism could provide useful information for future studies aiming to finding biomarkers of schizophrenia.

Keywords: Schizophrenia, Olfaction, Sex, Negative symptom, Positive symptom

* Correspondence: xujiajun120@126.com; junmeihu@hotmail.com
[†]Xiacan Chen and Jiajun Xu contributed equally to this work.
[2]Mental Health Center, West China Hospital, Sichuan University, Sichuan, China
[1]West China School of Basic Medical Sciences & Forensic Medicine, Sichuan University, Sichuan, China

Background

Schizophrenia, mainly defined by its psychotic symptoms, lacks physiological examination to diagnosis [1]. Many studies were conducted with the aim of finding biomarkers of schizophrenia and olfactory function has been one of the directions. Olfaction, an age- and sex-related function, is one of the most direct neural pathways between external environment and the central nervous system. There is overlap of some neuroanatomical structure with the impaired brain region in those with schizophrenia, such as the medial temporal lobe, amygdala and hippocampus [1–3]. Furthermore, the olfactory function examination was more convenient and reliable than a review of the patient symptom state which is subjective and always reported by patients themselves. Lastly, olfactory impairment was found in schizophrenia patients, and has been especially correlated with negative symptoms [4, 5]. Consequently, an understanding olfaction would be useful for the clinical practice of schizophrenia.

Olfaction is a multiple sensory process, and the deficit of it can be divided into peripheral and central abnormalities. Odour detection threshold (sensitivity) is more peripheral, while identification and discrimination are more central [6–8]. Olfactory dysfunction is well documented in schizophrenia patients and odour identification impairment has been suggested as a vulnerability marker of deficit syndrome in some studies [5, 9], while a meta-analysis failed to find evidence for considering olfaction identification as vulnerability marker of schizophrenia [10]; however, the absence of accounting for sex effect in the meta-analysis could profoundly influence the results, for sex difference in olfaction have been documented not only in healthy individuals, but also in schizophrenia patients [11, 12]. Many studies were conducted with small sample sizes and these multiple olfactory functions (e.g., threshold, identification and discrimination) were barely examined in same subjects, as *Moberg* noted [13]; in addition, odour threshold and discrimination were reported much less among patients with schizophrenia when comparing with odour identification [4, 7].

Sexual dimorphism is common in neuroscience and schizophrenia studies. The differences of manifestations, social function and brain structure have been addressed between male and female among schizophrenia [14–17]. Sex difference was also presented in olfactory performance among patients with schizophrenia, in that some researchers have reported that male schizophrenia patients show a strong relation between negative symptoms and odour identification, while female patients have failed to present this relation [12, 18]. However, the relation between psychotic symptoms and other odour domains (e.g., threshold and discrimination) has been rarely studied.

Meanwhile, olfaction was reported as an age-related function among general adults, but many studies did not include age as a confounding factor when detecting olfactory impairment among patients with schizophrenia [11, 19]. Even though many studies about olfactory impairment among patients with schizophrenia have been conducted, few studies aimed at reporting the relation between olfaction and schizophrenia in Chinese patients. Addressing these limitations, we want to conduct a case-control study with the aim of detecting three olfactory performances in Chinese schizophrenia patients compared with healthy control subjects, and elucidating the sexual dimorphism in the relationship between psychotic symptom and olfactory function among schizophrenia patients, with the consideration of age effect, to provide useful information for further olfactory study in schizophrenia and clinical practice.

Methods

Procedure and participates

The aim of this study was to detect differences in responses to three olfactory performances in Chinese schizophrenia patients compared with healthy control subjects and to examine the sexual dimorphism in the relationship between psychotic symptoms and olfactory function among schizophrenia patients, with the consideration of age effect.

For this study, we recruited 110 patients aged 18–35 years old who were diagnosed with schizophrenia (66 males, 44 females). The patients were diagnosed according to DSM-V; patients were excluded for neurological disorder, organic brain injury, any other mental illness, any major olfactory disturbance histories or general poor somatic health. These participants were all in the first-episode stage of schizophrenia and naive to any antipsychotic medication prior to the olfactory testing. Young adults (18–35 years old) were selected as participants for two reasons: one was that in previous studies of the "Sniffin' Sticks" test (SST) in a general population, a difference was found in olfactory performance among different adult age groups (e.g., young adult, middle-aged adult and older adult) [11, 19]; the other reason was that first-episode schizophrenia is most often seex in the young adult (18–35 years old) was the main age group.

Healthy controls, 110 community-based subjects aged 18–35 years, were recruited by advertising and were free of any psychotic disorders according to DSM-V. The exclusion criteria were in accordance with the schizophrenia group; additionally, individuals with a family history of psychosis were excluded. Age (±3 years) and sex were matched for each control. The demographic details are shown in Table 1. All healthy participants and guardians of patients provided written informed consent.

Psychotic symptom assessment

Psychotic symptoms were assessed by two psychiatrists using the Positive and Negative Syndrome Scale (PANSS) and the interrater reliability was 0.81. This scale included positive, negative and general psychopathy subscales [20].

Olfactory testing

The Sniffin' Sticks Test, with a high repeatability, was used to evaluate olfaction [21, 22]. It is composed of three tests—odour threshold, odour discrimination and odour identification. The odour threshold task consists of 16 types of n-butanol solution with different concentrations, which start from 4%. Triplet of felt-tipped pens is a group with two containing blank solvent and a third containing the odorant of n-butanol solution, and the triplets are presented to the subject in randomized order. The subject is asked to determine the odorant from the other two blank solvent.

The odour discrimination task comprises 16 groups as well. A group, consisting of a triplet of pens, includes two with the same odorant and a third with a different odorant. A triplet of pens is randomly presented to the subject. The subject has to identify which one smelled different.

During the odour identification test, 16 odours were presented to participants through the felt-tipped pen dispensers and each odour must be identified by the subject from a list of four descriptors.

In the three sub-tests, the interval between the presentation of each pen and each group was approximately 3 s and 20–30 s, respectively. As the score of each sub-test ranges from 0 to 16 and the total score, which was the TDI score comprising threshold, discrimination and identification, ranges from 0 to 48.

Statistical analyses

Continuous data were described by mean or median and compared between the schizophrenia and control groups by *t* test, or non-parametric test if the data did not meet normal distribution. The Kolmogorov–Smirnov test was used to assess the normality. Categorical data were compared by chi-square test between the two groups. Partial correlation was used to control confounding factors and

Table 1 Demographic characteristics and olfactory performance scores

	Schizophrenia	Healthy	*t*
	n = 110 (male: 66;female:44)	n = 110 (male:66;female:44)	
Age, mean (SD) in years	22.86 (4.61)	23.46 (4.18)	5265 (Mann-Whitney)
M	22.85 (4.69)	24.47 (4.80)	1737*
F	22.89 (4.56)	22.00 (2.40)	967
Sex, N (p)			
M	66	66	0 (χ^2)
F	44	44	
Smoking	21 (19.1)	8 (7.3)	6.7*(χ^2)
M	19 (28.79)	8 (12.12)	5.63*(χ^2)
F	2 (4.54)	0	2.05(χ^2)
SST, mean (SD) in score			
Threshold	5.98 (2.77)	8.75 (3.18)	6.89**
M	5.92 (3.08)	8.92 (3.28)	5.42**
F	6.07 (2.25)	8.50 (3.03)	4.26**
Discrimination	8.73 (3.55)	12.44 (1.79)	9.80**
M	8.62 (3.82)	12.55 (1.76)	7.58**
F	8.89 (3.13)	12.27 (1.84)	6.20**
Identification	10.60 (2.73)	13.02 (1.72)	7.12**
M	10.09 (3.00)	13.14 (1.76)	6.99**
F	11.36 (2.09)	12.84 (1.66)	3.67**
TDI	25.31 (6.65)	34.21 (4.98)	11.23**
M	24.64 (7.24)	34.61 (5.09)	9.15**
F	26.32 (5.58)	33.61 (4.81)	6.57**

SST the Sniffin' sticks test, *M* Male, *F* Female, *TDI* the total score of threshold, discrimination and identification

*: $P < 0.05$; **: $P < 0.01$

show the relationship between clinical scales (PANSS) and the SST scores. An alpha level of below 0.05 was defined as statistical significance. The significant P value was corrected by Bonferroni Correction for multiple testing. All data analyses were performed with the statistical package SPSS (version 16.0).

Results

Demographic factors, smoking status and the SST scores (including olfactory threshold, discrimination, identification and TDI score) are displayed in Table 1. The average age was 22.86 (SD = 4.61) and 23.46 (SD = 4.18) years for the schizophrenia and healthy group, respectively. There was no significant difference in the age and sex between the schizophrenia and healthy group. The schizophrenia participants showed lower mean scores of SST test than the control group among both males and females (Table 1 and Fig. 1). Among the schizophrenia group, the difference in smoking status shows statistical significance between male and female ($\chi^2 = 10.01$, $P < 0.01$).

The olfactory performances and psychotic symptoms for male and female schizophrenia patients are illustrated in Table 2. The positive, negative and general psychopathology subscale scores, and the five factor symptom scores did not show a statistical difference; the difference of the identification score had statistical significance ($t = -2.45$, $P < 0.05$), while the threshold, discrimination and TDI scores did not.

The threshold (KS Z = 1.69, $p < 0.05$), discrimination (KS Z = 1.85, $p < 0.05$), identification (KS Z = 1.75, $p < 0.05$) and TDI (KS Z = 1.14, $p < 0.05$) scores did not meet the normal distribution, nor did the positive symptom score (KS Z = 1.38, $p = 0.046$). The negative symptom score met the normal distribution (KS Z = 0.94, $p = 0.35$). Correlation between psychotic symptoms and olfactory performance in the schizophrenia group is illustrated in Fig. 2. Controlling for the confounding factor, in male schizophrenia participants, the negative subscale score showed a significant inverse correlation with discrimination ($\gamma = -0.37$, $p < 0.008$), identification ($\gamma = -0.45$, $p < 0.008$) and TDI ($\gamma = -0.50$, $p < 0.008$) scores; the general psychopathology subscale score was inversely and significantly correlated with identification ($\gamma = -0.47$, $p < 0.008$), and the TDI ($\gamma = -0.41$, $p < 0.008$) scores.

In contrast, among female schizophrenia patients, positive and general psychopathology subscale scores appeared to have a significant inverse correlation with the identification score (positive: $\gamma = -0.47$, $p < 0.008$; general psychopathology: $\gamma = -0.42$, $p < 0.008$).

Discussion

Considering the effect of age, we conducted this case-control study to explore the olfactory function of first-episode schizophrenia patients aged 18–35 in China and the sex effect on the relationship between olfaction and schizophrenia with the consideration of the smoking confounder. In this study, olfactory impairment was found among Chinese schizophrenia patients. In terms of psychotic symptoms, negative symptoms were correlated with odour discrimination and identification in male schizophrenia patients, whereas positive symptoms were correlated with odour identification in female schizophrenia patients. General psychopathy symptom was correlated with odour identification both in male and female schizophrenia patients.

In this study, matched by sex and age, schizophrenia patients showed poorer performance across all the measures of olfaction, compared with the healthy group. Although many researchers have reported olfactory impairment in schizophrenia since 20 years ago [23], few have reported about olfactory performance among those with schizophrenia. Recently, a study conducted in China reported an odour identification deficit in patients with schizophrenia [24]; unfortunately, this study only detected the odour identification performance instead of the whole olfactory function of Chinese patients with schizophrenia.

After adjusting for the smoking status, odour identification was correlated with negative and positive symptoms among male and female schizophrenia patients, respectively. The extant literature had noted a robust correlation between odour identification and negative symptoms in schizophrenia [25, 26] and many studies further showed sex effect on olfactory function both in schizophrenia [27, 28] and in general population [11, 22]. Further studies considering sex effect indicated a high correlation between negative symptoms and odour identification only in male schizophrenia patients [29]. Our study is strongly consistent with

Table 2 Comparison of PANSS scores and the SST scores between male and female schizophrenia

	Male $n = 66$	Female $n = 44$	t
SST score, mean (SD)			
Threshold	5.92 (3.08)	6.07 (2.25)	−.27
Discrimination	8.62 (3.82)	8.89 (3.13)	−.38
Identification	10.09 (3.00)	11.36 (2.09)	−2.45*
TDI	24.64 (7.24)	26.32 (5.58)	−1.30
PANSS score, mean (SD)			
Sub-scale score			
Positive	16.26 (4.97)	15.82 (4.60)	.47
Negative	16.80 (6.22)	15.89 (5.23)	.81
General Psychopathy	31.76 (8.40)	30.52 (7.49)	.79

PANSS the positive and negative syndrome scale, *SST* the Sniffin' sticks test, *TDI* the total score of threshold, discrimination and identification
*: $P < 0.05$; **: $P < 0.01$

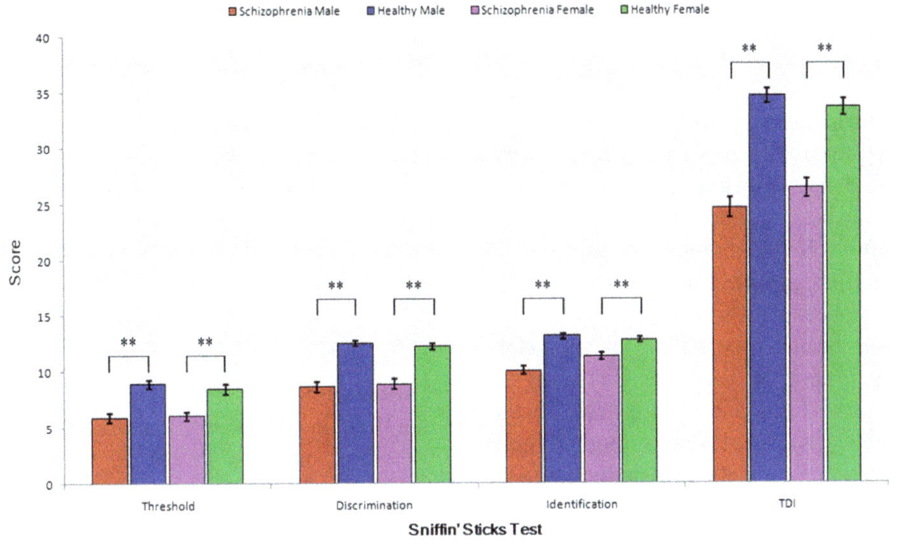

Fig. 1 Mean "Sniffin' Sticks" test scores with standard error bars by diagnosis and sex. Abbreviations TDI, the total score of threshold, discrimination and identification

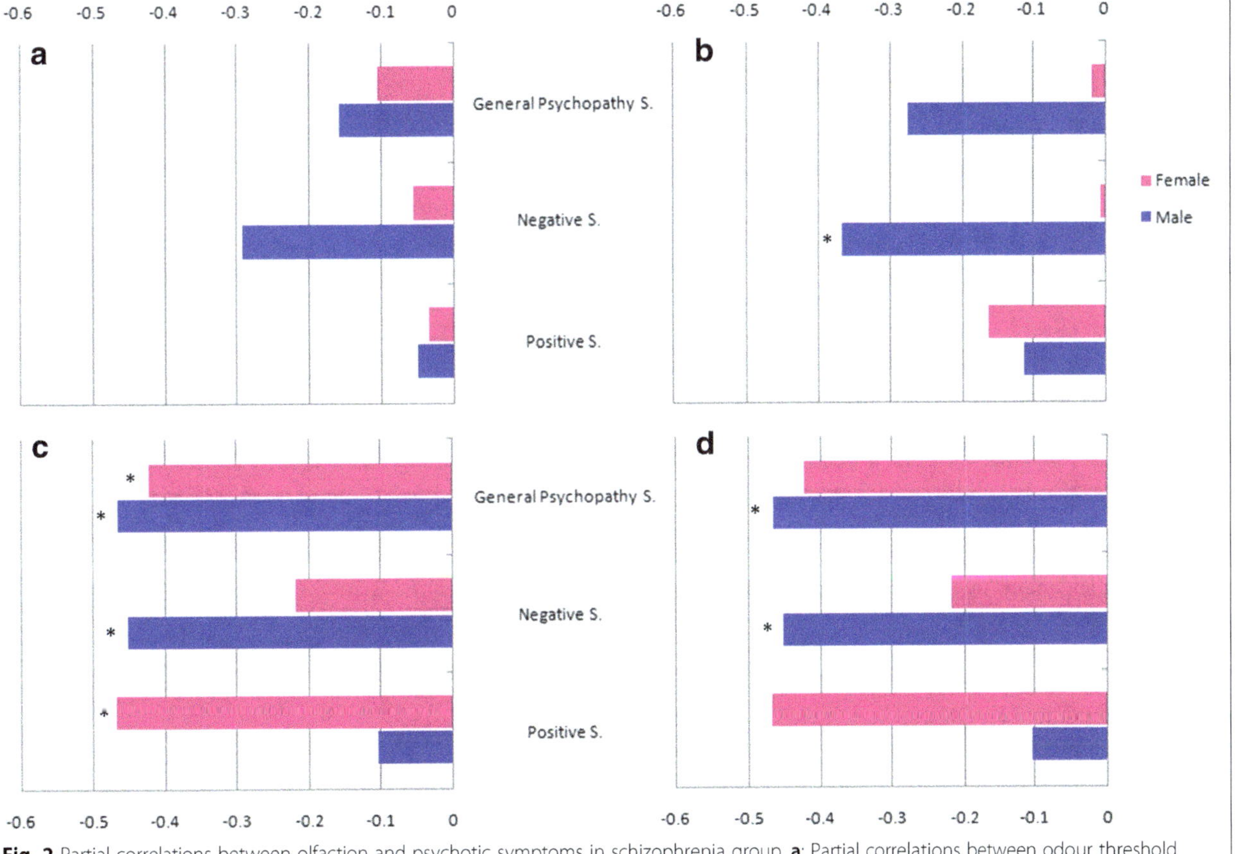

Fig. 2 Partial correlations between olfaction and psychotic symptoms in schizophrenia group. **a**: Partial correlations between odour threshold score and PANSS scores; **b**: Partial correlations between odour discrimination score and PANSS scores; **c**: Partial correlations between odour identification score and PANSS scores; **d**: Partial correlations between TDI and PANSS score. Adjusted for the smoking status. Abbreviations: General psychopathy S., general psychopathy subscale; Negative S., negative subscale; Positive S., positive subscale. PANSS, the Positive and Negative Syndrome Scale; TDI, the total score of threshold, discrimination and identification.*: Adjusted $P < 0.008$

this finding that poorer odour identification was only related to negative symptoms in male schizophrenia patients. In addition, a different finding that olfactory identification was correlated with positive symptoms among female schizophrenia patients still remains in this study. This was scarcely reported before. Only a recently study found fewer serious positive symptoms were associated with better odour detection threshold for citralva [30].We think whether considering the effect of sex or not might account for the different reporting. Moreover, because the negative symptom of schizophrenia have been reported to be correlated with olfactory impairment by researchers starting two decades ago [13], many following studies have focused on exploring negative symptoms and might neglect positive symptoms when detecting olfactory function in patients with schizophrenia [12].

Meanwhile, sex dimorphism exists in the symptomatology, antipsychotic response [28], social functioning [14], illness characteristics [15] and cerebral structure [16] of schizophrenia. It might be helpful to consider these factors, as well as hormone effect [28], when future studies try to elucidate the sex effect on olfaction. Meanwhile, odour identification has been described as a central process [31] and the limbic structure (e.g., amygdala and the orbitofrontal cortex) was the location of olfactory association cortex. The abnormality of limbic structure was not only connected with olfactory dysfunction [31] but also connected with negative symptomatology [32]. Furthermore, the orbitofrontal cortex to amygdala ratio presented sex dimorphism [33], and hyperfrontality and hypofrontality was correlated with positive and negative symptoms, respectively [34, 35]. Collectively, these might provide another possible explanation for the sex difference presented regarding the relationship between olfactory impairment and symptomatology. Moreover, the sex related difference of olfactory bulb [36] might also be a possible way to elucidate this result. In addition, Chinese patients were participants in this study, for whom the sex effect on olfaction was hardly reported. It might be possible that there is heterogeneity of olfactory impairment in Chinese schizophrenia patients.

Odour discrimination, studied much less than olfactory identification in previous research [8], was related to negative symptoms among male patients in this study. Odour discrimination being more central processing when compared with odour threshold, and its deficit is related to the hippocampus and amygdala, which are also the impaired brain region among schizophrenia [31]. Therefore, the relation between odour discrimination and negative symptoms in male schizophrenia patients should be detailed further. Expectedly, general psychopathy, including cognition, was correlated with odour identification. This was in consistent with previous studies that have found that olfactory identification was strongly related with cognition and it was considered to be a useful supplementary screening tool of Alzheimer's disease [37].

The limitation of this study was the lack of neuroimaging or electrophysiological studies to further explain why different sex shows different relationships between psychotic symptoms and olfactory impairment. This is the direction of our further studies.

Conclusion

Sex influenced the relationship between psychotic symptoms and olfactory impairment in first-episode schizophrenia patients aged 18–35 years. Negative and positive symptoms were associated with odour identification deficit in male and female schizophrenia, respectively. The odour discrimination deficit was correlated with negative symptom among male schizophrenia patients. The effect of sex on olfactory impairment among patients with schizophrenia should be studied more profoundly.

Abbreviations

PANSS: Positive and Negative Syndrome Scale; SST: The Sniffin' Sticks Test; TDI: The total score of threshold, discrimination and identification

Acknowledgements

We thank Professor Xiehe Liu, who kindly provided guidance on this research.

Funding

The design of the study, and collection, analysis and interpretation of data are supported by the National Natural Science Foundation of China (No. 81401132). The publication of the paper was supported by the Key Research and Development Project of Province Science and Technology Department, Sichuan (No. 2017SZ0062).

Authors' contributions

XC and JX contributed equally. Study concept and design: JX, XC and JH. Data collection: JX, XC. Analysis and interpretation of data: XC, JX. Drafting of the manuscript: XC and JX. Critical revision of the manuscript for important intellectual content: JH, WG, BL, JZ. All authors reviewed and approved the manuscript.

Consent for publication

Not applicable.

Competing interests

The authors declare that they have no competing interests.

References

1. Kahn RS, Keefe RSE. Schizophrenia is a cognitive illness: time for a change in focus. Jama Psychiatry. 2013;70(10):1107.
2. Turetsky BI, Hahn CG, Borgmann-Winter K, Moberg PJ. Scents and nonsense: olfactory dysfunction in schizophrenia. Schizophr Bull. 2009;35(6):1117–31.
3. Nolte J, S J. The human brain: an introduction to its functional anatomy. 6th ed. Philadelphia: Mosby; 2008.
4. Ugur T, Weisbrod M, Franzek E, Pfuller U, Sauer H. Olfactory impairment in monozygotic twins discordant for schizophrenia. Eur Arch Psychiatry Clin Neurosci. 2005;255(2):94–8.
5. Ishizuka K, Tajinda K, Colantuoni C, Morita M, Winicki J, Le C, Lin S, Schretlen D, Sawa A, Cascella NG. Negative symptoms of schizophrenia correlate with impairment on the University of Pennsylvania smell identification test. Neurosci Res. 2010;66(1):106–10.
6. Amsterdam JD, Settle RG, Doty RL, Abelman E, Winokur A. Taste and smell perception in depression. Biol Psychiatry. 1987;22(12):1481–5.
7. Rupp CI, Fleischhacker WW, Kemmler G, Oberbauer H, Scholtz AW, Wanko C, Hinterhuber H. Various bilateral olfactory deficits in male patients with schizophrenia. Schizophr Bull. 2005;31(1):155–65.
8. Nguyen AD, Shenton ME, Levitt JJ. Olfactory dysfunction in schizophrenia: a review of neuroanatomy and psychophysiological measurements. Harv Rev Psychiatry. 2010;18(5):279–92.
9. Pelka-Wysiecka J, Wronski M, Bienkowski P, Murawiec S, Samochowiec A, Samochowiec J. Odors identification differences in deficit and nondeficit schizophrenia. Pharmacol Rep. 2016;68(2):390–5.
10. Cohen AS, Brown LA, Auster TL. Olfaction, "olfiction", and the schizophrenia-spectrum: an updated meta-analysis on identification and acuity. Schizophr Res. 2012;135(1–3):152–7.
11. Hummel T, Kobal G, Gudziol H, Mackaysim A. Normative data for the "Sniffin' sticks" including tests of odor identification, odor discrimination, and olfactory thresholds: an upgrade based on a group of more than 3,000 subjects. Eur Arch Otorhinolaryngol. 2007;264(3):237–43.
12. Malaspina D, Goetz R, Keller A, Messinger JW, Bruder G, Goetz D, Opler M, Harlap S, Harkavy-Friedman J, Antonius D. Olfactory processing, sex effects and heterogeneity in schizophrenia. Schizophr Res. 2012;135(1–3):144–51.
13. Moberg PJ, Agrin R, Gur RE, Gur RC, Turetsky BI, Doty RL. Olfactory dysfunction in schizophrenia : a qualitative and quantitative review. Neuropsychopharmacol Official Publ Am Coll europsychopharmacol. 1999; 21(3):325–40.
14. Andia AM, Zisook S, Heaton RK, Hesselink J, Jernigan T, Kuck J, Morganville J, Braff DL. Gender differences in schizophrenia. J Nerv Ment Dis. 1995; 183(8):522–8.
15. Ochoa S, Usall J, Cobo J, Labad X, Kulkarni J. Gender differences in schizophrenia and first-episode psychosis: a comprehensive literature review. Schizophrenia Res Treat. 2012;2012:916198.
16. Crow TJ, Chance SA, Priddle TH, Radua J, James AC. Laterality interacts with sex across the schizophrenia/bipolarity continuum: an interpretation of meta-analyses of structural MRI. Psychiatry Res. 2013;210(3):1232–44.
17. Beery AK, Zucker I. Sex bias in neuroscience and biomedical research. Neurosci Biobehav Rev. 2011;35(3):565–72.
18. Good KP, Leslie RA, McGlone J, Milliken HI, Kopala LC. Sex differences in olfactory function in young patients with psychotic disorders. Schizophr Res. 2007;97(1–3):97–102.
19. Sorokowska A, Schriever VA, Gudziol V, Hummel C, Hähner A, Iannilli E, Sinding C, Aziz M, Seo HS, Negoias S. Changes of olfactory abilities in relation to age: odor identification in more than 1400 people aged 4 to 80 years. Eur Arch Otorhinolaryngol. 2015;272(8):1937–44.
20. Kay SR, Opler LA, Lindenmayer JP. Reliability and validity of the positive and negative syndrome scale for schizophrenics. Psychiatry Res. 1988;23(1):99–110.
21. Kobal G, Klimek L, Wolfensberger M, Gudziol H, Temmel A, Owen CM, Seeber H, Pauli E, Hummel T. Multicenter investigation of 1,036 subjects using a standardized method for the assessment of olfactory function combining tests of odor identification, odor discrimination, and olfactory thresholds. Eur Arch Otorhinolaryngol. 2000;257(4):205–11.
22. Kobal G, Hummel T, Sekinger B, Barz S, Roscher S, Wolf S. "Sniffin' sticks": screening of olfactory performance. Rhinology. 1996;34(4):222–6.
23. Hurwitz T, Kopala L, Clark C, Jones B. Olfactory deficits in schizophrenia. Biol Psychiatry. 1988;23(2):123–8.
24. Zou LQ, Zhou HY, Lui SSY, Wang Y, Wang Y, Gan J, Zhu XZ, Cheung EFC, Chan RCK. Olfactory identification deficit and its relationship with hedonic traits in patients with first-episode schizophrenia and individuals with schizotypy. Prog Neuro-Psychopharmacol Biol Psychiatry. 2018;83:137–41.
25. Good KP, Whitehorn D, Rui Q, Milliken H, Kopala LC. Olfactory identification deficits in first-episode psychosis may predict patients at risk for persistent negative and disorganized or cognitive symptoms. Am J Psychiatr. 2006; 163(163):932–3.
26. Good KP, Tibbo P, Milliken H, Whitehorn D, Alexiadis M, Robertson N, Kopala LC. An investigation of a possible relationship between olfactory identification deficits at first episode and four-year outcomes in patients with psychosis. Schizophr Res. 2010;124(1–3):60–5.
27. Highley JR, DeLisi LE, Roberts N, Webb JA, Relja M, Razi K, Crow TJ. Sex-dependent effects of schizophrenia: an MRI study of gyral folding, and cortical and white matter volume. Psychiatry Res. 2003;124(1):11–23.
28. Abel KM, Drake R, Goldstein JM. Sex differences in schizophrenia. Int Rev Psychiatry. 2010;22(5):417–28.
29. Urban M, Rabe-Jablonska J. Olfactory dysfunctions in patients with schizophrenia. Psychiatr Pol. 2007;41(4):503–12.
30. Kamath V, Lasutschinkow P, Ishizuka K, Sawa A. Olfactory functioning in first-episode psychosis. Schizophr Bull. 2017;44(3):672–80.
31. Rupp CI, Fleischhacker WW, Kemmler G, Kremser C, Bilder RM, Mechtcheriakov S, Szeszko PR, Walch T, Scholtz AW, Klimbacher M, et al. Olfactory functions and volumetric measures of orbitofrontal and limbic regions in schizophrenia. Schizophr Res. 2005;74(2–3):149–61.
32. Rahm C, Liberg B, Reckless G, Ousdal O, Melle I, Andreassen OA, Agartz I. Negative symptoms in schizophrenia show association with amygdala volumes and neural activation during affective processing. Acta Neuropsychiatrica. 2015;27(4):213–20.
33. Gur RE, Kohler C, Turetsky BI, Siegel SJ, Kanes SJ, Bilker WB, Brennan AR, Gur RC. A sexually dimorphic ratio of orbitofrontal to amygdala volume is altered in schizophrenia. Biol Psychiatry. 2004;55(5):512–7.
34. Semkovska M, Bedard MA, Stip E. Hypofrontality and negative symptoms in schizophrenia: synthesis of anatomic and neuropsychological knowledge and ecological perspectives. Encephale. 2001;27(5):405–15.
35. Shinto AS, Kamaleshwaran KK, Srinivasan D, Paranthaman S, Selvaraj K, Pranesh MB, Lakshminarayanan GN, Prakash B. "Hyperfrontality" as seen on FDG PET in unmedicated schizophrenia patients with positive symptoms. Clin Nucl Med. 2014;39(8):694–7.
36. Oliveira-Pinto AV, Santos RM, Coutinho RA, Oliveira LM, Santos GB, Alho AT, Leite RE, Farfel JM, Suemoto CK, Grinberg LT, et al. Sexual dimorphism in the human olfactory bulb: females have more neurons and glial cells than males. PLoS One. 2014;9(11):e111733.
37. Quarmley M, Moberg PJ, Mechanic-Hamilton D, Kabadi S, Arnold SE, Wolk DA, Roalf DR. Odor identification screening improves diagnostic classification in incipient Alzheimer's disease. J Alzheimers Dis Jad. 2016;55(4):1497–507.

10

Subjective well-being, drug attitude, and changes in symptomatology in chronic schizophrenia patients starting treatment with new-generation antipsychotic medication

Christian G. Widschwendter*, Georg Kemmler, Maria A. Rettenbacher, Nursen Yalcin-Siedentopf and Alex Hofer

Abstract

Background: Non-adherence to medication remains a major challenge in the long-term management of patients with schizophrenia. Next to lack of insight into the illness, adverse effects of antipsychotic drugs, cognitive deficits, poor therapeutic alliance, reduced quality of life, missing social support, and negative attitudes toward medication are predictors of non-adherence. This study examined potential correlations between attitudes toward antipsychotic drug therapy, subjective well-being, and symptom change in patients with chronic schizophrenia.

Methods: 30 patients with schizophrenia starting monotherapy with a new-generation antipsychotic were included into the study. The Drug Attitude Inventory (DAI) and the Subjective Well-being under Neuroleptic Treatment Scale, short form (SWN-K), were administered after 2, 4, and 12 weeks of treatment. At the same points in time and at baseline, psychopathological symptoms were rated by means of the Positive and Negative Syndrome Scale (PANSS), and functioning was assessed by means of the Global Assessment of Functioning Scale (GAF). Antipsychotic induced side effects were evaluated by using the Udvalg for Kliniske Undersogelser (UKU) Side Effect Rating Scale.

Results: Study participants had a mean age of 37.5 ± 9.7 years, baseline symptoms were mild. The PANSS total score improved significantly from baseline to weeks 4 ($p = .003$) and 12 ($p = .001$), respectively. Neither the DAI total score nor the SWN-K total score changed significantly over the course of time. The severity of symptoms was not correlated with drug attitude at any time point but was negatively correlated with wellbeing at weeks 2 ($r = -.419$, $p = .021$) and 4 ($r = -.441$, $p = .015$). There was no significant correlation between DAI and SWN-K total scores at any time point.

Conclusions: Next to showing that the DAI and the SWN-K measure different aspects of subjective experiences during antipsychotic treatment these findings emphasize the use of both instruments to optimize adherence to medication.

Background

Despite advances in the pharmacotherapy of schizophrenia poor-adherence to antipsychotic medication remains a major challenge in the long-term treatment of patients. Most studies reported on high frequencies of partial and non-adherence in this patient group with different factors being relevant in this context [1]: next to lack of insight into the illness negative attitudes towards the illness and the medication, negative past experiences with the illness and its treatment, and the lack of support systems are known to be strong predictors of non-adherence [2–5]. This is of particular relevance, since non-adherence is one of the most important risk factors for relapse, rehospitalization, and treatment resistance as well as for substance abuse, violence, arrests, suicide attempts, and impaired long-term functioning [6]. During the era of first generation antipsychotics, the emphasis of treatment lay

* Correspondence: christian.widschwendter@i-med.ac.at
Medical University Innsbruck, Department of Psychiatry,Psychotherapy, and Psychosomatics. Division of Psychiatry I, Anichstrasse 35, 6020 Innsbruck, Austria

on objective outcome parameters, e.g., a reduction of positive symptoms, and little research was done with regard to the patients' subjective perspective [7]. With the introduction of new generation antipsychotics treatment goals became more ambitious and more attention was paid to patients' complaints, e.g., cognitive slowing, affective blunting or loss of spontaneity and volition [8, 9]. Next to that, the interest in the patients' view of quality of life has significantly increased over the last decades [10].

Most patients with schizophrenia, if not acutely psychotic or experiencing severe cognitive impairments, are able to complete self-rating scales in a meaningful way, and it has been shown that patients' and psychiatrists' perspectives on antipsychotic treatment differ considerably [11–13]. Several scales have been developed to assess quality of life in patients with schizophrenia [7] and both the impact of pharmacological therapy on quality of life and the relationship between subjective experience and attitudes and adherence to medication attracted attention over the past decades. In 1983, Hogan et al. developed the Drug Attitude Inventory (DAI) with the objective to quantify patient's subjective experience of treatment with antipsychotic drugs [14]. Importantly, positive attitudes towards medication have been associated with lower symptom levels, and treatment response has been demonstrated to be positively correlated with a positive drug attitude [3, 15–19]. Later, Naber et al. developed the "Subjective Well-being under Neuroleptic Treatment" scale (SWN), which captures the subjective experiences of patients during antipsychotic drug treatment [12, 20] and has inconsistently been shown to correlate with current symptomatology or changes in psychopathology [20–22].

Although some authors claimed that both instruments examine quality of life [7, 23], merely the SWN is highly correlated with this subjective outcome variable [12]. Initially designed to predict drug compliance, the DAI focuses on the subjective effects of antipsychotic medication and on values and attitudes toward the illness and health without differentiating between these issues [24]. The SWN, on the other hand, measures quality of life rather than experiences attributed to antipsychotic medication without distinguishing between pharmacogenic or morbogenic components [7]. However, consensus on a uniform definition of the multidimensional and partially subjective concept of quality of life [25–27] is still missing. In contrast to "overall quality of life", the term "health-related quality of life" is used in the context of medical treatment and research and includes three major determinants: subjective well-being, functioning in daily life, and external resources. Consequently and in contrast to the concept of "well-being", which can be seen as a psychological and emotional state, the concept of quality of life also encompasses physical, social, cognitive and functional aspects [24, 28].

The aim of this study was to assess the associations between subjective well-being and attitudes towards antipsychotic medication as well as the interrelations between these issues and both symptoms and functioning in patients with chronic schizophrenia starting monotherapy with a new-generation antipsychotic drug.

Methods

Subjects and experimental design

Patients aged between 18 and 65 years and starting treatment with a new-generation antipsychotic drug were included into a prospective longitudinal study to build a drug monitoring register. Subjects were recruited via a specialized outpatient service for patients with psychotic disorders or they were inpatients. They met the diagnostic criteria of schizophrenia, schizotypal and delusional disorders according to ICD-10 and signed informed consent forms as approved by the local ethics committee. They did not suffer from any other axis I disorder, including substance abuse. Diagnoses were confirmed using chart information and reports from clinicians who had treated these patients. Patients who had previously been receiving antipsychotic medication underwent a washout period of 3–5 days. Antipsychotics were chosen by the psychiatrists treating the patients, dosing followed clinical needs within the recommended labeled dose ranges.

At baseline as well as after 2, 4, and 12 weeks of treatment, psychopathology was rated by means of the Positive and Negative Syndrome Scale (PANSS) [29]. At the same points in time, the severity of illness and overall level of functioning were assessed using the Global Assessment of Functioning Scale (GAF) [30, 31]. Additionally, side effects were quantified using the Udvalg for Kliniske Undersogelser (UKU) Side Effect Rating Scale [32] at weeks 2, 4, and 12. The UKU comprises a total of 48 symptoms, arranged into four groups: psychic, neurological, autonomic and other side effects. Each symptom is scored on a severity scale from 0 to 3, and the rater assesses whether the report is best attributed to a side effect (rated as improbable, possible or probable) or related to the disease. Only adverse effects with scores ≥1 on any UKU item and a causal relationship of possible or probable, were considered as antipsychotic induced side effects.

After 2, 4, and 12 weeks of treatment, the patients' subjective well-being as well as their subjective response to and their attitudes towards medication were assessed by means of the short form of the SWN (SWN-K) and the DAI, respectively.

The SWN-K represents a self-rating Likert scale with 6 response categories (1 = not at all, 6 = very much) [20]. It consists of 20 statements (10 positive and 10 negative) on 5 subscales ("mental functioning", "emotional regulation", "social integration", "physical functioning", "self-control") with a minimum total score of 20 and a maximum total score of 120; higher scores indicate better well-being. In accordance with the guidelines, scoring of negatively worded items was reversed (1 → 6, 2 → 5, ..., 6 → 1) before total score and subscores were calculated [20]. The criterion for adequate subjective well-being is met if an SWN-K total score ≥ 80 is achieved [33, 34].

The DAI, on the other hand, is a 30-item self-report questionnaire consisting of statements about perceived effects and benefits of antipsychotics with which the patient can agree or disagree. It is divided into 7 factors: (1) subjective positive feelings related to antipsychotics (e.g., feeling happier), (2) subjective negative feelings attributed to the drugs (e.g., feeling tired and sluggish), (3) health/illness-dependent drug intake: patients' model of health (e.g., believing it is unnatural to take medication), (4) patients' confidence in the physician (e.g., believing it is up to the doctor when one stops taking medication), (5) control: patients' attitudes toward the locus of control in taking medication (e.g, feeling pressured to ingest medication), (6) prevention: patients' belief in the effect of antipsychotics in forestalling relapse (e.g., antipsychotics can prevent getting sick), and (7) harm: patients' concerns with potential toxic effects (e.g., believing medication is a slow acting poison). Each item oft the DAI is scored 1 or 2, depending on whether the answer selected by the patient indicates a negative or positive view of medication. Raw scores of the DAI (total score and subscales) were linearly transformed to a common range from 0 to 100 to facilitate interpretation [35]. For the total score and for those DAI subscales addressing positive aspects, higher scores reflect a more positive drug attitude. For DAI subscales dealing with negative aspects higher scores indicate a more negative drug attitude.

Statistical methods and power analysis

Prior to the analysis all metric variables were checked for deviations from normality by investigating their skewness, G_1. Values of G_1 above 0.5 or below − 0.5 were regarded as sizable deviation from normality indicating the need for non-parametric testing. Changes of PANSS, GAF, SWN-K and DAI over the course of time were analyzed by repeated-measures ANOVA or by Friedman test and subsequent Wilcoxon matched-pairs tests, depending on the variable type (normally or non-normally distributed, respectively). Missing observations were omitted listwise in the repeated-measures analyses (i.e., if one time point was missing the patient as a whole was disregarded in the respective analysis). However, missing values were very rare as all patients completed the SWN-K and 29 of 30 (96.7%) completed the DAI at all planned assessment times (week 2, 4 and 12). Associations of SWN-K and DAI scores with patient characteristics, symptomatology (PANSS), side effects (UKU) and GAF were investigated by means of the Spearman rank correlation coefficient, as part of the variables involved were non-normally distributed.

The sample size of $n = 30$ patients provides sufficient power ($1-\beta = 0.8$) to detect in a repeated-measures ANOVA under standard assumptions (type-one error $\alpha = 0.05$; correlations among repeated measures, $r = 0.5$; non-sphericity correction, $\varepsilon = 0.9$) effect sizes of $f = 0.236$ for the comparison of 4 assessments and $f = 0.258$ for comparing 3 assessments. These are medium effect sizes according to Cohen's classification [36]. Moreover, the sample size of $n = 30$ is sufficient to detect with a power of $1-\beta=0.8$ and a two-tailed type-one-error of 0.05, Spearman rank correlation coefficients $r \geq 0.49$ a in a non-parametric correlation analysis. This is a medium to large correlation according to Cohen's classification (close to the threshold of 0.5 indicating large correlations).

Results

Demographic and clinical characteristics of the study sample are summarized in Table 1. Data of 30 patients were available for analysis at baseline, week 2 and 4. At week 12, the DAI evaluation was missing for one subject, and the GAF evaluation for another one. None of the patients withdrew within the 12 weeks observation period. They had a mean age of 37.5 ± 9.7 years and a mean duration of illness of 8.7 ± 6.7 years with a range from 2 to 21 years. 57% were male. At baseline, the mean PANSS total score was 59.7 ± 16.5, indicating mild symptom severity. The mean baseline GAF score was 56.7 ± 16.4, thereby indicating a moderate impairment. At baseline, 40% of study participants were inpatients, while the others were treated at a specialized outpatient clinic. All patients started monotherapy with a new-generation antipsychotic drug (amisulpride: $n = 7$, aripiprazole: n = 7, clozapine: $n = 6$, olanzapine: $n = 3$, quetiapine: n = 3, ziprasidone: $n = 2$, sertindole: n = 2). The mean doses and ranges of antipsychotic medication were as follows: amisulpride 428.6 ± 138 mg (200–600 mg), aripiprazole 19.3 ± 15.5 mg (15–30 mg), clozapine 366.7 ± 75.3 mg (300–500 mg), olanzapine 16.7 ± 5.8 mg (10–20 mg), quetiapine 700 ± 173.2 mg (600-900 mg), ziprasidone 140 ± 28.3 mg (120–160 mg), and sertindole 16 ± 0 mg.

The time course of disease severity as indicated by PANSS scores, subjective well-being (SWN-K total score), and attitudes toward medication (DAI total score) is depicted in Table 2. The PANSS total score improved significantly from baseline to weeks 4 and 12, respectively. There was no significant improvement from baseline to week 2. Both the PANSS positive and general psychopathology subscores improved from baseline to weeks 2, 4, and 12, whereas the PANSS negative

Table 1 Demographic and Clinical Patient Characteristics (n = 30)

Age, mean ± SD, years	37.5 ± 9.7
Sex, n (%), female/male	13(43.3)/17(56.7)
Duration of illness, mean ± SD, years	8.7 ± 6.7
PANSS score at baseline, mean ± SD	
Total score	59.7 ± 16.5
Positive symptoms	12.1 ± 5.1
Negative symptoms	17.0 ± 7.1
General psychopathology	30.6 ± 8.1
GAF score at baseline, mean ± SD	56.7 ± 16.4

PANSS = Positive and Negative Syndrome Scale; GAF = Global Assessment of Functioning Scale

subscore remained virtually unchanged. The GAF score improved from baseline to weeks 4 and 12. At any assessment, SWN-K and DAI scores reflected both adequate subjective well-being and positive attitudes toward antipsychotic treatment, respectively. Neither SWN-K nor DAI total scores changed significantly over the course of time.

Correlations between SWN-K and DAI and the interrelations between these scales and both symptom level (PANSS) and functioning (GAF) are depicted in Table 3. There was no correlation between SWN-K and DAI total scores at any time point. A significant negative correlation was found between the SWN-K total score and both the total score and the general psychopathology subscore of the PANSS at weeks 2 and 4, but not at week 12. Moreover, the SWN-K total score correlated negatively with the PANSS positive subscore at week 4, whereas no significant correlation was found between the SWN-K total score and the PANSS negative subscore. The DAI total score did neither correlate with the PANSS total score or any of its subscales nor with the GAF score at any point in time. In contrast, the SWN-K total score correlated positively with the GAF score at all time points.

Regarding correlations of patient characteristics, i.e. age, gender, duration of illness, and inpatient vs. outpatient, with SWN-K and DAI scores, no significant correlation was found. Side effects that were most frequently reported within the observation period of 12 weeks (found in ≥10% of patients) were as follows: increased salivation (18.3%), concentration difficulties (15.8%), asthenia (15.8%), weight gain (15%), tension/ inner unrest (15%), hypokinesia (12.5%), failing memory (11.7%), akathisia (10%), and diminished sexual desire (10%). The item tension/ inner unrest was negatively correlated with the SWN-K total score at weeks 2 (r = −.362, p = .05) and 12 (r = −.454, p = .012), and with the DAI total score at week 2 (r = −.377, p = .04). Additionally, the side effect failing memory was negatively correlated with the SWN-K total score at week 12 (r = −.367, p = .046). No further correlation between side effects and both subjective well-being and drug attitude was found.

Discussion

The aim of the current study was to assess a potential association between subjective well-being and attitudes toward antipsychotic medication as well as the interrelations between these issues and both symptom severity and functioning in chronic schizophrenia patients starting treatment with a new-generation antipsychotic drug. As expected, both symptoms and global functioning improved over the course of antipsychotic treatment. Most previous studies reported on an improvement of patients' subjective well-being over the course of treatment [37–39]. In our sample, however, the SWN-K total score did not change over time. Next to a limited sample size this seemingly contradictive finding could be a result of patient selection, since we investigated chronically ill patients experiencing mild baseline symptomatology and a generally positive attitude toward medication as indicated by high mean DAI total scores. Of note, four distinct clusters of subjective well-being have been described in individuals with schizophrenia: 16% of "patients moderate" "stable high", 31% "stable moderate", 33% "stable low", and merely 20% improving "subjective well-being over the course of treatment" [40]. According to this classification, the patients included into the current study may be seen to have had a stable high subjective well-being, since they consistently achieved a mean SWN-K total score of ˃80. Following Larsen and Gerlach, we hypothesize that the relatively long mean duration of illness of approximately 9 years may have enabled them to accept their illness [41]. In line with previous studies, we did not find consistent correlations between the PANSS or its subscales and the SWN-K total score [23].

The negative correlation between the SWN-K total score and both the PANSS total score and the general psychopathology subscore is in line with the literature [42, 43], and can be explained by the fact that they contain items that include symptoms of anxiety and depression, which may be more critical in influencing subjective well-being rating than any other symptom of schizophrenia.

Our finding of a significant correlation of global functioning with patients' subjective well-being corroborates the results of previous studies [44, 45]. Accordingly, subjective well-being may directly impact upon a patient's social, psychological, and occupational functioning and vice versa.

Similar to the SWN-K total score and in line with a previous report [46], the DAI total score did not change over

Table 2 Time course of disease severity, global functioning, subjective wellbeing, and attitudes toward antipsychotic medication

	Observation time								Comparison (Repeated measures ANOVA)				
	Baseline (0)		Week 2 (1)		Week 4 (2)		Week 12 (3)		Overall		(0) vs. (1)	(0) vs. (2)	(0) vs. (3)
	Mean	SD	Mean	SD	Mean	SD	Mean	SD	F	*p*-value	p-value	p-value	p-value
PANSS total score	59.71	16.51	56.40	15.36	53.07↓	15.90	52.33↓	14.41	6.10	0.001	0.078	0.003	0.001
PANSS positive	12.13	5.14	10.63↓	3.83	9.80↓	3.34	9.53↓[#]	3.07	9.02	< 0.001	0.015	0.001	0.001
PANSS negative	17.00	7.07	17.03	6.87	16.30	7.09	16.17	7.47	0.53	0.629	0.964	0.493	0.333
PANSS general	30.58	8.12	28.74↓	7.36	26.97↓	7.11	26.63↓[#]	6.15	7.81	< 0.001	0.042	0.001	0.001
GAF	56.67	16.40	59.03	15.34	62.43↑[x]	16.46	61.52↑	17.36	5.80	0.004	0.078	0.004	0.011
SWN-K total	-[a]	-[a]	83.45	18.63	85.91	17.92	87.56	17.14	1.47	0.253	-[a]	0.984[b]	0.512[b]
SWN-K mental	-[a]	-[a]	16.47	5.19	17.14	4.41	17.43	3.87	1.85	0.173	-[a]	0.190[b]	0.121[b]
SWN-K self-control	-[a]	-[a]	15.03	3.61	16.08	3.89	16.00	4.35	1.94	0.156	-[a]	0.072[b]	0.139[b]
SWN-K emotional	-[a]	-[a]	17.63	5.08	17.93	4.80	18.53	4.51	1.58	0.217	-[a]	0.621[b]	0.088[b]
SWN-K physical	-[a]	-[a]	17.47	4.70	17.23	4.45	17.94	4.51	0.70	0.476	-[a]	0.744[b]	0.470[b]
SWN-K spcial	-[a]	-[a]	16.87	4.68	17.53	4.49	17.69	4.25	1.31	0.276	-[a]	0.115[b]	0.209[b]
DAI total score	-[a]	-[a]	79.93	16.31	81.83	15.88	79.93	16.34	0.29	0.747	-[a]	0.528[b]	0.999[b]
DAI positive	-[a]	-[a]	70.83	29.60	71.13	33.49	71.67	33.79	0.02	0.975	-[a]	0.937[b]	0.844[b]
DAI negative	-[a]	-[a]	18.33	31.36	15.56	26.60	21.39	28.17	0.94	0.397	-[a]	0.524[b]	0.499[b]
DAI illness-related	-[a]	-[a]	33.89	35.15	27.78	34.00	23.33↓	32.93	3.00	0.061	-[a]	0.118[b]	0.032[b]
DAI doctor	-[a]	-[a]	93.33	21.71	91.67	23.06	91.38	23.41	0.49	0.570	-[a]	0.326[b]	0.330[b]
DAI control	-[a]	-[a]	8.33	26.53	6.67	25.37	11.67	28.42	2.45	0.110	-[a]	0.326[b]	0.161[b]
DAI prevention	-[a]	-[a]	91.67	26.53	90.00	30.51	93.10	25.79	0.59	0.489	-[a]	0.663[b]	0.343[b]
DAI harm	-[a]	-[a]	28.33	38.69	25.00	36.55	28.33	38.69	0.44	0.649	-[a]	0.423[b]	0.999[b]

PANSS = Positive and Negative Syndrome Scale; GAF = Global Assessment of Functioning Scale; SWN-K = Subjective Well-being under Neuroleptic Treatment Scale, short form, DAI = Drug Attitude Inventory
↓ Significantly lower than at baseline
↑ Significantly higher than at baseline
[#]Significantly lower than at week 2
[x]Significantly higher than at week 2
[a]Not assessed at day 0
[b]Comparison with day 14

Table 3 Correlation of subjective well-being and drug attitude with symptomatology and global functioning. Spearman rank correlation

			PANSS positive	PANSS negative	PANSS general	PANSS total	GAF	DAI total
Week 2	SWN-K total	r Spearman (p-value)	−.274 (.143)	−.323 (.082)	−.419* (.021)	−.375* (.041)	.559** (.001)	.196 (.299)
	DAI total	r Spearman (p-value)	−.017 (.93)	−.095 (.616)	−.206 (.276)	−.197 (.297)	−.006 (.976)	-
Week 4	SWN-K total	r Spearman (p-value)	−.415* (.022)	−.235 (.210)	−.441* (.015)	−.480** (.007)	.642** (.000)	.128 (.5)
	DAI total	r Spearman (p-value)	.084 (.66)	.161 (.394)	.09 (.637)	.19 (.314)	−.203 (.283)	-
Week 12	SWN-K tota	r Spearman (p-value)	−.238 (.205)	−.238 (.206)	−.324 (.081)	−.318 (.087)	.576** (.001)[a]	.068 (.727)[a]
	DAI total	r Spearman (p-value)	−.069 (.721)[a]	−.102 (.598)[a]	−.095 (.625)[a]	−.114 (.555)[a]	−.095 (.63)[b]	-

SWN-K = Subjective Well-being under Neuroleptic Treatment Scale, short form; PANSS = Positive and Negative Syndrome Scale; DAI = Drug Attitude Inventory

[a] $N = 29$

[b] $N = 28$

time. Moreover, drug attitude did not correlate with symptom change. Generally, drug adherence has been reported to be predicted by the patients' subjective responses to and attitudes toward antipsychotics [14]. The high mean DAI total score in our sample reflects a general positive attitude toward antipsychotic medication and underscores once more, that we investigated a selected patient sample. It clearly has to be noted that adherence is generally higher among study samples than in routine care and that our findings are therefore not attributable to all individuals suffering from schizophrenia [1].

Notably and in contrast to our finding of a consistent association between patients' subjective well-being and functioning, the DAI total score did not correlate with the GAF score at any time point, which corroborates previous findings [47]. However, in contrast to previous reports we did not find a correlation between the SWN-K and DAI total scores [48, 49]. Next to differences in the patient samples studied, this contradictory result can be explained by the scales‘ varying scopes. The DAIs‘ strength lies in measuring compliance and attitudes towards antipsychotic treatment, whereas the SWN-K can be seen as an alternative for a quality of life instrument in patients using antipsychotic medication [48]. One previous study [49] examined a very heterogeneous sample encompassing patients receiving first- and new-generation antipsychotics in different formulations (oral versus long-acting injectable drugs) with 60% of patients having been on the current medication for at least one year. Furthermore, symptom severity has not been reported in this study. Another longitudinal study [48] investigated patients experiencing more severe symptoms at baseline than our sample. Accordingly, these studies are not entirely comparable with ours.

Regarding the impact of antipsychotic-induced side effects on subjective well-being and drug attitude, inconsistent correlations have been found for tension/ inner unrest and failing memory. This finding is supported by previous research that found that the psychiatrists' beliefs about the tolerance of a particular antipsychotic drug do not necessarily reflect patients' well being and attitude toward medication [50]. \Additionally, this effect can be interpreted as the intense efforts in both inpatient units and specialized outpatient clinic to actively elicit adverse events and to respond to patients' concerns quickly.

When interpreting our data, one has to consider a number of limitations. First of all, the sample size was rather small and early noncompliers, who usually stop attending mental health services, have not been included. Furthermore, the fact that only patients with a generally good attitude toward medication took part in the study limits the generalizability of our findings. Lastly, we did not thoroughly assess the reason for switching antipsychotic medication in patients who had previously been receiving antipsychotic drugs.

Conclusions

In summary, our findings emphasize that, particularly in chronic schizophrenia patients experiencing mild symptoms, the differences between the SWN and DAI may give good reason for the use of both instruments during antipsychotic treatment in clinical practice and/ or research to systematically monitor and adjust treatment with antipsychotic medication. In so doing it may help finding the optimal dosage and type of antipsychotic medication for an individual patient and therefore enhance adherence.

Abbreviations

DAI: Drug Attitude Inventory; GAF: Global Assessment of Functioning Scale; PANSS: Positive and Negative Syndrome Scale; SWN: Subjective Well-being under Neuroleptic Treatment Scale; SWN-K: Subjective Well-being under Neuroleptic Treatment Scale, short form

Acknowledgements

The authors wish to thank the study participants for their contribution to the study.

Authors' contributions

AH and CGW initiated, designed and coordinated the study. CW, MAR, NY-S, and AH conducted data collection, GK helped in analyzing the data, CGW wrote the manuscript, AH and G critically revised and approved the final manuscript. All authors read and approved the final manuscript.

Consent for publication

No patient identifiable information has been reported.

Competing interests

Christian Widschwendter, Georg Kemmler, and Nursen Yalcin-Siedentopf have no actual or potential conflict of interest. Maria A. Rettenbacher is member of a advisory board of Eli Lilly and has received speaker's or consultancy fees from Eli Lilly. Alex Hofer has received a research grant from Janssen-Cilag. He has received speaker's or consultancy fees from Bristol-Myers Squibb, Janssen-Cilag and Lundbeck as well as reimbursements for travel and meeting expenses from Janssen-Cilag and Lundbeck.

References

1. Kane JM, Kishimoto T, Correll CU. Non-adherence to medication in patients with psychotic disorders: epidemiology, contributing factors and management strategies. World Psychiatry. 2013;12(3):216-226; doi: https://doi.org/10.1002/wps.20060.

2. Brain C, Allerby K, Sameby B, Quinlan P, Joas E, Karilampi U, Lindström E, Eberhard J, Burns T, Waern M. Drug attitude and other predictors of medication adherence in schizophrenia: 12 months of electronic monitoring (MEMS(®)) in the Swedish COAST-study. Eur Neuropsychopharmacol. 2013; 23(12):1754–62. 0.1016/j.euroneuro.2013.09.001.
3. Hofer A, Kemmler G, Eder U, Honeder M, Hummer M, Fleischhacker WW. Attitudes toward antipsychotics among outpatient clinic attendees with schizophrenia. J Clin Psychiatry. 2002;63(1):49–53.
4. Rettenbacher MA, Hofer A, Eder U, Hummer M, Kemmler G, Weiss EM, Fleischhacker WW. Compliance in schizophrenia: psychopathology, side effects, and patients' attitudes toward the illness and medication. J Clin Psychiatry. 2004;65(9):1211–8.
5. Acosta FJ, Hernández JL, Pereira J, Herrera J, Rodríguez CJ. Medication adherence in schizophrenia. World J Psychiatry. 2012;2(5):74-82. https://doi.org/10.5498/wjp.v2.i5.74.
6. Hofer A, Fleischhacker WW. Compliance with treatment and its relevance for the management of schizophrenia. Hot Topics Neurol Psychiatry. 2011;11:7–13.
7. Karow A, Naber D. Subjective well-being and quality of life under atypical antipsychotic treatment. Psychopharmacology. 2002;162(1):3–10.
8. Windgassen K. Treatment with neuroleptics: the patient's perspective. Acta Psychiatr Scand. 1992;86(5):405–10.
9. Lewander T. Neuroleptics and the neuroleptic-induced deficit syndrome. Acta Psychiatr Scand Suppl. 1994;380:8–13.
10. de Millas W, Lambert M, Naber D. The impact of subjective well-being under neuroleptic treatment on compliance and remission. Dialogues Clin Neurosci. 2006;8(1):131–6.
11. Lambert M, Schimmelmann BG, Karow A, Naber D. Subjective well-being and initial dysphoric reaction under antipsychotic drugs - concepts, measurement and clinical relevance. Pharmacopsychiatry. 2003;36(Suppl 3):181–90.
12. Naber D. A self-rating to measure subjective effects of neuroleptic drugs, relationships to objective psychopathology, quality of life, compliance and other clinical variables. Int Clin Psychopharmacol. 1995;10(Suppl 3):133–8.
13. Voruganti L, Heslegrave R, Awad AG, Seeman MV. Quality of life measurement in schizophrenia: reconciling the quest for subjectivity with the question of reliability. Psychol Med. 1998;28(1):165–72.
14. Hogan TP, Awad AG, Eastwood R. A self-report scale predictive of drug compliance in schizophrenics: reliability and discriminative validity. Psychol Med. 1983;13(1):177–83.
15. Freudenreich O, Cather C, Evins AE, Henderson DC, Goff DC. Attitudes of schizophrenia outpatients toward psychiatric medications: relationship to clinical variables and insight. J Clin Psychiatry. 2004;65(10):1372–6.
16. Mohamed S, Rosenheck R, McEvoy J, Swartz M, Stroup S, Lieberman JA. Cross-sectional and longitudinal relationships between insight and attitudes toward medication and clinical outcomes in chronic schizophrenia. Schizophr Bull. 2009; https://doi.org/10.1093/schbul/sbn067.
17. Mintz AR, Dobson KS, Romney DM. Insight in schizophrenia: a meta-analysis. Schizophr Res. 1995;18(1):21–8.
18. Kemp RA, Lambert TJ. Insight in schizophrenia and its relationship to psychopathology. Schizophr Res. 2003;61(1):75–88.
19. Hofer A, Rettenbacher MA, Edlinger M, Kemmler G, Widschwendter CG, Fleischhacker WW. Subjective response and attitudes toward antipsychotic drug therapy during the initial treatment period: a prospective follow-up study in patients with schizophrenia. Acta Psychiatr Scand. 2007;116(5):354–61.
20. Naber D, Moritz S, Lambert M, Pajonk FG, Holzbach R, Mass R, Andresen B. Improvement of schizophrenic patients' subjective well-being under atypical antipsychotic drugs. Schizophr Res. 2001;50(1–2):79–88.
21. Putzhammer A, Perfahl M, Pfeiff L, Hajak G. Correlation of subjective well-being in schizophrenic patients with gait parameters, expert-rated motor disturbances, and psychopathological status. Pharmacopsychiatry. 2005;38(3):132–8.
22. Lee Y-W, Kim J-H, Ann J-H, Cho S-E, Lee J, Kim M-J, Cho S-J, Cho I-H, Kim SJ, Lee Y-J, Bae S-M. Subjective well-being in patients with schizophrenia treated with atypical antipsychotics: the impact of psychopathology and adverse drug effects. Clinical psychopharmacology and Neuroscience. 2010; 8(3):149–55.
23. Vothknecht S, Schoevers RA, de Haan L. Subjective well-being in schizophrenia as measured with the subjective well-being under neuroleptic treatment scale: a review. Aust N Z J Psychiatry. 2011;45(3): 182–92. https://doi.org/10.3109/00048674.2010.545984.
24. Awad AG, Voruganti LN. Measuring quality of life in patients with schizophrenia: an update. PharmacoEconomics. 2012;30(3):183–95. https://doi.org/10.2165/11594470-000000000-00000.
25. Spilker B. Quality of life and pharmacogenomics in clinical trials. New York: Lippincott-Raven Press; 1996.
26. Katschnig H. Schizophrenia and quality of life. Acta Psychiatr Scand. 2000;407:33–7.
27. Diener E. Subjective well-being. Psychol Bull. 1984;95:542–75.
28. Awad AG, Voruganti LN, Heslegrave RJ. Measuring quality of life in patients with schizophrenia. PharmacoEconomics. 1997;11(1):32–47.
29. Kay SR, Fiszbein A, Opler LA. The positive and negative syndrome scale (PANSS) for schizophrenia. Schizophr Bull. 1987;13(2):261–76.
30. Endicott J, Spitzer RL, Fleiss JL, Cohen J. The global assessment scale: a procedure for measuring overall severity of psychiatric disturbance. Arch Gen Psychiatry. 1976;33(6):766–71.
31. Hall RC. Global assessment of functioning. A modified scale Psychosomatics. 1995;36(3):267–75.
32. Lingjaerde O, Ahlfors UG, Bech P, Dencker SJ, Elgen K. The UKU side effect rating scale – a new comprehensive rating scale for psychotropic drugs and a cross-sectional study of side effects in neuroleptic-treated patients. Acta Psychiatr Scand. 1987;334:1–100.
33. Lambert M, Schimmelmann BG, Naber D, Schacht A, Karow A, Wagner T, Czekalla J. Prediction of remission as a combination of symptomatic and functional remission and adequate subjective well-being in 2960 patients with schizophrenia. J Clin Psychiatry. 2006;67:1690–7.
34. Lambert M, Naber D, Eich FX, Schacht M, Linden M, Schimmelmann BG. Remission of severely impaired subjective wellbeing in 727 patients with schizophrenia treated with amisulpride. Acta Psychiatr Scand. 2007;115:106–13.
35. Hofer A, Kemmler G, Eder U, Honeder M, Hummer M, Fleischhacker WW. Attitudes toward antipsychotics among outpatient clinic attendees with schizophrenia. J Clin Psychiatry. 2002 Jan;63(1):49–53.
36. Cohen J. A power primer. Psychol Bull. 1992;112(1):155–9.
37. Schennach-Wolff R, Seemüller F, Obermeier M, Messer T, Laux G, Pfeiffer H, Naber D, Schmidt LG, Gaebel W, Klosterkötter J, Heuser I, Maier W, Lemke MR, Rüther E, Buchkremer G, Gastpar M, Jäger M, Möller HJ, Riedel M. Response and remission of subjective well-being in patients suffering from schizophrenia spectrum disorders. Eur Psychiatry. 2011; 26(5):284–92. https://doi.org/10.1016/j.eurpsy.2009.11.005.
38. Wehmeier PM, Kluge M, Schacht A, Helsberg K, Schreiber W, Schimmelmann BG, Lambert M. Patterns of physician and patient rated quality of life during antipsychotic treatment in outpatients with schizophrenia. J Psychiatr Res. 2008;42(8):676–83.
39. Lambert M, Schimmelmann BG, Naber D, Eich FX, Schulz H, Huber CG, Karow A. Early- and delayed antipsychotic response and prediction of outcome in 528 severely impaired patients with schizophrenia treated with amisulpride. Pharmacopsychiatry. 2009;42(6):277–83. https://doi.org/10.1055/s-0029-1234105.
40. Lambert M, Schimmelmann BG, Schacht A, Karow A, Wagner T, Wehmeier PM, Huber CG, Hundemer HP, Dittmann RW, Naber D. Long-term patterns of subjective wellbeing in schizophrenia: cluster, predictors of cluster affiliation, and their relation to recovery criteria in 2842 patients followed over 3 years. Schizophr Res. 2009;107(2-3):165–72. https://doi.org/10.1016/j.schres.2008.08.035.
41. Larsen EB, Gerlach J. Subjective experience of treatment, side-effects, mental state and quality of life in schizophrenic outpatients treated with depot neuroleptics. Acta Psychiatr Scand. 1996;93(5):381–8.
42. Dan A, Kumar S, Avasthi A, Grover S. A comparative study on quality of life of patients of schizophrenia with and without depression. Psychiatry Res. 2011;189(2):185–9. https://doi.org/10.1016/j.psychres.2011.02.017.
43. Solanki RK, Singh P, Midha A, Chugh K. Schizophrenia: impact on quality of life. Indian J Psychiatry. 2008;50:181–6. https://doi.org/10.4103/0019-5545.43632.
44. Mas-Expósito L, Amador-Campos JA, Gómez-Benito J, Lalucat-Jo L. Research Group on Severe Mental Disorder. The World Health Organization quality of life scale brief version: a validation study in patients with schizophrenia. Qual Life Res. 2011;20(7):1079–89. https://doi.org/10.1007/s11136-011-9847-1.
45. Hosseini SH, Karkhaneh Yousefi M. Quality of life and GAF in schizophrenia correlation between quality of life and global functioning in schizophrenia. Iran J Psychiatry Behav Sci. 2011;5(2):120–5.
46. Campbell AH, Scalo JF, Crismon ML, Barner JC, Argo TR, Lawson KA, Miller A. Attitudes Toward Medications and The Relationship To Outcomes in Patients with Schizophrenia. Clin Schizophr Relat Psychoses. 2015; https://doi.org/10.3371/CSRP.CASC.070415.

47. Nielsen RE, Lindström E, Nielsen J, Levander S. DAI-10 is as good as DAI-30 in schizophrenia. Eur Neuropsychopharmacol. 2012;22(10):747–50. https://doi.org/10.1016/j.euroneuro.2012.02.008.
48. Wolters HA, Knegtering H, van den Bosch RJ, Wiersma D. Effects and side effects of antipsychotic treatment in schizophrenia: pros and cons of available self-rating scales. Schizophr Res. 2009;112(1-3):114–8. https://doi.org/10.1016/j.schres.2009.03.026.
49. Mauri M, Mauri MC, Adami M, Reggiardo G, Giulio C. Efficacy and tolerability of paliperidone ER in patients with unsatisfactorily controlled schizophrenia by other antipsychotics: a flexible-dose approach. Int Clin Psychopharmacol. 2015;30(6):329–37. https://doi.org/10.1097/YIC.0000000000000092.
50. Marder SR. Subjective experiences on antipsychotic medications: synthesis and conclusions. Acta Psychiatr Scand Suppl. 2005;427:43–6.

11

Clinical practice guidelines for diagnosis of autism spectrum disorder in adults and children in the UK

Jennie Hayes[*], Tamsin Ford, Hateem Rafeeque and Ginny Russell

Abstract

Background: Research suggests that diagnostic procedures for Autism Spectrum Disorder are not consistent across practice and that diagnostic rates can be affected by contextual and social drivers. The purpose of this review was to consider how the content of clinical practice guidelines shapes diagnoses of Autism Spectrum Disorder in the UK; and investigate where, within those guidelines, social factors and influences are considered.

Methods: We electronically searched multiple databases (NICE Evidence Base; TRIP; Social Policy and Practice; US National Guidelines Clearinghouse; HMIC; The Cochrane Library; Embase; Global health; Ovid; PsychARTICLES; PsychINFO) and relevant web sources (government, professional and regional NHS websites) for clinical practice guidelines. We extracted details of key diagnostic elements such as assessment process and diagnostic tools. A qualitative narrative analysis was conducted to identify social factors and influences.

Results: Twenty-one documents were found and analysed. Guidelines varied in recommendations for use of diagnostic tools and assessment procedures. Although multidisciplinary assessment was identified as the 'ideal' assessment, some guidelines suggested in practice one experienced healthcare professional was sufficient. Social factors in operational, interactional and contextual areas added complexity to guidelines but there were few concrete recommendations as to how these factors should be operationalized for best diagnostic outcomes.

Conclusion: Although individual guidelines appeared to present a coherent and systematic assessment process, they varied enough in their recommendations to make the choices available to healthcare professionals particularly complex and confusing. We recommend a more explicit acknowledgement of social factors in clinical practice guidelines with advice about how they should be managed and operationalised to enable more consistency of practice and transparency for those coming for diagnosis.

Keywords: Autism spectrum disorder, Diagnosis, Clinical guideline, Narrative review, Social factors, Diagnostic uncertainty, Clinical judgement

Background

The diagnosis of autism poses particular challenges for healthcare professionals (HCPs) as, in common with other neurodevelopmental disorders and most psychiatric disorders, there are no biomarkers utilised in clinical practice [1–3]. In addition, the condition is heterogeneous, with wide ranging levels of severity and symptom expression and characteristics common to autism may occur in people with other conditions [4]. Those coming for diagnosis may also have symptoms of other conditions such as epilepsy, learning disability or sleep disorders, for example, complicating diagnosis further, with some arguing for a de-compartmentalisation of these conditions in younger children [5]. The 'gold standard' of diagnosis is considered to be consensus agreement within a multi-agency team [6, 7]. However, negotiating consensus between HCPs with different training, professional roles, experience and knowledge can be challenging and time consuming. Finally, a review of the accuracy, reliability, validity and utility of reported diagnostic tools and assessments found that many diagnostic instruments for autism

* Correspondence: Jennie.Hayes@exeter.ac.uk
University of Exeter Medical School, St Luke's Campus, University of Exeter, Exeter EX1 2LU, UK

lack a high-quality independent evidence base [6]. For example, only three instruments - the Autism Diagnostic Observation Schedule (ADOS), Autism Diagnostic Interview Revised (ADI-R) and the Childhood Autism Rating Scale (CARS) - had a strong supporting evidence base [6].

Given the potential challenges, clinical practice guidelines (CPGs) perform an important role in informing HCPs of best practice. CPGs are 'systematically developed statements to assist practitioner and patient decisions about appropriate health care for specific clinical circumstances' [8]. National CPGs in the UK help to provide evidence-based recommendations to support Autism Strategies and Action Plans [9] and form the guidance framework for HCPs undertaking assessment and diagnosis of autism in the UK. In addition to CPGs produced by specialist, government supported healthcare associations, for example, the Scottish Intercollegiate Guidelines Network (SIGN) [10], professional clinical bodies also publish discipline-specific practice parameters or position papers, for example, the Royal College of Psychiatrists (RCPsych) [11].

Social factors

Although CPGs aim to inform diagnostic practice, research suggests that diagnostic and assessment procedures vary in practice [9]. Diagnosis is dependent on observing socially-based behaviours that are arguably not necessarily characteristic of the person under assessment but arise from two-way social relationships and social context. Assessment mechanisms include drawing information from a range of sources, including clinician observation, reporting from family members and wider contexts such as school or workplace. This means that assessments are contextual and inter-relational and symptoms may change according to context or interpersonal relationship, making different assessment sources potentially contradictory.

Some studies show that social factors such as individual patient preference, availability of resources or local organisational factors can shape diagnostic practice, in, for example, heart disease [12]. Studies in autism have also shown how diagnostic rates can be affected by contextual and social drivers, such as diagnostic resources [13] or diffusion of information about autism through social networks [14]. Where there is diagnostic uncertainty clinicians may 'upgrade' to a diagnosis of autism if they believe it would be in the best interests of the patient; if the diagnosis would trigger appropriate services and funding; or counteract the limitations of diagnostic tools, particularly in atypical presentations [15, 16]. It seems, in practice, clinicians may adopt a pragmatic, practical or functional approach.

Socio-economic and cultural factors

Research has shown that lower social economic status (SES) is associated with increased parent-reported prevalence [17], contrasting with the US where higher SES and parental education is linked to increased likelihood of diagnosis [14, 18]. Research also suggests that people with autism from Black, Asian and Minority Ethnic (BAME) communities are less likely to be diagnosed with autism or access appropriate services [19] despite research which shows that behaviours associated with autism are likely to be consistent across cultures and countries [20].

Prior to diagnosis, social factors can also determine who comes forward for diagnosis and who is referred for further assessment. Research examining a longitudinal UK cohort study identified that with the severity of autistic traits held constant, younger mothers and mothers of first-born children were significantly less likely to have children diagnosed with ASD [21]. In addition, boys were more likely to receive a diagnosis than girls, and maternal depression was linked with a lack of diagnosis [21]. These findings suggest both cultural and economic influences impact the diagnostic pathway.

Biomarkers in autism diagnosis

There is a great deal of research that explores the underlying neurobiological, genetic, chemical and cognitive factors that may, in future, provide biomarkers which could be utilised in autism diagnosis (see [22] for a review of genetic, metabolic and brain focused biomarkers). For example, a recent research study has identified a link between damage to proteins in blood plasma and autism symptoms [23]; while another found shared brain activity between boys diagnosed with ASD and those with obsessive-compulsive disorder (OCD) which in turn differed from a non-diagnosed control group [24]. However, it has been argued that the heterogeneous and interactive nature of autism symptoms makes the identification of clinically useful biomarker tests problematic [25]. Furthermore, findings from biomarker research have yet to be integrated with clinical practice and none currently have enough evidence to support routine clinical use [22]. For the foreseeable future, therefore, these developments are unlikely to change diagnostic practice [26].

Purpose of the review

Although a few studies have begun to explore health professionals' views of autism diagnosis [16, 27, 28], to our knowledge there are few studies that examine how clinical guidelines may inform assessment. One exception is a recent systematic review of English speaking guidelines undertaken by Penner et al. [29] which reported that guidelines varied considerably in quality, content and recommendations but included guidelines working across incomparable health systems in different countries. We therefore carried out a focussed narrative review of guidelines that impact on UK-based practice.

Penner et al. suggest that in the face of disparate clinical guidance clinicians should 'be mindful of local resources and wait times, eligibility requirements for ASD services...and the wishes of families when deciding on how best to assess for ASD' [29]. Our narrative review responds to this call for a pragmatic approach by investigating where, within guidelines, social factors and influences such as those suggested are considered.

Method

Scoping search

A scoping search was undertaken to check there was no similar review published. A search was made in the following databases; PsychARTICLES; Embase; Global health; HMIC; Ovid (books; medline; journals); PsychINFO; Social policy and practice. One relevant article was retrieved [29], as discussed above.

Inclusion and exclusion criteria

Full inclusion and exclusion criteria are in Table 1. Whilst we took a broad approach to CPGs, including, for example, journal articles summarizing national CPGs and the diagnostic process, as well as national CPGs, the researchers acknowledge that each of these type of guidelines have different purposes (see Table 2). However, we argue that each may have an impact on HCP's process of diagnosis to a greater or lesser extent and for the purposes of this study all were included under the term clinical practice guidelines.

Table 1 Inclusion and Exclusion Criteria

Inclusion Criteria
Documents with guidance-based status for HCPs working in secondary care in the UK; or were published papers, aimed at HCPs, with the aim of reviewing CPGs
Documents related to autism diagnosis and assessment for either children, adults or both
Documents produced either by or through government or professional clinical bodies or published in a journal aimed at HCPs
Documents related to diagnosis and assessment in UK (England, Scotland, Wales and N Ireland)
Documents dated from 2009 (reflecting publication of the first UK specific Autism Act) or were the most recent CPG published by a key professional body
Exclusion Criteria
Documents related solely to referral, treatment, prognosis or support services
Reviews of diagnostic criteria and other academic papers
Guidelines related to primary care as we were interested in diagnosis rather than referral
Narrative reviews, editorials and opinions
Documents related to parliament or legislature; national or regional strategies as they are not the primary source for clinicians
Local guidance
Guidance provided by private providers of diagnostic services
International professional body guidelines (other than ICD/DSM)

Identification of CPGs

We did not set out to undertake a comprehensive systematic review, as it was not a requirement of our study that we consider risk of bias either within or across studies [30]. However, we took a PRISMA approach to our search strategy, borrowing from systematic review methodology in terms of screening titles and abstracts and data extraction techniques [31]. A systematic search was conducted in June 2017 using the following databases: NICE Evidence Base; TRIP; Social Policy and Practice; US National Guidelines Clearinghouse; HMIC; The Cochrane Library. In addition, searches were made of government related websites and relevant professional bodies as well as NICE and SIGN. We used the following search terms to search all databases and websites: 'autism', 'diagnosis', 'guidance', 'statutory', 'clinical', 'practice', 'guideline', 'protocol', 'strategy', 'policy', 'bill', 'act', and 'parameter'. A full search strategy is in Fig. 1.

Study selection

The first reviewer (JH) removed duplicates and screened titles for relevance. Full text copies of the potentially relevant documents were downloaded for screening. The first reviewer screened full text documents and excluded those not relevant. The remaining titles were independently checked by the clinical specialist (TF) using pre-specified inclusion/exclusion criteria (outlined in Table 1). Discrepancies were resolved by discussion, with involvement of a third reviewer (GR). Twenty-eight documents were considered for analysis, with seven being withdrawn at full analysis stage. See Fig. 2 for full details.

Guidelines from the International Classification of Mental and Behavioural Disorders (Tenth edition) (ICD-10) [32] and the Diagnostic and Statistical Manual of Mental Disorders (Fifth edition) (DSM-5) [33] were considered alongside UK relevant guidelines as they are considered authoritative sources for the definition of symptoms utilized in autism diagnosis, as well as other neurological conditions.

Data extraction

A data extraction framework was created to draw key characteristics from the guidelines (year, author, geographical remit, target audience, age range, range of diagnoses covered, age at which symptoms are recognised, diagnostic criteria referred to); as well as key elements in the diagnostic process (recommended tools, role and composition of the multidisciplinary team (MDT), who can diagnose, assessment targets and key features of assessment). This framework was piloted with

Table 2 Purpose of Diagnostic Guidelines

Type of guideline	General purpose of type of guideline
Diagnostic Criteria	To assist clinicians in the diagnosis of mental conditions by providing descriptions of the main clinical features in each category
National Clinical Guidelines	To offer best practice advice and guidance for professionals and service users and their families
Guidelines from Professional Bodies	To offer profession specific advice to clinicians and healthcare professionals in their specialist area
Journal Articles	To summarise clinical guidelines in clinician-facing publications to keep clinicians up to date and/or alert them to changes in good practice

four reviewers (JH, GR, RW and DE) in a comparison of analysis of three guidelines. The framework was amended accordingly and is included in Additional file 1. Data were independently extracted by two reviewers (JH and HR) from 21 CPGs and disagreements were resolved by discussion and further checks. Data were tabulated and analysed.

Analysis of social factors

A modified form of narrative review, as described by Popay et al. [34] and Ferrari [35], was adopted whereby data extraction enabled synthesis of key data, whilst also allowing rich narrative description [35]. Narrative review was selected as it enabled the telling of the 'story' of CPGs, and consideration of how guidelines, as a set of texts, shape diagnosis [34].

A process of inductive analysis was undertaken based on social factors and influences. These were defined, for the purpose of this review, as contextual factors that influence diagnosis but are not based on symptoms of autism. We drew from the concept of a social model of diagnosis as developed by Jutel and Nettleton [36]. This model considers how diagnostic classifications and medical diagnoses are socially created and how social forces – including technological, professional, cultural and economic forces – contribute to shaping aspects of the diagnostic process including those related to classification, the consequences of diagnosis and the process of diagnosis itself [36]. Overall, a social model challenges the idea of diagnosis as 'a moment of clinical purity' [37] or as a way simply to identify underlying biological problems. We included factors that were relevant to multidisciplinary working or parental/family influence (the process of diagnosis); the potential outcomes of diagnosis for the patient and how HCPs may take this into account (the consequences of diagnosis); and how issues around classification shape the diagnostic process such as how borderline cases are dealt with (diagnosis as a category). This was a dynamic process whereby data extracts were considered in relation to each other via conceptual mapping and clustering [34].

Terminology

For the purposes of this review and in line with the Autism Strategy [38] we use the term 'autism' throughout.

Results

Characteristics of guidelines

A total of 236 documents were retrieved, and 21 were included in the final narrative review (see Table 3 for full list of included documents and guideline characteristics).

Scoping search:

- PsychARTICLES; Embase; Global health; HMIC; Ovid (books; medline; journals; PsychINFO; Social policy and practice

Main Review Search Strategy:

- Organic **web searching** starting from Government Health and Professional Bodies sites: The Scottish Government; Gov.UK; The Welsh government; The Northern Ireland Executive; NHS Scotland; NHS England; NHS Northern Ireland; NHS Wales; National Institute for Health and Care Excellence (NICE); Scottish Intercollegiate Guidelines Network (SIGN); British Psychological Society; American Academy of Child and Adult Psychiatry (AACAP); American Academy of Paediatrics (AAP); American Academy of Neurology (AAN); Royal College of Child Health Practitioners (RCCHP); Royal College of Psychiatrists (RCP); Royal College of Paediatrics and Child Health; Royal College of Nursing; British Medical Journal; Royal College of General Practitioners; Royal College of Physicians

- **Databases:** NICE Evidence Base; TRIP; Social Policy and Practice; US National Guidelines Clearinghouse; HMIC; The Cochrane Library

Search terms:

1. autis*
2. strateg*
3. statutory
4. policy
5. protocol
6. diagnos*
7. bill
8. act
9. guideline
10. 1 and 2 or 3 or 4 or 5 or 6 or 7 or 8 or 9
11. parameter
12. 1 and clinical and 9
13. 1 and practice and 11

Fig. 1 Full Search Strategy

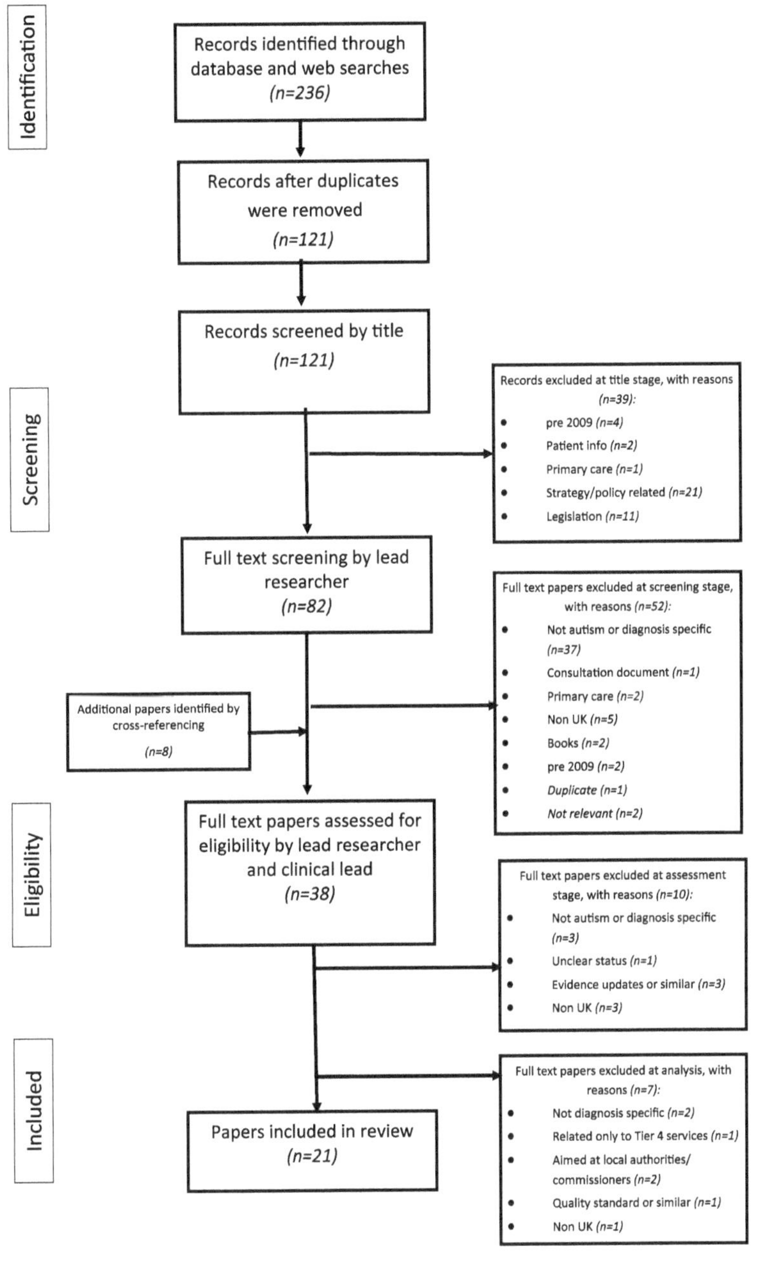

Fig. 2 Study selection flow diagram

The documents studied are grouped into four types: a) International Diagnostic Criteria ($n = 2$); b) National Clinical Guidelines ($n = 5$); c) Journal articles that summarize National Clinical Guidelines and the diagnostic process, published in key clinical journals ($n = 10$); d) Guidelines from professional bodies ($n = 4$). It should be noted that journal articles, in some cases, are designed to give an update rather than a full guideline therefore the lack of detail in some areas should not necessarily be seen as a weakness.

Of the 21 guidelines considered, six dealt with diagnosis of adults, seven with children and eight with all ages. Of those, two guidelines were international but key to diagnostic practice in the UK (ICD-10 and DSM-5), five related to the UK as a whole, five to England and Wales, one to Scotland, two to Northern Ireland and one to outside the US and Canada (and therefore included the UK). Five guidelines did not specify a geographical remit but were published in the UK in clinician-facing journals. All guidelines were aimed at HCPs, with six aimed at particular specialist roles that included psychiatrists, psychologists, speech and language therapists, community practitioners and paediatricians.

Table 3 Key characteristics of guidelines

Title	Year	Author(s)	Publisher/ Journal	Geographical remit	Target audience	Age range	Range of diagnoses covered	Diagnostic criteria referred to	Age at which symptoms are recognised
DIAGNOSTIC CRITERIA									
The ICD-10 Classification of Mental and Behavioural Disorders: clinical descriptions and diagnostic guidelines [32]	1993	N/A	World Health Organisation	International	Clinical, educational and service use	All ages	Pervasive development disorders	N/A	Before age of 3 years (childhood autism); after age 3 (atypical autism).
Diagnostic and Statistical Manual of Mental Disorders (Fifth Edition) [33]	2013	N/A	American Psychiatric Association	International	Clinicians, students, practitioners, researchers	All ages	Autism Spectrum Disorder	N/A	During 2nd year of life (12–24 months) or earlier than 12 months if developmental delays are severe
NATIONAL CLINICAL GUIDELINES									
NICE Autism in under 19 s: recognition, referral and diagnosis (NICE CG128) [39]	2011	National Collaborating Centre for Women's and Children's Health	National Institute for Health and Care Excellence (NICE)	England and Wales	Healthcare professionals	From birth up to 19 years	Pervasive developmental disorder (PDD)	ICD-10 or DSM-IV	May be uncertainty before 24 months, or with developmental age of less than 18 months
Six Steps of Autism Care for children and young people in Northern Ireland (RASDN) [44]	2011	Regional Autistic Disorder Network for Northern Ireland	Health and Social Care Board	Northern Ireland	Health care and education professionals, parents, carers, service users and providers.	Up to the age of 18 years	Autism spectrum disorder	ICD-10, DSM-IV, NICE, SIGN, NZ Guidelines, NHS Map of Medicine	Pre-school. Language delay by the age of two years.
Autism Spectrum Disorder in adults: diagnosis and management (NICE CG142) [9]	2012	National Collaborating Centre for Mental Health	National Institute for Health and Care Excellence (NICE)	England and Wales	Health and social care providers and commissioners	Adults aged 18 and over	Autism spectrum disorders	N/S *ICD-10 specified in full version of CG142 [62]	N/A
Autism Adult Care Pathway (RASDN) [54]	2013	Regional Autistic Spectrum Disorder Network	Health and Social Care Board	Northern Ireland	Professionals, adults and families	Adults from age 18	Autism spectrum disorders	DSM-5 and ICD-10, NICE guidance CG142.	N/S
Assessment, diagnosis and interventions for autism spectrum disorders: A national clinical guideline (SIGN 145) [10]	2016	N/A	Scottish Intercollegiate Guidelines Network	Scotland	Healthcare professionals	Whole age range	Autism spectrum disorder	ICD-10 and DSM-5	Autism can be reliably diagnosed between the ages of 2–3.

Table 3 Key characteristics of guidelines *(Continued)*

Title	Year	Author(s)	Publisher/ Journal	Geographical remit	Target audience	Age range	Range of diagnoses covered	Diagnostic criteria referred to	Age at which symptoms are recognised
GUIDELINES FROM PROFESSIONAL BODIES									
RCSLT (Royal College of Speech and Language Therapists Clinical Guidelines (Autism) [41][a]	2005	N/A	Royal College of Speech and Language Therapists	UK	Speech and language therapists	Children and adults	Autism spectrum disorder	ICIDH-2 *(for general clinical assessment)*	N/S
Good practice in the management of autism (including Asperger syndrome) in adults (RCPych CR191) [11]	2014	Royal College of Psychiatrists	Royal College of Psychiatrists	UK	Psychiatrists working with adults of at least normal intellectual ability	Adults from age 18	Autism	ICD-10, DSM-5, NICE, 2012.	N/S
Autism Spectrum Disorders: Guidance for Psychologists (BPS) [40][b]	2016	Stuart-Hamilton, Dillenburger, Hood & Austin	British Psychological Society	UK	Psychologists	All ages	Autism Spectrum Disorder	ICD-10 and DSM-5, NICE, 2011.	Both diagnostic manuals consider ASD indicators to be present by the age of 36 months although some children can be identified under the age of 24 months.
BMJ Best Practice online resource [43]	2017	Parr &Woodbury-Smith	British Medical Journal	Outside US and Canada	Medical Practitioners	All ages	Autism Spectrum Disorder	DSM-IV, DSM-5 & ICD-10. NICE, SIGN, AACAP, AAP, NZ ASD guideline, AAN	More than 80% of children with ASD show clear behavioural signs by the age of 24 months, some indicators in 12–18 months
JOURNAL ARTICLES									
Diagnosis and management of autism in childhood [47]	2011	Blenner, Reddy & Augustyn	British Medical Journal	N/S	General clinicians	Children	Autism Spectrum Disorder	DSM-IV TR or ICD-10	N/S
Diagnosis and assessment in autism spectrum disorders [48]	2012	Carpenter	Advances in Mental Health and Intellectual disabilities	N/S	Those designing and providing diagnostic services	All ages	Autism Spectrum Disorder	DSM-IV TR or ICD-10. Gillberg's for AS. There are others but few use them (Kopra et al., 2008; Chiappedi et al., 2010).	N/S
Autism spectrum disorder in adults: clinical features and the role of the psychiatrist [49]	2013	Garland, O'Rourke & Robertson	Advances in Psychiatric Treatment	UK	Psychiatrists	Adults	Autism Spectrum Disorders	ICD-10 and DSM-5, NICE	To satisfy ICD-10 criteria for childhood autism, impairments must manifest before the age of 3 years

Table 3 Key characteristics of guidelines *(Continued)*

Title	Year	Author(s)	Publisher/ Journal	Geographical remit	Target audience	Age range	Range of diagnoses covered	Diagnostic criteria referred to	Age at which symptoms are recognised
Recognising, referring and diagnosing autism [45]	2012	Howlett & Richman	Every Child Journal	England and Wales	Professionals working with children and young people	Children and young people	Autism	NICE	The core autism behaviours are typically present in early childhood; but features can appear different with age or change with circumstances
Autism [50]	2013	Lai, Lombardo & Baron-Cohen	The Lancet	N/S	N/S	All ages	Autism or the autism spectrum	DSM-5, ICD-10	N/S
Autism [51]	2009	Levy, Mandell & Schultz	The Lancet	N/S	N/S	N/S but primarily talks about children	Autism Spectrum Disorder	DSM-IV and ICD-10	Parents often aware from age 18 months, a diagnosis is often not made until 2 years after the initial expression of parental concern.
Autism spectrum disorder: diagnosis and management [53]	2009	O'Hare	Archives of Disease in Childhood: Education and Practice Edition	N/S but relates primarily to SIGN guidelines	Paediatricians	Children and young people	Autism Spectrum Disorder	ICD-10 and DSM-IV, SIGN	N/S
Recognition, referral, diagnosis, and management of adults with autism: summary of NICE guidance [58]	2012	Pilling, Baron-Cohen, Megnin-Viggars, Lee & Taylor	British Medical Journal	England and Wales	N/S	Adults	Autism	N/S	N/S
Autism Spectrum Disorders in childhood: a clinical update [46]	2011	Reynolds	Community Practitioner	UK	Community practitioners	Children	Autism Spectrum Disorder	ICD-10, DSM-IV	N/S
The NICE guideline on recognition, referral, diagnosis and management of adults on the autism spectrum [52]	2014	Wilson, Roberts, Gillan, Ohlsen, Robertson & Zinkstok	Advances in Mental Health and Intellectual Disabilities	England and Wales	Health care professionals, service managers, service users, practitioners	All adults	Autism spectrum disorder	N/S	N/S

[a]Pre 2009 but constitutes current guideline in use from RCSLT
[b]Currently under review but represents the most recent published guideline from BPS

Guidelines acknowledged that there is variation in rates of identification, assessment criteria and practice [9]; that there is increasing demand for diagnostic services [39]; and that increased awareness of autism is likely to lead to a rise in people presenting for assessment [40].

Definitions of autism

Definitions of autism in ICD-10 and DSM-5 differed. ICD-10 took a categorical approach with a definition of Pervasive Development Disorders that included sub-diagnoses within it; whilst DSM-5 used the overarching dimensional concept of Autism Spectrum Disorder. Some inconsistencies were present related to the differences in classification in ICD-10 and DSM-5, therefore, for example, Rett's Syndrome and Asperger's Syndrome were sub-diagnoses of Pervasive Development Disorders in ICD-10, but were encompassed in the overarching diagnosis of Autism Spectrum Disorder in DSM-5 [32, 33]. Definitions of autism in all other guidelines considered in this study were broadly consistent with the idea of a 'spectrum'.

Most guidelines ($n = 14$) referred to symptom criteria from both ICD-10 and the (then) current version of DSM (DSM-IV up to 2012 and DSM-5 from 2013), with eight guidelines recommending that HCPs should use the current version of DSM or ICD criteria for diagnosis. Exceptions were NICE CG142, which was based on ICD-10, [9]; Royal College of Speech and Language Therapists (RCSLT) [41], which drew on the International Classification of Functioning, Disability and Health (ICIDH-2) for general clinical assessment [42]; and journal articles describing NICE guidelines which made no mention of DSM/ICD ($n = 3$).

Overall, therefore, the guidelines were mixed in their recommended sources for symptom criteria due to the current differences in the two classification systems.

Narrative review of social factors

We used three inter-related elements as an organising framework to describe the social factors identified in clinical guidelines: operational, interactional and contextual. These factors do not stand alone from each other, indeed, they appear to have a dynamic and inter-dependent relationship, however, organising them provides a way to map their range and scope (see Fig. 3).

Operational factors

Operational factors included how different assessment processes impact on the diagnostic decision, such as which tools and processes are engaged and when; what constitutes an assessment; and whether the decisions take place as part of diagnosis or formulation. Table 4 outlines some of these operational factors.

The assessment process

One guideline suggested that clinical practice varies greatly [43] and we found this to be mirrored in CPGs with a wide range of potential assessment processes included. DSM-5 recommended that a diagnostic assessment should include gathering multiple sources of information from clinician's observations, caregiver

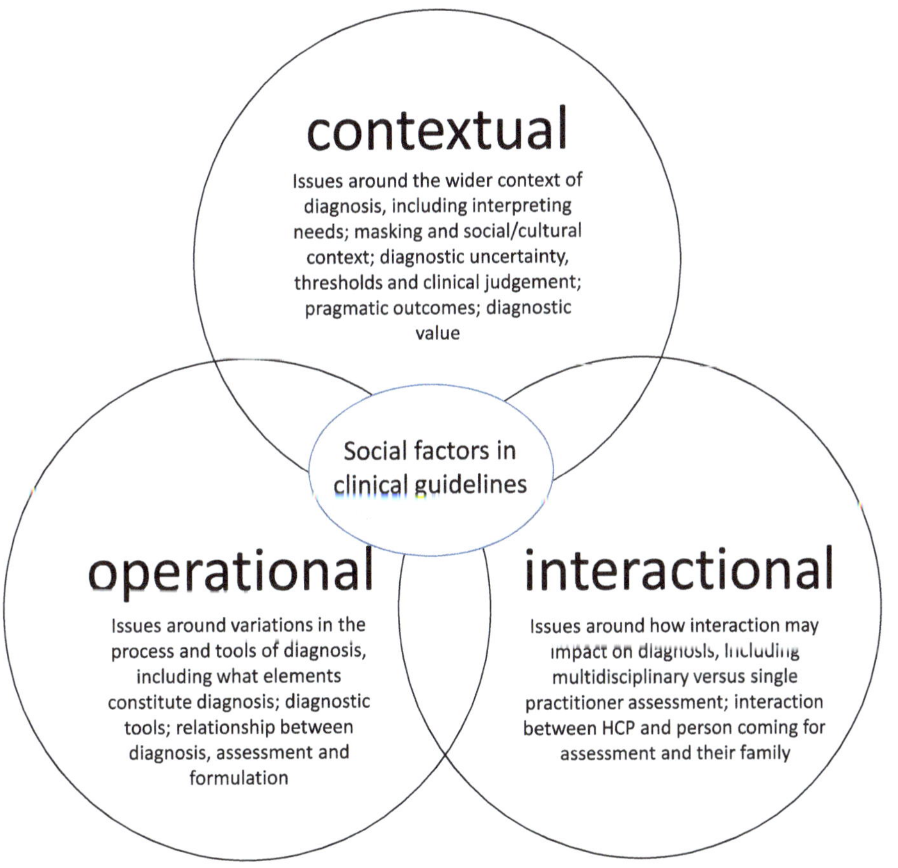

Fig. 3 Social factors in clinical guidelines

history and self-report (where possible). National guidelines, although providing far greater detail, tended to include these areas and additionally suggested various other detailed assessments such as gathering wider functional/assessment information [10]; using documentary evidence, assessing risks, and assessment of challenging behaviour [9]; assessing for co-conditions [9, 39]; physical examination [39]; comprehensive educational assessment [44]; assessment of communication, neuropsychological functioning, motor and sensory skills, and adaptive functioning [10]. Professional guidelines added other factors such as comprehensive cognitive assessment [40] and impact of individual's mental health [41], accounts of relationships in different settings [11] and observation in school or another setting [43]. Journal articles tended to reflect national guidelines and varied in the level of detail outlined for assessment factors. Two articles gave little detail of assessment processes but one referred readers directly to NICE guidelines for further detail [45] and the other was aimed at community practitioners who would be more likely to be involved in referral than diagnosis [46]. Articles also included assessment of co-occuring conditions (e.g. [47–52]) and a physical or medical examination (e.g. [47, 50]). Additional assessment areas included assessment of specific domains such as family stressors and coping abilities [47]. In one guideline [48] it was suggested that some clinicians bypass ICD/DSM criteria and instead undertake:

> '...testing for specific underlying difficulties such as lack of theory of mind or lack of central coherence and then using these to decide the presence of the behavioural criteria' [48].

The RCSLT guideline [41] differed from most by suggesting consideration of theories relating to the triad of social impairments, such as executive functioning deficits, motivation, memory and central coherence, as well as social interaction and communication. However, some (e.g. [40]) suggested cognitive or neuropsychological testing whilst SIGN guidelines stated that such assessments are 'useful for individual profiling but are not diagnostic instruments' [10]. This anomaly may reflect the specialist role of SLTs in the diagnostic process.

Overall, we would concur with a reflection in one guideline, which noted how the HCP may be faced with 'possible uncertainty as to where to go next in their investigation framework as this could be potentially enormous' [53].

Diagnostic tools

Recommendations about the use of diagnostic tools were mixed. One third of the guidelines ($n = 7$) did not specify any particular tool for diagnostic assessment. Other CPGs tended to suggest the consideration of a range of tools without specifically recommending any particular instrument(s), although regular references were made to ADOS ($n = 13$), ADI-R ($n = 11$), DISCO ($n = 9$) and 3di ($n = 6$). The NICE guideline for children and young people emphasised use of DSM/ICD criteria rather than tools; the NICE guideline for adults did the opposite [9, 39]. Overall, findings concurred with Penner et al. in that guidelines varied substantially in their recommendations for use of diagnostic tools [29].

Diagnosis and formulation

There were differences in the way guidelines described the relationship between, or referred to, diagnosis, assessment, profiling, needs assessment and wider formulation. All guidelines encompassed the concept of a wider (needs related) assessment but few explicitly separated out these processes or discussed how this related to a diagnostic assessment. One exception to this was the Regional Autistic Spectrum Disorder Network (RASDN) children's guideline, which separated the diagnostic from the formulation process, describing the latter as including examination of the person's wider environment:

> 'The outcome of the formulation should be to understand an individual in a more global holistic way rather than merely in terms of signs and symptoms, as in the case of diagnosis' [44].

The RCPsych guideline suggested that diagnosis is only one component of the wider multidisciplinary exercise [11]. Some guidelines did not mention formulation but suggested a profile of strengths, abilities and weaknesses should be carried out alongside a diagnostic assessment (e.g. [10, 39]). Adult guidelines from RASDN separated out a diagnostic assessment from a full needs assessment [54]; NICE guidelines for adults considered comprehensive assessment to include diagnostic, needs and risk assessment [9]; whilst the full children's guidelines similarly brought together the diagnostic and needs elements under 'autism diagnostic assessment', explaining that:

> '..the label of autism does not constitute a complete diagnostic assessment and a profile of the child or young person's strengths and weaknesses is also essential. This requires a multidisciplinary team which has the skills to undertake the assessments necessary for profiling' [55].

Operationally, therefore, there were contradictions between guidelines about what constitutes the diagnostic process, how it should be structured and which diagnostic tools should be used.

Table 4 Key diagnostic recommendations

CPG	Recommended tools	MDT recommended	MDT membership	Assessment targets	Key features of assessment
DIAGNOSTIC CRITERIA					
ICD-10 (1993) [32]	N/S	N/S	N/S	N/S	Diagnose on the basis of behavioural features
DSM-5 (2013) [33]	No specific tool	N/S	N/S	N/S	Careful clinical history & summary of social, psychological & biological factors. Multiple sources of information: • clinician's observations • caregiver history • self-report (where possible) Clinical judgement
NATIONAL CLINICAL GUIDELINES					
NICE CG128 (2011) [39]	No specific tool recommended	Autism team members should carry out assessment (short version). A diagnosis can be made by a single experienced HCP; profile of strengths & weaknesses is essential, and requires MDT [55] (full version).	Autism team made up of Paediatrician &/or Child & Adolescent Psychiatrist, SLT, Clinical &/or Educational Psychologist & access to paediatrician/paediatric neurologist, Child & Adolescent Psychiatrist, Educational Psychologist, Clinical Psychologist, OT, if not in team. Also consider specialist health visitor or nurse, specialist teacher or social worker.	Start the autism diagnostic assessment within 3 months of referral. Follow up appointment within 6 weeks of assessment.	Seek report from the pre-school or school; gather additional health or social care information. Include in every autism diagnostic assessment: • questions about parent/carer/child's concerns • details of the child's experiences of home life, education and social care • developmental history, focusing on developmental and behavioural features • assessment (through interaction with and observation of the child or young person) of social and communication skills and behaviours • medical history, including prenatal, perinatal and family history, and past and current health conditions • physical examination • consideration of the differential diagnosis • systematic assessment for conditions that may coexist with autism • development of a profile of the child's or young person's strengths, skills, impairments and needs that can be used to create a needs-based management plan, taking into account family and educational context • communication of assessment findings to the parent/carer/child

Table 4 Key diagnostic recommendations *(Continued)*

CPG	Recommended tools	MDT recommended	MDT membership	Assessment targets	Key features of assessment
RASDN (2011) [44]	No specific tool	The use of MDT approach is necessary	Involving at least two disciplines: paediatrician; child psychiatrist; SLT, OT, clinical psychologist; specialist health visitor; mental health practitioner (CAMHS); social worker; nurse; ed. psych. Teacher; other trained professionals	Referral screened within 5 days. Info provided within 4 weeks. 13 weeks to first appointment. Feedback within 4 weeks, report within 6 weeks of formulation.	Step one: Initial directed conversation. Step two: Integrated multidisciplinary team assessment (leads to diagnosis/ non-diagnosis) includes: • medical history inc: birth history, family history, & general medical concerns • developmental history focusing on developmental & behavioural concerns • observational assessment of the child/young person • further assessment/observations in another setting (school/home) • physical exam in some groups • specific assessments may be required, e.g. SLT assessment • educational assessment Step three: Integrated MDT formulation (leads to wider understanding of difficulties) Step four: family feedback and care planning
NICE CG142 (2012) [9]	Identification: Consider AQ-10 (without LD); Brief assessment (with LD). Diagnosis and assessment: AAA including AQ and EQ; ADI-R; ADOS-G; ASDI; RAADS-R (without LD). ADOS-G; ADI-R (with LD); DISCO, ADOS-G, ADI-R	Comprehensive assessment should be team based (short version). At a minimum by a qualified clinician usually a clinical psychologist, psychiatrist or neurologist [62] (full version).	Specialist autism team made up of: Clinical Psychologists, Nurses, OTs, Psychiatrists, Social Workers, SLTs, Support Staff	N/S	During a comprehensive assessment, enquire about and assess the following: • core autism signs and symptoms that have been present in childhood and continuing into adulthood • early developmental history, where possible • behavioural problems • functioning at home, in education or in employment • past and current physical and mental disorders • other neurodevelopmental conditions • hyper- and/or hypo-sensory sensitivities and attention to detail. Direct observation of core autism signs and symptoms especially in social situations. Assess for possible differential diagnoses and coexisting disorders Assess risks; Develop care plan, provide health passport, consider

Table 4 Key diagnostic recommendations *(Continued)*

CPG	Recommended tools	MDT recommended	MDT membership	Assessment targets	Key features of assessment
					24 h crisis management plan; Assess challenging behaviour Consider further investigations on individual basis
RASDN (2013) [54]	Screening: GADS, GARS-2, AASQ, ASAS, NAS, AQ-10 History: ADI-R, DISCO, ASDI, RAADS-R; Direct assessment: ASIT, HSST, SSQ, Observation: ADOS-G	Diagnosis must be team based & draw on a range of professionals.	At least two of: clinical psychology (core), psychiatry, SLT, LD/MH nursing; OT, other appropriately trained professionals.	Final report to be provided within 6 weeks of assessment.	As an absolute minimum, elements 2, 3 & 4 *must* be included in the assessment. 1. Neurodevelopmental history, corroborated via relative/family; 2. Direct autism specific assessment with individual; 3. Observational recording of assessment sessions; 4. Clinical judgement. May also include; standardized measure of adaptive functioning; assessment of language & communication skills; functional assessment of problematic behaviour; full needs assessment
SIGN 145 (2016) [10]	Identification: AQ-10 Diagnosis and Assessment: E.g. ADI-R, DISCO, 3di, CARS, CARS-2, ADOS-G. NAPC and RCPsych guides.	MDT … should be considered as the optimum approach	Experienced professionals	N/S	• History taking (informant interview): prenatal, perinatal & developmental history; description of the current problems experienced; family history; description of who is in family; coexisting conditions and differential diagnoses • Clinical observation/assessment (individual assessment/interview): directly observe & assess the individual's social & communication skills and behaviour • Contextual and functional information from a variety of settings and people • Profile of the individual's strengths and difficulties: communication, cognitive, neuropsychological and adaptive functioning; motor and sensory skills • Biomedical investigations on an individual basis when clinically relevant • Assessment of mental health needs, wellbeing and risk should be considered

Table 4 Key diagnostic recommendations *(Continued)*

CPG	Recommended tools	MDT recommended	MDT membership	Assessment targets	Key features of assessment
GUIDELINES FROM PROFESSIONAL BODIES					
RCSLT (2005) [41]	N/S	Should always be multidisciplinary & multi-agency to achieve optimum benefit.	This may include SLT, child psychology, child psychiatry, clinical psychology, paediatrician, EdPsych., OT & teacher	N/S	During assessment, consideration must be given to the triad of social impairments, as well as theories relating to the triad, for example sensory sensitivity and integration; intersubjectivity; executive functioning deficits; motivation; memory and central coherence. • Joint attention • Readiness & ability to focus & shift attention • Social interaction • Use of communicative strategies • Evaluation of child's play • Info about learning potential • Impact of individual's mental health
RCPsych (2014) [11]	Identification: AQ, RAADS-R. RPsych Guide. Questionnaires: ASAS, GARS, GARS-2, SCQ, SRS-2, AQ, AQ-10, RAADS-R, SCDS, ABC. Diagnostic interviews: ADI-R, ADOS-2, DISCO, 3Di, AAA, RPsych Guide, PDD-MRS, ASDI, CARS-2, HBS, WADIC Assessment for associated dev disabilities: AQ, EQ, SQ, Faces test, eyes test, Faux Pas Recognition Test, SSQ, Dewey's Social Stories, Adult/Adolescent sensory profile	NICE advocates multidisciplinary exercise, but psychiatrists might be expected to diagnose straightforward cases & be alert to indications for a more specialist assessment.	MDT usually includes psychology & nursing as core membership	N/S	• Speak with informant • Take neurodevelopmental history • Consider obtaining early health records Might include assessment for; cognitive ability, functional ability, coexistent neurodevelopmental disabilities, coexistent psychiatric disorders, mental capacity, risk of harm/offending, medical problems Wherever possible, it is essential that the clinician gets accurate accounts of relationships in different settings (e.g. at work & at home), particularly where they might be more demanding for that individual.
BPS (2016) [40]	e.g. ADOS, ADI, DISCO, ADI-R	It is recommended that assessment is multidisciplinary.	At least one psychologist, in addition to other relevant personnel, such as OTs, mental health workers etc.	It is recommended that assessment is timely.	The taking of a developmental history with carers as well as observation across different settings. Information from a range of sources. Psychologists contribution to identification and assessment may include: • Assessment of protective factors, strengths and abilities • Assessment of associated mental health issues • Comprehensive developmental and family history • Assessment of learning styles • Assessment of strengths and of barriers to learning

Table 4 Key diagnostic recommendations *(Continued)*

CPG	Recommended tools	MDT recommended	MDT membership	Assessment targets	Key features of assessment
					• Assessment of environmental conditions for learning • Functional behavioural assessment • Assessment of social communication style • Assessment of the needs of families. • Comprehensive cognitive assessment, which may include psychometrics if deemed necessary
BMJ (2017) [43]	Screening: CHAT, M-CHAT Parental questionnaires: SCQ, CAST CARS; for adults, the SRS, ASQ. Diagnosis and Assessment: eg ADOS-G, ADI-R; 3di; DISCO	Diagnosis should be confirmed or made by an appropriately trained professional, ideally working as part of MDT	Paediatricians, child psychiatrists, adult psychiatrists or psychologists, & other professionals	N/S	A combination of: • neurodevelopmental history • standardised interview, & • observational assessment Gather information about functioning in more than one environment; A full neurological examination including measurement of head circumference is routinely performed in all children.
JOURNAL ARTICLES					
Blenner et al (2011) [47]	Screening: CHAT, PDDST, STAT, CHAT-23, M-CHAT, ITC, SCQ. Diagnosis: ADOS.	Paediatric neurologists, developmental & behavioural paediatricians, child psychiatrists or psychologists, or, ideally, MDT.	N/S	N/S	Comprehensive evaluation that includes • lifetime & family history • review of medical & educational records • behavioural observation • physical examination • administration of standardised instruments such as the autism diagnostic observation schedule • cognitive & adaptive assessment • review of established DSM or ICD diagnostic criteria • Assessment of specific domains, such as communication skills, sensory and motor problems, and family stressors and coping abilities • Look for causes & co-occuring conditions (further tests)
Carpenter (2012) [48]	Screening: ASDASQ, AQ and EQ, AAA. AQ-10, RAADS-R. RCPsych guide. Observation: PDD-MRS (with ID) ADOS-G. Interview: ADI-R DISCO, 3Di. AAA to provide structure.	Diagnosis can be made by one clinician. Wider assessment requires a team. A variety of professionals can diagnose.	N/S	Labour intensive - up to 8 h to make & document diagnosis.	Three elements (judged against criteria of ICD-10 or DSM-4): • interview with person • observation • interview with an informant Some clinicians bypass the criteria & test, for example, theory of mind, central coherence. Consider possible co-morbidities

Table 4 Key diagnostic recommendations *(Continued)*

CPG	Recommended tools	MDT recommended	MDT membership	Assessment targets	Key features of assessment
					Holistic assessments needs to be structured around: • Need for social support and for help with employment • Sensory and processing difficulties • Medical issues • Neuro-psychiatric conditions • Practical skills, including motor difficulties • Social interaction skills • Emotional understanding (of self and others) and personal coping strategies • Interests and preoccupations • Sexual interests and future desires • Insight and future desires and motivation • Psychiatric concerns • Other behaviours that may get person into contact with the law • Support for carers
Garland et al. (2013) [49]	Screening: AQ-50, AQ-10 Diagnosis: ADI-R, ADOS = G, RCPsych Diagnostic Interview Guide	When mental health difficulties also exist, the expertise of the wider MDT is likely to be engaged.	Outlines psychiatrist's role.	Enough time should be set aside	• History of presenting complaint • Psychiatric history • Family history • Medical history • Developmental history • Personal & social history • Mental state examination • Assess for comorbid disorders inc. neurodevelopment disorders • Physical assessment • Functional level assessment • Assess risk • Assessment of care & support needs • Consideration of need in areas of education & employment
Howlett & Richman (2011) [45]	No specific tool	If the local autism team does not have the skills to assess these children themselves, they should liaise with professionals who are able to do so	Minimum, paediatrician &/or child & adolescent psychiatrist, SLT & clinical &/or Ed.Psych. Other professionals … specialist health visitor, nurse, specialist teacher, social worker	Timely & appropriate. Follow up appointment within six weeks of assessment	Should provide detailed developmental profile. Based on NICE guidance.
Lai et al...... (2013) [50]	Screening: CHAT, ESAT, M-CHAT, ITC, Q-CHAT, STAT (for young children); SCQ, SRS, SRS-2, CAST, ASSQ, AQ (for older children and adolescents); AQ, RAADS-R (FOR ADULTS). Diagnosis and assessment: ADI-R, DISCO, 3Di (for structured interview); ADOS,	Assessment needs to be multidisciplinary	N/S	N/S	• Interview with the parent or caregiver • Interaction with the individual • Collection of information about behaviour in community settings • Cognitive assessments • Medical examination • Co-occurring conditions

Table 4 Key diagnostic recommendations *(Continued)*

CPG	Recommended tools	MDT recommended	MDT membership	Assessment targets	Key features of assessment
	ADOS-2, CARS, CARS-2 (observational measure).				
Levy et al (2009) [51]	SCREENING: Q-CHAT, M-CHAT, FYI, ECI-4, CSI-4, SCQ, ASDS, KADI, AQ-Child, A (AUTISM) ABC (autism), PDDRS, PDD-MRS, DBC, DBC-ES, PDDBI, ABC (aberrant), CCC, SRS, RBS-R, SCDC. Diagnosis and assessment: PIA-CV, DISCO, ADI-R, 3Di. CHAT, STAT, AOSI, ADOS CARS	These assessments should be multidisciplinary	The MDT should include clinicians skilled in speech & language therapy, occupational therapy, education, psychology, & social work.		• Use ICD or DSM criteria • Core and comorbid symptoms, cognition, language, & adaptive, sensory, & motor skills. • Review of caregiver concerns, descriptions of behaviour, medical history, & questionnaires. • Include stage 1 data. • Observations across settings • Cognitive, communication, & ASD-specific assessment • Medical assessment • Differential diagnosis
O'Hare (2009) [53]	Screening: M-CHAT, NAPC Checklist Diagnosis: ADOS-G, SRS	A multidisciplinary diagnostic approach is recommended	Paediatricians are essential members.	N/S	• Direct clinical structured observations • Critical that information is gathered from different settings, outwith the clinic – there are structured questionnaires for parents/teachers • Physical exam and other specialist tests as required
Pilling et al. (2012) [58]	Identification: AQ-10.	N/S	N/S	N/S	Inquire about & assess the following: • Core autism signs & symptoms • Early developmental history • Behavioural problems • Functioning at home, education, employment • Past & current physical & mental disorders • Other neurodevelopmental conditions • Neurological disorders (for example, epilepsy) • Communication difficulties • Hypersensory &/or hyposensory sensitivities & attention to detail • Carry out direct observation of core autism signs & symptoms especially in social situations • Functional analysis
Reynolds (2011) [46]	No specific tool	N/S	N/S	N/S	Observed behaviours with patient presenting symptoms from 'Triad of Impairments': social interaction, social communication, social imagination
	Identification: AQ-10	Should be carried out by MDT consisting of professionals who have	N/S	N/S	

Table 4 Key diagnostic recommendations *(Continued)*

CPG	Recommended tools	MDT recommended	MDT membership	Assessment targets	Key features of assessment
Wilson et al (2013) [52]	Diagnosis and assessment: ADI-R; ADOS-G. AAA, ADI-R, ADOS-G, ASDI, RAADS-R (without ID). ADI-R and ADOS-G (with ID). DISCO, ADI-R, or ADOS-G.	experience in diagnosing autism (from NICE).			A comprehensive assessment of autism should involve an assessment of • core autism signs and symptoms • early developmental history, where possible, and in the absence of an informant written information, such as school reports may be used • behavioural problems • functioning at home, in education, or in employment • past and current physical and mental disorders • other neurodevelopmental conditions • neurological disorders (e.g. epilepsy) • sensory processing and sensory sensitivity issues Assess coexisting mental health disorders. Risk assessment. Functional analysis for challenging behaviour

Key OT Occupational Therapist, *SLT* Speech and Language Therapist, *HCP* Healthcare professional, *MDT* Multidisciplinary team, Ed.Psych Educational Psychologist

Interactional factors

Interactional factors related to how the dialogue between HCPs and between HCPs and families impacts on the assessment process. These include how consensus is reached, how disagreement is resolved and how the views of the person and family are integrated into the decision-making process.

Multidisciplinary assessment versus single practitioner assessment

Where specified, all guidelines advocated for diagnosis to take place within a multidisciplinary setting with various guidelines suggesting this was 'necessary' [44], the 'optimum approach' [10] or 'ideal' [43] (See Table 4). Some suggested ($n = 4$) that an appropriately trained and experienced single professional is sufficient to diagnose in particular cases, but to be alert for indications for a more specialist assessment [11] and with access to multidisciplinary support if required [48].

Despite this almost universal recommendation, the extended version of NICE children's guidelines (and cited by SIGN [10] and Carpenter [48]) questioned the evidence base for multidisciplinary assessment reporting a study [56] that showed moderate agreement between an individual HCP and an MDT in making a diagnosis, but stating that it was a low quality study [55]. These guidelines also suggested in practice that a diagnosis can be made by a single experienced HCP but that a comprehensive profile of the patient requires a multidisciplinary approach [55]. SIGN guidelines also cited research [57] which demonstrates that parents value a multidisciplinary assessment [10].

None of the guidelines in this review dealt with how HCPs come to a consensus within a multi-disciplinary context, although Northern Ireland guidelines recommended that training should include the promotion of collaborative and innovative working [44] and that clinicians must understand the profession specific roles and responsibilities of the overall team [44, 54].

Therefore, most guidelines referred to MDTs as best practice, but lacked recommendations about how roles within MDTs are negotiated, how disagreement is resolved (other than second opinion outside the team); or how teams should work together, a factor that is acknowledged by NICE adults guideline [9].

Interaction with the person and their family

Many guidelines ($n = 9$) outlined the importance of keeping the person/family informed and involved throughout the process or recommended a person-centred approach. Some described the relationship with the person coming for diagnosis and their family as a partnership (e.g. NICE adult guideline [9]) or as person-centred (e.g. RASDN adult guideline [54]). Some guidelines ($n = 6$) acknowledged that the person or family may disagree with or be reluctant to accept a diagnosis or, alternatively desire one [46] and be determined on a particular outcome, which can lead to misleading results [11]. Carpenter asserted that some people may begin to see diagnosis as a desirable outcome and pre-prepare answers based on structured interviews published on the internet [48]. The potential for disagreement or desire for diagnosis, therefore, may impact on the interaction with the person or their family. So, although the relationship with the patient/family is considered within CPGs, there is little guidance as to how HCPs might deal with patient/family desire or disagreement.

Contextual factors

There were factors related to the way in which HCPs interpret symptoms in different settings, how diagnostic thresholds are judged against criteria and included considerations around the impact and consequences of a diagnosis.

Interpreting needs

All national guidelines ($n = 5$) outlined the requirement to consider the needs, preferences and values of the individual and their family and/or support them to communicate their needs and concerns. Most guidelines ($n = 17$) described elements of diagnosis that relate to either family environment, family needs and concerns, circumstances, relationships, functioning, experiences in different settings, contextual information or level of support needs. Many guidelines reflected the need to consider assessment of support required. Enquiries should be made about how symptoms impact on function within the family, at home, school or work [9, 39, 47, 54, 58]. Overall, therefore, there was a focus not only on the assessment of symptoms, and the way in which these affect the daily life of the person and their family, but the wider environmental and social context of the person and the way in which they are supported, or not, by that context.

Masking and social context

Some guidelines ($n = 6$) reported the difficulties of diagnosing autism when compensation strategies may 'mask' difficulties in some contexts, particularly as an adult [33], and in girls [50] where autism may go unrecognised. Some suggested that individuals may come forward for diagnosis when their circumstances change and/or stressors increase (e.g. [10, 45, 54]). Some guidelines ($n = 5$) noted that cultural differences will exist in norms for social interaction or that cultural variations can deliver misleading signs and symptoms. DSM-5 suggested that the boundaries between normality and pathology differ between cultures and the level at which experience may become problematic may differ [33].

SIGN suggested that those with autism may not have met 'normal' adult milestones in work, relationships or independence and contained extensive information on how females can present with a different symptom profile [10]. Others warned that behaviours might be the result of disruptive home experiences, carer illness [39] or complex psychosocial or child protection backgrounds [53].

Despite research showing links between diagnostic rates and SES, there was very little mention of the impact of SES in CPGs. DSM-5 stated that cultural and socioeconomic factors may affect age at recognition or diagnosis [33] but generally guidelines failed to consider how this might be considered in practice, other than to be aware that 'cultural variations can deliver misleading signs and symptoms' [45] or that autism is 'not restricted to particular ethnic or economic backgrounds' [40]. RCSLT guidelines considered assessment of bilingual individuals [41] and some suggested that ethnicity may delay engagement in the diagnostic process [11] or may increase difficulty in accessing services [54].

Overall, guidelines suggested it was the responsibility of the HCP to make a judgement about which behaviours appear to be 'normal' in complex social and family circumstances, as well as against norms for behaviour.

Diagnostic uncertainty, thresholds and the role of clinical judgement

Overall the general focus of guidelines was to outline a framework to find the best way to decide whether autism is present or not around a threshold of symptom severity. However, many guidelines problematized this, for example, one guideline discussed how definitions of autism have changed with DMS-5 [11] and others suggested that social factors, such as an upbringing characterized by lack of boundaries [45] or symptoms amplified by distress [11] may cause diagnostic difficulties.

All national guidelines considered uncertainties around diagnosis, particularly with very young children or those with co-existing disorders [39]; when there may be disagreement within the diagnosing team or between the team and the patient or family, or when there is a lack of local expertise [9]. Many warned of diagnostic difficulties, or 'obscuring' [11, 53] that can take place if there is an intellectual disability or other complex coexisting condition and several considered the difficulties of overlapping diagnostic criteria [33, 50, 51, 53]. Further uncertainty was outlined when individuals may not reach the diagnostic threshold [39] or when children with autism score below the cut-off as determined by the diagnostic instrument [43].

Despite this uncertainty, CPGs generally proposed a systematic approach to diagnosis and, in some cases, asserted that progress has been achieved in establishing consensus around a behavioural definition and established systematic clinical assessments (e.g. [50]) even whilst recognizing that the 'boundaries between disorders are more porous than originally perceived' [33].

Eight guidelines stressed the key role of clinical judgement in the diagnostic process. DSM-5 outlined that the use of diagnostic criteria should be informed by clinical judgement [33] and ICD-10 suggested that guidelines should be used flexibly in clinical work [32]. The full version of NICE children's guideline recommended: 'Use information from all sources, together with clinical judgement, to diagnose autism based on ICD-10 or DSM-IV criteria' [55]. One guideline suggested that clinicians may depend on the 'feel' of the interaction with the patient for diagnosis [48]. The RCPsych guideline stated that:'...much will depend on the extent of the clinician's experience, their rigour in applying standard criteria and their ability to recognise alternative diagnoses' [11]. Uncertainty, clinical judgement and clinician experience, therefore, were all identified as important factors in the diagnostic process.

Pragmatic outcomes and diagnostic value

Most guidelines ($n = 17$) discussed the need for HCPs to have knowledge of local support and resources available to deliver appropriate advice when required. The value of the diagnosis was generally described as a way to provide appropriate support, intervention and resources. NICE guidelines for children and young people clarified this:

> 'Diagnosis and the assessment of needs ...can open doors to support and services...all of these can improve the lives of the child or young person and their family' [39].

However, NICE guidelines for adults acknowledged that adults who are diagnosed may receive no support due to lack of services [9] and Pilling et al. stated that whilst care for children and young people is generally well coordinated, this is not always the case for adult services [58].

Although some guidelines acknowledged that people may not want a diagnosis and the label it brings with it (e.g. [44, 54]) or that it can be stigmatising or damaging to career plans [11], generally guidelines described the benefits of a diagnosis primarily as relating to improved quality of life, creating an opportunity to have needs met, greater understanding and reassurance about one's own situation and access to interventions and services. Some guidelines considered that diagnosis can provide relief, understanding or an opportunity to move on with increased support [11, 39, 45].

Many guidelines stressed the importance of early diagnosis as this enables early intervention which leads to improved health outcomes (e.g. [41, 44, 47, 50]). However, the BMJ guideline asserted that the, '...efficacy of early intervention varies from child to child' [43], and that 'consideration of the direct financial costs, indirect costs... and the impact on relationships within the family... must be balanced against likely and possible improvements in outcome for the person with ASD' [43], bringing uncertainty into the benefits of diagnosis. Furthermore, O'Hare asserted that it is difficult to prove that earlier intervention is more effective [53].

Overall, guidelines reflected a concern about the potential impact or benefits on the child or adult receiving a diagnosis and considered positive factors such as access to support and intervention, increased understanding or relief; as well as potential negative impacts such as stigma. Carpenter, however, questioned the relationship between need and diagnosis, by asking whether diagnosis is influenced by what intervention the person needs or '...explicitly determined by the person's need to have the label to access a service... rather than their fitting strict diagnostic criteria?' [48].

To conclude, whilst CPGs appeared to frame a methodical and clinical diagnostic process, they also rehearsed a number of subjective dilemmas that HCPs have to negotiate along the way. Some CPGs themselves drew attention to social issues that muddle the process: the difficulties of establishing a clear threshold in a condition where symptoms are impacted by the stressors of environment [11]; the problem of relying on mechanistic assessments or algorithms [11, 48]; the crucial role of clinical judgement [54]; the possibility of diagnostic uncertainty through disagreement, lack of local expertise or when a complex coexisting condition is present [9]; the complexity caused by interaction with co-occurring conditions; masking of autism by comorbid conditions in secondary care [58]; the impact of good (or poor) social support and coping strategies on how symptoms present [33], to name a few.

Discussion

We found that CPGs varied in how they described the diagnostic process in relation to use of diagnostic tools, key elements and structure of the diagnostic process (for example how diagnosis related to wider needs assessment) and how autism was classified, defined either by current versions of DSM or ICD. In addition, whilst some recommendations were clear and universal, for example, recommendations for multidisciplinary working, there was little guidance as to how this should work in practice.

In addition, we found that uncertainty was central to many diagnostic decisions, placing a great emphasis on clinical judgement. This uncertainty included questions around the benefits of early intervention, the shifting nature of the diagnostic threshold, the difficulties of interpreting needs in different social contexts, the problems of interpreting 'masking' or coping strategies, the differences in presentation across age and breadth of symptoms, the inter-relationship with co-conditions and sharing of symptoms, the impact of stressors on symptoms as well as interpretation of symptoms and needs in different cultural contexts.

Overall, therefore, our narrative review found that although individual guidelines appeared to present a coherent and systematic assessment process, they varied enough in their recommendations to make the choices available to healthcare professionals particularly complex and confusing; and presented a context of uncertainty which appeared to be central to the diagnosis of autism. We argue that clinical guidelines for autism diagnosis illuminate the process of diagnosis as social rather than straightforwardly clinical, and that judgement is required to consider a number of sometimes contradictory and complex social factors.

Social factors in CPGs

Organising the narrative review findings in relation to operational, interactional and contextual factors enabled consideration of the influence of social factors throughout the diagnostic process.

In the wide range of inter-related assessment processes that HCPs negotiate in order to make the diagnostic decision, the factors considered appear to be both social and medical. Social factors include: how the category of 'autism' is defined and boundaried; operational and interactional factors present in the process of diagnosis; to the consequences of diagnosis including how diagnosis is valued (see Fig. 3). Each of these factors had a place in clinical guidelines to a greater or lesser extent but in many cases they were not operationalized to enable a clear and transparent framework. For example, although there were many references to individuals masking symptoms, family 'scaffolding' of social impairment and coping strategies, there was little guidance about how HCPs can judge the impact of these on need, behavioural symptoms or functioning.

CPGs, therefore, tended to mask (whilst paradoxically acknowledging) the existence of social factors in the diagnostic process. A more explicit acknowledgement of social factors and how to manage them might problematize the nature of autism diagnosis altogether: if all these factors have a place in diagnosis, how do they relate to clinical factors and what does it mean for descriptions of symptoms? Whilst it is not our intention to undermine the utility of diagnostic categories in relation to access to resources or support, there appears to be a need for balance in CPGs between a clinical approach which both recognises and acknowledges the uncertainty of the diagnostic threshold; and a pragmatic or functional approach which responds to individual and wider needs and takes account of social factors.

Diagnostic tools and process

Clinical guidelines for autism varied in aspects of their key recommendations in operational factors. Ambiguities around which tools to use, the key elements in the diagnostic process and the relationship between diagnosis, assessment and formulation suggest that local practice may be shaped by other factors, such as available resources, experience and professional roles. Which tools are used, whether different elements of the process are considered together, sequentially or inconsistently, and the specific aims of each part of the assessment process may have an impact on diagnostic outcomes. A clearer framework would help HCPs to consider which elements of the process are relevant and when.

MDT working and views of the family

Guidance about how HCPs can reach a consensus with others in a multidisciplinary context or deal with patient/family disagreement or desire was lacking, leaving interactional factors as key to the process but largely unexplained. Whilst it might not appear to be in the remit of CPGs to make specific recommendations about how teams are organised and configured, particularly across different health systems, we argue that team functioning as a key shaping factor in diagnosis requires more attention in CPGs, to ensure clarity of roles and transparency for those coming for diagnosis. Similarly, as acknowledged by some CPGs, desire of the patient/family can influence the diagnostic process, therefore CPGs should offer guidance about how that might be managed.

Diagnostic uncertainty and judgement

Uncertainty about diagnostic thresholds and differences in diagnostic criteria make clinical judgement key to the diagnostic process and yet how this comes about was not clearly defined. The extent to which diagnosis should be based on underlying symptoms versus contextual factors such as wider needs or circumstances of the individual was unclear. In addition, how HCPs consider the consequences of the diagnosis for the patient and their family was unclear, although there was a strong link described between diagnosis and access to support.

Ambiguities in CPGs suggest that guidelines have limitations in how far they are able to promote consistency across practice especially given the lack of a biomarker for autism, the reliance on observed behaviour and family narratives for diagnosis, and the differences across health systems. However, adults, children and families coming for diagnosis might expect a consistent process of assessment in keeping with a framework outlined in CPGs, as CPGs become a fixed reference point both for HCPs and the lay public. There is, therefore, a tension between potential expectations of those coming for diagnosis that there should be a uniform process; and the flexibility HCPs require to respond to individual need.

Given the social nature of diagnosis as argued in this article, biomarker use in clinical practice, if and when it is successfully developed, is likely to remain only one aspect of an interactive diagnostic process, and therefore may not necessarily alleviate some of the difficulties and complexities of diagnosis that we describe. However, as biomarker research develops, it is likely that it will produce important evidence to be considered in the development of future CPGs.

Building on previous work

Whilst our narrative review differed in purpose to the systematic review undertaken by Penner et al. [29], there were some similar findings across the two studies. We found, as did the authors of this previous review, that guidelines were inconsistent in their recommendations around diagnostic assessment. For example, whilst guidelines generally recommended MDT assessment, some suggested that a single experienced clinician could diagnose [11, 39, 48] and there was little cited evidence for the efficacy of MDT assessment. In addition, CPGs did not provide guidance as to how waiting times (where specified) would be achieved and we would add that they provided little operational guidance as to how MDT decision-making should operate to be most effective. We found, as did Penner et al., that guidelines varied substantially in recommended tools and personnel; and that none of the professional guidelines provided target waiting times for assessment (See Table 4). Whilst we did not assess guidelines for quality, we agree that there are multiple guidelines that HCPs might access, and that they vary in their level of detail and their recommendations.

We built on Penner et al.'s findings in a number of ways. Our review of the range of assessment processes that HCPs involved in autism diagnosis may undertake (See Table 4) suggested a wide range of choices in assessment processes. We also found that using different classification criteria (ICD-10 and DSM-5) further increases complexity in CPGs. Finally, we found that consideration of factors such as interaction with the patient and family, how needs might be defined and assessed, and issues of masking, social context, uncertainty and clinical judgement highlighted the way in which social processes and factors might impact on diagnostic decision-making. We also found that, despite the CPGs in our study operating within comparable health systems across the UK, CPGs did not make consistent recommendations around how diagnosis might release post-diagnostic resources, and what that means for the process of diagnosis itself.

Overall we agree with Penner et al.'s findings that CPGs should incorporate flexibility to ensure that individual needs are met. Additionally, we suggest that guidelines should acknowledge more explicitly the social framing of diagnosis and support clinicians with a framework which enables them to act pragmatically in the best interests of the patient. We would argue that inconsistencies and lack of operational guidance around social factors in CPGs suggests that local factors such as access to resources and HCP expertise are likely to shape diagnosis more than is explicitly outlined in CPGs.

Unlike Penner et al., we do not think that a formal approach to decision-making such as the Delphi method would help HCPs in the assessment process; rather it might simply add another layer of complexity to a process which is already challenging. Our experience is that HCPs already struggle to find time to meet together in the context of an ever-increasing workload; an extra administrative burden may make this even more difficult.

Finally, unlike Penner et al., we included in our review CPGs for adult diagnosis and children over 6 years old, which enabled us to consider factors common across age groups. Whilst we did not specifically look for differences between children's and adult's CPGs we are aware that the different pathways for children's and adult's assessment [3, 59], may well impact on an individual's ability to access diagnostic services, the process of assessment itself as well as potential support post-diagnosis. We would consider these differences as social organisational factors that may impact the assessment process and merit further consideration in the development of future CPGs.

Guidelines, therefore, appear to offer a relatively linear and straightforward pathway towards a diagnostic decision in their presentation, with DSM-5 asserting that criteria facilitate an objective assessment of symptom presentations in a variety of settings [20]. However, comparing individual guidelines suggests inconsistencies in this framework and close analysis reveals a more fluid process, disrupting the apparent clinical purity of diagnosis [37].

Conclusion

Overall, there was a bewildering range of options for HCPs in the assessment process, and a number of different emphases in guidelines which might lead a clinical team one way or another. Navigating this framework in practice is, therefore, likely to be less systematic than the guidelines might suggest, allowing for, as it must, social and contextual influences. In reality, the clinical pathway for autism diagnosis differs across health systems and trusts across the UK [3] leading to the potential for a great deal of variation in diagnostic decision-making.

Strengths and limitations

Although there has been a recent systematic review of clinical guidelines [29], we consider our narrative approach to be helpful to understand the complex and sometimes contradictory nature of the diagnostic process. Methodologically, we undertook a systematic search and included a transparent but pragmatic selection of documents. This is, to our knowledge, the first review which strives to consider where social factors are considered in clinical guidelines for autism diagnosis. One limit was that as it was a review of current guidelines, changes through time were not exposed. Our review was limited to the UK context because health care settings vary widely in international contexts. In addition, we only examined the content of guidelines rather than how they are used. Whilst CPGs are intended to assist clinical decision-making by improving effectiveness and decreasing variations in clinical practice [60], one review of guidelines for psychiatric diagnoses suggested that CPGs are not implemented enough in clinical practice due to either lack of agreement or ambiguity between guidelines [61]. It is likely that there is wide variation in how CPGs are used in practice in autism diagnosis and we plan further studies to consider this.

Implications and recommendations for future research

Social factors were not only explicit in guidelines, but were central to them. However, an observer might be forgiven for assuming these are subsidiary factors in diagnosis, with the more 'medical' 'symptom checklist' at its core. HCPs are expected, as outlined in DSM-5, to integrate the social, psychological and biological in case formulation, however, greater clarity about how this should operate would be helpful. Our findings suggest that more detail about how clinical judgement should consider social factors in diagnosis would provide a more transparent guideline for HCPs.

We would not recommend greater rigidity within CPGs when evidence for best diagnostic practice is inconsistent (e.g. use of diagnostic tools), and which may restrict HCPs in making decisions that are in the best interest of the person coming for diagnosis. Rather we recommend a more explicit acknowledgement of social factors in CPGs with advice about how they should be managed and operationalised to enable more consistency of practice and transparency for those coming for diagnosis.

Specifically, greater clarification is required related to the sequence and timing of the diagnostic, assessment and formulation processes. The recognition and assessment of needs is both part of the assessment process and inextricably linked to the consequences of diagnosis; guidelines might attempt to consider how these might be reconciled. A greater acknowledgement of the active role of the patient, client or patient's family in the diagnostic process would help to place potentially competing narratives into context. It would be useful to consider whether guidelines are culturally specific to health services and setting and we would recommend that further narrative reviews should be conducted to examine CPGs in other countries. In addition, greater clarity is required around how multidisciplinary interaction might operate to support consensus decision-making. Further research creating an evidence base on best practice for multidisciplinary decision-making and the use of different diagnostic tools in practice is required, taking into account the complexity of social factors in diagnosis.

Abbreviations

3di: The Developmental, Dimensional and Diagnostic Interview; ADI-R: Autism Diagnostic Interview Revised; ADOS: Autism Diagnostic Observation Schedule; BMJ: British Medical Journal; BPS: The British Psychological Society; CPG: Clinical Practice Guideline; DISCO: The Diagnostic Interview for Social and Communication Disorders; DSM-5: Diagnostic and Statistical Manual of Mental Disorders (Fifth Edition); HCP: Healthcare Professional; HMIC: The Healthcare Management Information Consortium; ICD-10: International Classification of Mental and Behavioural Disorders (Tenth edition) ICIDH-2International Classification of Functioning, Disability and Health; MDT: Multidisciplinary Team; NICE: The National Institute for Health and Care Excellence; RASDN: The Regional Autistic Spectrum Disorder Network; RCPsych: Royal College of Psychiatrists; RCSLT: Royal College of Speech and Language Therapists; SIGN: The Scottish Intercollegiate Guidelines Network; SLT: Speech and Language Therapist

Acknowledgements

The authors thank Daisy Elliott and Rhianna White for their help with piloting this project.

Funding

The study is part of the Exploring Diagnosis project made possible by a Wellcome Trust Investigator Award http://blogs.exeter.ac.uk/exploringdiagnosis/

Authors' contributions

JH undertook the systematic search, analyzed and interpreted the data. TF and GR were major contributors in conception and design, reviewed the data selection and revised the manuscript for important intellectual content. HR supported with data collection and initial analysis. All authors read and approved the final manuscript.

Consent for publication

Not applicable.

Competing interests

The authors declare that they have no competing interests.

References

1. Kobeissy F, Alawieh A, Mondello S, Boustany RM, Gold MS. Biomarkers in psychiatry: how close are we? Frontiers in Psychiatry. 2013;3
2. Klin A, Lang J, Cichetti D, Volkmar F. Brief Report: Interrater reliability of clinical diagnosis and DSM-IV criteria for autistic disorder: results of the DSM-IV Autism field trial. J Autism Dev Disord. 2000;30:163–7.
3. Vllasaliu L, Jensen K, Hoss S, Landenberger M, Menze M, Schütz M, et al. Diagnostic instruments for autism spectrum disorder (ASD) (protocol). 2011.
4. Huerta M, Lord C. Diagnostic evaluation of autism spectrum disorders. Pediatr Clin N Am. 2012;59:103–11.
5. Gillberg C. The ESSENCE in child psychiatry: Early Symptomatic Syndromes Eliciting Neurodevelopmental Clinical Examinations. Res Dev Disabil. 31: 1543–51. https://doi.org/10.1016/j.ridd.2010.06.002.
6. Falkmer T, Anderson K, Falkmer M, Horlin C. Diagnostic procedures in autism spectrum disorders: a systematic literature review. Eur Child Adolesc Psychiatry. 2013;22:329–40. https://doi.org/10.1007/s00787-013-0375-0.
7. Woolfenden S, Sarkozy V, Ridley G, Williams K. A systematic review of the diagnostic stability of Autism Spectrum disorder. Res Autism Spectr Disord. 2011;6:345–54.
8. Field M, Lohr K. Guidelines for clinical practice: from development to use. Washington DC: Institute of Medicine. Washington, D.C: National Academy Press; 1992. https://www.ncbi.nlm.nih.gov/books/NBK234504/#ddd00035
9. NICE. Autism Spectrum disorder in adults: diagnosis and management. 2012. https://www.nice.org.uk/guidance/cg142/resources/autism-spectrum-disorder-in-adults-diagnosis-and-management-pdf-35109567475909.
10. Scottish Intercollegiate Guidelines Network. SIGN 145: assessment, diagnosis and interventions for autism spectrum disorders: a national clinical guideline. 2016. http://www.sign.ac.uk/assets/sign145.pdf. Accessed 27 Mar 2017.
11. Royal College of Psychiatrists. Good practice in the management of autism (including Asperger syndrome) in adults: College Report CR191. 2014. http://www.rcpsych.ac.uk/files/pdfversion/CR191.pdf. Accessed 7 Jun 2017.
12. Fuat A, Hungin APS, Murphy JJ. Barriers to accurate diagnosis and effective management of heart failure in primary care: qualitative study. Br Med J. 2003;326:196–201. https://doi.org/10.1136/bmj.326.7382.196.
13. Mazumdar S, Winter A, Liu KY, Bearman P. Spatial clusters of autism births and diagnoses point to contextual drivers ofincreased prevalence. Soc Sci Med. 2013;95:87–96.
14. Liu K-Y, King M, Bearman PS. Social influence and the autism epidemic. Am J Sociol. 2010;115:1387–434.
15. Skellern C, Schluter P, McDowell M. From complexity to category: responding to diagnostic uncertainties of autistic spectrum disorders. J Paediatr Child Health. 2005;41:407–12. https://doi.org/10.1111/j.1440-1754.2005.00634.x.
16. Rogers CL, Goddard L, Hill EL, Henry LA, Crane L. Experiences of diagnosing autism spectrum disorder: a survey of professionals in the United Kingdom. Autism. 2016;20:820–31. https://doi.org/10.1177/1362361315611109.
17. Russell G, Rodgers LR, Ukoumunne OC, Ford T. Prevalence of parent-reported ASD and ADHD in the UK: findings from the millennium cohort study. J Autism Dev Disord. 2014;44:31–40. https://doi.org/10.1007/s10803-013-1849-0.
18. King M, Bearman P. Socioeconomic status and the increased prevalence of Autism in California. Am Sociol Rev. 2011;76:320–46. https://doi.org/10.1177/0003122411399389.
19. The National Autistic Society. Diverse perspectives: the challenges for families affected by autism from black. London: Asian and Minority Ethnic Communities; 2014.
20. Norbury CF, Sparks A. Difference or disorder? Cultural issues in understanding neurodevelopmental disorders. Dev Psychol. 2013;49:45–58.
21. Russell G, Steer C, Golding J. Social and demographic factors that influence the diagnosis of autistic spectrum disorders. Soc Psychol Psychiatr Epidemiol. 2011;46:1283–93.
22. Goldani AAS, Downs SR, Widjaja F, Lawton B, Hendren RL. Biomarkers in autism. Front psychiatry. 2014;5:100. https://doi.org/10.3389/fpsyt.2014.00100.

23. Anwar A, Abruzzo PM, Pasha S, Rajpoot K, Bolotta A, Ghezzo A, et al. Advanced glycation endproducts, dityrosine and arginine transporter dysfunction in autism - a source of biomarkers for clinical diagnosis. Mol Autism. 2018;9 https://doi.org/10.1186/s13229-017-0183-3.
24. Carlisi CO, Norman L, Murphy CM, Christakou A, Chantiluke K, Giampietro V, et al. Disorder-specific and shared brain abnormalities during vigilance in Autism and obsessive-compulsive disorder. Biol Psychiatry Cogn Neurosci Neuroimaging. 2017;2:644–54. https://doi.org/10.1016/j.bpsc.2016.12.005.
25. Anderson GM. Autism biomarkers: challenges, pitfalls and possibilities. J Autism Dev Disord. 2015;45:1103–13. https://doi.org/10.1007/s10803-014-2225-4.
26. NHS Choices. New blood test for Autism a long way off. 2018. https://www.nhs.uk/news/pregnancy-and-child/new-blood-test-autism-long-way/. Accessed 3 May 2018.
27. Imran N, Chaudry MR, Azeem MW, Bhatti MR, Choudhary ZI, Cheema MA. A survey of Autism knowledge and attitudes among the healthcare professionals in Lahore, Pakistan. BMC Pediatr. 2011;11:107. https://doi.org/10.1186/1471-2431-11-107.
28. Taylor LJ, Eapen V, Maybery MT, Midford S, Paynter J, Quarmby L, et al. Diagnostic evaluation for autism spectrum disorder: a survey of health professionals in Australia. BMJ Open. 2016;6:e012517. https://doi.org/10.1136/bmjopen-2016-012517.
29. Penner M, Anagnostou E, Andoni LY, Ungar WJ. Systematic review of clinical guidance documents for autism spectrum disorder diagnostic assessment in select regions. Autism. 2017:136236131668587. https://doi.org/10.1177/1362361316685879.
30. Moher D, Liberati A, Tetzlaff J, Altman DG, Group TP. Preferred reporting items for systematic reviews and meta-analyses: the PRISMA statement (reprinted from annals of internal medicine). Phys Ther. 2009;89:873–80. https://doi.org/10.1371/journal.pmed.1000097.
31. Liberati A, Altman DG, Tetzlaff J, Mulrow C, Gøtzsche PC, Ioannidis JPA, et al. The PRISMA statement for reporting systematic reviews and meta-analyses of studies that evaluate health care interventions: explanation and elaboration. PLoS Med. 2009;6 https://doi.org/10.1371/journal.pmed.1000100.
32. World Health Organization. The ICD-10 Classification of Mental and Behavioural Disorders: diagnostic criteria for research. 1993.
33. APA. Diagnostic and statistical manual of mental disorders. Fifth ed. Washington DC: American Psychiatric Association; 2013.
34. Popay J, Roberts H, Sowden A, Petticrew M, Arai L, Rodgers M, et al. Guidance on the Conduct of Narrative Synthesis in Systematic Reviews: A Product from the ESRC Methods Programme. 2006. https://www.researchgate.net/profile/Lisa_Arai/publication/242311393_Guidance_on_the_conduct_of_narrative_synthesis_in_systematic_reviews_a_comparison_of_guidance-led_narrative_synthesis_versus_meta-analysis/links/5532159f0cf2f2a588ad67fd.pdf. Accessed 20 Jun 2017.
35. Ferrari R. Writing narrative style literature reviews. Med Writ. 2015;24:230–5. https://doi.org/10.1179/2047480615Z.000000000329.
36. Jutel A, Nettleton S. Towards a sociology of diagnosis: reflections and opportunities. Soc Sci Med. 2011;73:793–800.
37. Latimer J. The gene, the clinic and the family: diagnosing dysmorphology, reviving medical dominance. Oxfordshire: Routledge; 2013.
38. Department of Health. "Fulfilling and rewarding lives": The strategy for adults with autism in England. 2010. http://webarchive.nationalarchives.gov.uk/20130107105354/http://www.dh.gov.uk/prod_consum_dh/groups/dh_digitalassets/@dh/@en/@ps/documents/digitalasset/dh_113405.pdf. Accessed 19 Jun 2017.
39. NICE. Autism spectrum disorder in under 19s: recognition, referral and diagnosis. 2011. https://www.nice.org.uk/guidance/cg128/resources/autism-spectrum-disorder-in-under-19s-recognition-referral-and-diagnosis-pdf-35109456621253. Accessed 2 Nov 2016.
40. British Psychological Society. Autistic Spectrum Disorders: Guidance for Psychologists. Br Psychol Soc. 2016; www.bps.org.uk. Accessed 27 Mar 2017 Available at https://blogs.exeter.ac.uk/exploringdiagnosis/.
41. RCSLT. Royal College of Speech & Language Therapists Clinical Guidelines. Oxon: Speechmark; 2005. p. 63–71.
42. World Health Organisation. International classification of functioning, Disability and health. 2001.
43. Parr J, Woodbury-Smith M. Autism spectrum disorder. BMJ Best Pract. 2017: 59–83. https://bestpractice.bmj.com/topics/en-gb/379.
44. RASDN. Six Steps of Autism Care. 2011. http://www.belfasttrust.hscni.net/pdf/Six_Steps_of_Autism_Care_Pathway_Report.pdf. Accessed 25 Mar 2018.
45. Howlett D, Richman S. Recognising, referring and diagnosing autism. Every Child J. 2011;2:44–9.
46. Reynolds KE. Autism spectrum disorders in childhood: a clinical update. Community Pr. 2011;84:36–8.
47. Blenner S, Reddy A, Augustyn M. Diagnosis and management of autism in childhood. BMJ. 2011; https://doi.org/10.1136/bmj.d6238.
48. Carpenter P. Diagnosis and assessment in autism spectrum disorders. Adv Ment Heal Intellect Disabil. 2012;6:121–9. https://doi.org/10.1108/20441281211227184.
49. Garland J, O'Rourke L, Robertson D. Autism spectrum disorder in adults: clinical features and the role of the psychiatrist. Adv Psychiatr Treat. 2013;19: 378–91. https://doi.org/10.1192/apt.bp.112.010439.
50. Lai M-C, Lombardo MV, Baron-Cohen S. Autism. Lancet. 2014;383:896–910. https://doi.org/10.1016/S0140-6736(13)61539-1.
51. Levy SE, Mandell DS, Schultz RT. Autism. Lancet. 2009;374:1627–38. https://doi.org/10.1016/S0140-6736(09)61376-3.
52. Wilson CE, Roberts G, Gillan N, Ohlsen C, Robertson D, Zinkstok J. The NICE guideline on recognition, referral, diagnosis and management of adults on the autism spectrum. Adv Ment Heal Intellect Disabil. 2014;8:3–14. https://doi.org/10.1108/AMHID-05-2013-0035.
53. O'Hare A. Autism spectrum disorder: diagnosis and management. Arch Dis Child - Educ Pract. 2009;94:161–8. https://doi.org/10.1136/adc.2008.150490.
54. Regional Autistic Spectrum Disorder Network. Autism Adult Care Pathway. 2013. http://www.hscbusiness.hscni.net/pdf/Adult_Care_PAthway_Reviewed_August_2013.pdf. Accessed 21 Jun 2017.
55. National Collaborating Centre for Women's and Children's Health. Autism: recognition, referral and diagnosis of children and young people on the autism spectrum: NICE Clinical Guideline. 2011. https://www.ncbi.nlm.nih.gov/pubmed/22624178. Accessed 17 Feb 2017.
56. Mahoney WJ, Szatmari P, MacLean JE, Bryson SE, Bartolucci G, Walter SD, Jones MB, Zwaigenbaum L. Reliability and accuracy of differentiating pervasive developmental disorder subtypes. J Am Acad Child Adolesc Psychiatry. 1998;37(3):278–85.
57. Moore V, Titcomb J, Johnson C, Cronk E, Baker S, Thysson L, et al. Developing an autism assessment service II: analysis of the first 81 cases seen. Child Psychol Psychiatr Rev. 1998;3(3):121–7.
58. Pilling S, Baron-Cohen S, Megnin-Viggars O, Lee R, Taylor C. Recognition, referral, diagnosis, and management of adults with autism: summary of NICE guidance. BMJ. 2012;344(jun27 1):e4082. https://doi.org/10.1136/bmj.e4082.
59. Baird G, Douglas HR, Murphy MS. Recognising and diagnosing autism in children and young people: summary of NICE guidance. BMJ. 2011; 343:–d6360.
60. Kredo T, Bernhardsson S, Machingaidze S, Young T, Louw Q, Ochodo E, et al. Guide to clinical practice guidelines: the current state of play. Int J Qual Heal Care. 2016;28:122–8. https://doi.org/10.1093/intqhc/mzv115.
61. Saddichha S, Chaturvedi SK. Clinical practice guidelines in psychiatry: more confusion than clarity? A critical review and recommendation of a unified guideline. ISRN Psychiatry. 2014;2014:828917. https://doi.org/10.1155/2014/828917.
62. National Collaborating Centre for Mental Health. Autism: the NICE guideline on recognition, referral, diagnosis and management of adults on the autism spectrum. In: The British Psychological Society and the Royal College of Psychiatrists; 2012. https://www.nice.org.uk/guidance/cg142/evidence/full-guideline-186587677.

12

Health-related quality of life and burden of illness in adults with newly diagnosed attention-deficit/hyperactivity disorder in Sweden

E. Ahnemark[1*], M. Di Schiena[2], A.-C. Fredman[2,8], E. Medin[3,4], J. K. Söderling[5] and Y. Ginsberg[6,7]

Abstract

Background: This observational, cross-sectional, retrospective chart review aimed to identify factors determining health-related quality of life (HRQoL) in adults with newly diagnosed attention-deficit/hyperactivity disorder (ADHD) in Sweden.

Methods: Adult participants with a new clinical diagnosis of ADHD were enrolled from two specialist outpatient clinics in Stockholm, Sweden, from 2013 to 2015. Data extracted from patient records included demographics, clinical characteristics and comorbid psychiatric diagnoses identified using the Mini International Neuropsychiatric Interview (MINI). Depression severity was assessed using the Montgomery–Åsberg Depression Rating Scale – Self-reported (MADRS-S). The self-rated five-dimension EuroQol questionnaire (EQ-5D) was used to measure HRQoL. Predictors of EQ-5D index score were identified using multivariate linear regression adjusting for age, sex, education level, and main income source.

Results: The mean age of the 189 enrolled patients was 35.2 years (standard deviation [SD], 12.3), and 107 (57%) were female. Psychiatric comorbidities were present in 92 patients (49%), with anxiety and depression being the most common diagnoses. The mean EQ-5D index score was 0.63 (SD, 0.28). Low EQ-5D index scores were significantly associated with high MADRS-S scores, multiple comorbid psychiatric disorders, low educational achievement, female sex, and not having a main income derived from employment or self-employment.

Conclusions: These findings suggest that adults with newly diagnosed ADHD experience low HRQoL, which may often be exacerbated by psychiatric comorbidities such as anxiety and depression. Patients presenting with ADHD and psychiatric comorbidities in adulthood may require particular care and resources in the management of their ADHD.

Keywords: ADHD, HRQoL, Psychiatric comorbidities

Background

Attention-deficit/hyperactivity disorder (ADHD) is estimated to affect between 2.5 and 5.0% of adults worldwide [1–3]. Although originally considered to be a disorder of childhood, ADHD is now recognized to persist into adulthood in approximately 65% of cases [4–7]. While many adults with newly diagnosed ADHD may have experienced symptoms as children [6], two recent studies have suggested that, in some cases, ADHD symptoms may not manifest until adulthood [8, 9]. Results from a study in Sweden demonstrated that the number of adults diagnosed with ADHD increased year on year from 2006 to 2011 [10], and in 2013 ADHD was diagnosed in 2.7% of adult psychiatric patients in Sweden [11]. Despite the increasing recognition of ADHD in the adult Swedish population, a recent registry study reported that patients with psychiatric symptoms may undergo years of treatment before receiving an ADHD diagnosis [11]. Nylander et al. found that diagnosis of ADHD in adults took, on average,

* Correspondence: eahnemark@shire.com
[1]Shire, Vasagatan 7, SE-111 20 Stockholm, Sweden
Full list of author information is available at the end of the article

3 years from the initial point of contact with psychiatric services, although in some cases diagnoses were delayed for as long as 10 years [11]. Delays in diagnosis were particularly apparent if the signs and symptoms of ADHD were attributed to other psychiatric disorders, for example, anxiety disorders, which often co-occur with ADHD [11]. These findings highlight the need for increased recognition and understanding of ADHD as an adult psychiatric disorder. Similarly, the European Network Adult ADHD published a consensus document in 2010, with the aims of increasing awareness of ADHD in adults and improving patient care across Europe [12].

The effects of ADHD can have a significant negative impact on many aspects of adult life, from social and emotional well-being to professional development and financial security [13, 14]. Despite this, few studies have investigated the burden of disease in adult patients with ADHD. Swedish patient records and archives provide a rich source of data for investigating burden of illness in adults with newly diagnosed ADHD. The diagnostic procedure for adults comprises a clinical interview to assess the frequency and duration of ADHD symptoms, as well as a full neuropsychiatric investigation of functional impairments from both clinical and social perspectives. This retrospective chart review study utilized the five-dimension EuroQol questionnaire (EQ-5D) [15] to develop a predictive model of health-related quality of life (HRQoL) in adults with newly diagnosed ADHD, based on their ADHD symptoms, psychiatric comorbidities, and socioeconomic characteristics.

Methods

Study design and conduct

This study was an observational, cross-sectional, retrospective chart review of adult patients with newly diagnosed ADHD at one of two specialist neuropsychiatric outpatient clinics (Liljeholmen or Danderyd) in Stockholm, Sweden, between 2013 and 2015. The study was conducted in accordance with the ethical standards of the World Medical Association Declaration of Helsinki. The study was approved by the Regional Ethical Review Board in Stockholm and the need for consent was waived due to the retrospective nature of the study.

Participants

The study population was identified from electronic medical records (EMRs) and archives of patients' neuropsychiatric investigations from the two study sites. Only patients aged 18 years and above who underwent neuropsychiatric investigation and received a new and confirmed diagnosis of ADHD (International Statistical Classification of Diseases and Related Health Problems – 10th Revision, Swedish modification [ICD-10-SE] diagnosis code F90) [16] were enrolled in the study.

Diagnostic investigations at Liljeholmen and Danderyd

Extensive diagnostic investigations were conducted at outpatient clinics for all enrolled patients. Patients were interviewed alongside any family members or companions (usually parents or spouse), and details of their medical history, developmental history, coexistent disorders, and current condition were recorded. A medical examination, including blood tests and drug screening, was also part of the diagnostic process. During the neuropsychiatric investigation, the frequency and duration of patients' psychiatric symptoms were recorded, their functional impairments and cognitive and executive functioning were assessed, and routine diagnostic tests for psychiatric disorders were completed. Several different self-report scales, psychological tests, and structured interviews were used to provide a comprehensive neuropsychiatric evaluation and confirm the ADHD diagnosis (Table 1). ADHD-specific instruments included the Diagnostic Interview for ADHD in Adults, second edition (DIVA 2.0), and the Adult ADHD Self-Report Scale version 1.1 (ASRS-v1.1).

Data extraction

All patient-related information, including findings from the neuropsychiatric investigations, were accessed through EMRs and patient archives. Clinical researchers with knowledge and experience of treating patients with ADHD extracted anonymized patient data using data-gathering forms specifically designed for the study. The data-gathering form was based on the recommendations for neuropsychiatric investigations of patients with suspected ADHD described in recent guidelines (www.psykiatristod.se) and validated by a clinical expert.

The information extracted included social and clinical characteristics, patient and family histories, and details of any prescribed medication. Adult scores from the DIVA 2.0 and ASRS-v.1.1 Screener (6 items) and Symptom checklist (18 items) were also obtained (Table 1) [17].

Full details of any psychiatric diagnoses, made using the Mini International Neuropsychiatric Interview (MINI) Swedish version 6.0.0 [18], were also extracted from the databases. The MINI comprises a short structured interview in which patient symptoms and signs are assessed against diagnostic criteria given in the Diagnostic and Statistical Manual of Mental Disorders, fourth edition (DSM-IV) [19]. MINI-identified depression includes depressive episodes and recurrent depression (ICD-10-SE diagnosis codes F32–F33). MINI-identified anxiety includes phobias, other anxiety disorders and obsessive–compulsive disorder (ICD-10-SE, F40–F42). Autism was diagnosed separately as part of the neuropsychiatric investigation.

Other extracted data included patient-reported indications of drug and alcohol abuse, depression, and HRQoL (Table 1). HRQoL was assessed using the EQ-5D, and the Montgomery–Åsberg Depression Rating

Table 1 Data extracted from electronic medical records and archives

Basic characteristics	Age, sex, type of referral, confirmed ADHD diagnosis, other psychiatric diagnoses (confirmed using MINI)
Social status	Marital status, parental status (biological), age of children, housing, education, main source of income
Patient history	Psychiatric history, previous confirmed psychiatric diagnoses, current registered somatic diagnoses
Family history	General and specific psychiatric and neuropsychiatric disorders in the family
Risk assessment	Previous suicide attempts, previous or current self-destructive, aggressive, or criminal behaviour
ADHD diagnostic interview	DIVA 2.0 (symptoms of attention deficit [A1] and hyperactivity/impulsivity [A2])
Patient-reported measures	Scores for ASRS-v.1.1 Screener and Symptom checklist and AUDIT, DUDIT, MADRS-S, and EQ-5D
Intelligence assessment	WAIS-IV score
Pharmacological treatments	Current psychiatric and somatic medications, recommended ADHD medication after neuropsychiatric investigation

ADHD attention-deficit/hyperactivity disorder, *ASRS-v.1.1* Adult ADHD Self-Report Scale version 1.1, *AUDIT* Alcohol Use Disorders Identification Test, *DIVA 2.0* Diagnostic Interview for ADHD in Adults, second edition, *DUDIT* Drug Use Disorders Identification Test, *EQ-5D* five-dimension EuroQol questionnaire, *MADRS-S* Montgomery–Åsberg Depression Rating Scale – Self-reported, *MINI* Mini International Neuropsychiatric Interview, *WAIS-IV* Wechsler Adult Intelligence Scale IV

Scale – Self-reported (MADRS-S) screening instrument [20] was used to evaluate the presence and severity of depressive symptoms. For patients enrolled from the Liljeholmen clinic, MADRS-S scores were calculated from Patient Health Questionnaire 9 (PHQ-9) scores using a published regression equation (MADRS-S = [1.206 × PHQ-9] + 4.062) [21].

Linear regression models

Potential predictors of HRQoL were identified using a linear regression model of EQ-5D index score, adjusting for age (18–29, 30–39, 40–49, or ≥ 50 years), sex, education (secondary/university or other), and main source of income (full- or part-time employment or other). A linear regression model with the same covariates was used to predict differences in EQ-5D index score between subgroups of patients with or without comorbid psychiatric diagnoses.

A multiple imputation model was employed to estimate values for missing data using five iterations per value. Covariates included in the imputation model were age, sex, study site, education, source of income, MINI-identified comorbid diagnoses, previously confirmed psychiatric disorders, previous suicide attempts, somatic diagnoses, current psychiatric medications, recommended ADHD medication after neuropsychiatric investigation, DIVA 2.0 scores, ASRS-v.1.1 scores, MADRS-S scores, and both EQ-5D index and visual analogue scale scores. Missing EQ-5D index scores were replaced for 27 patients (Additional file 1: Table S1). Patients aged 50 years or older and those recruited in Liljeholmen (as opposed to Danderyd) were more likely to have missing EQ-5D values. Although imputed values for these patients tended to be below the mean, the distributions of the observed and imputed EQ-5D index score data were similar. Multiple imputation was performed using SAS v9.3 software (SAS Institute, Cary, NC, USA).

Statistical analysis

Differences between study sites in mean patient age and the ratio of male to female patients were analysed using t-tests and χ^2 tests, respectively ($\alpha = 0.05$). Data were analysed using SAS v9.3 (SAS Institute, Cary, NC, USA).

Results

Demographics and patient characteristics

The study enrolled 189 adult patients with newly diagnosed ADHD, of whom 57% were women (Table 2). The mean patient age was 35.2 years (standard deviation [SD], 12.3), and ages ranged from 18 to 72 years. There was no statistically significant difference in mean patient age between the two clinics, but a significantly larger proportion of female participants were enrolled from Danderyd than from Liljeholmen ($p = 0.04$; Table 2).

The majority of patients (114/189 [60%]) had diagnoses of 'combined type' ADHD, while 49/189 (26%) had 'predominantly inattentive type' and 26/189 (14%) had 'unspecified type' (which includes either 'combined' type or 'predominantly inattentive' type; Table 2). Of the 189 patients, most did not reach a level of education beyond secondary school; 13% had a university education. Fewer than half of the patients listed employment as their main source of income, with 37% in full- or part-time employment and 10% self-employed (either full- or part-time; Table 2).

Clinical characteristics and treatment history

Data extracted from the MINIs revealed that almost half of patients (92/189 [49%]) had a psychiatric comorbidity (Table 3). Anxiety and depression were the most common, affecting 65/189 patients (34%) and 37/189 patients (20%), respectively. Both anxiety and depression were frequently registered alongside other MINI-identified diagnoses, but few patients had anxiety or depression diagnosed as a single comorbidity (25/189 [13%] and 11/189 [6%], respectively; Table 3). An autism diagnosis was recorded in 30/189 patients (16%).

The majority of patients (108/189 [57%]) had been prescribed pharmacological treatments for psychiatric

Table 2 Patient demographics and clinical characteristics

Characteristic	Danderyd ($n = 101$)	Liljeholmen ($n = 88$)	Overall ($N = 189$)
Sex, *n* (%)			
Female	61 (60)	46 (52)	107 (57)
Male	40 (40)	42 (48)	82 (43)
p value[a]			0.04
Age, years			
Mean (SD)	33.7 (12.4)	36.9 (12.0)	35.2 (12.3)
Median (range)	30 (18–72)	36 (18–66)	33 (18–72)
p value[b]			0.08
Confirmed ADHD diagnosis, *n* (%)			
Combined type[c]	57 (56)	57 (65)	114 (60)
Predominantly inattentive type[d]	37 (37)	12 (14)	49 (26)
Unspecified type[e]	7 (7)	19 (21)	26 (14)
DIVA 2.0, mean number of symptoms (SD)			
Attention deficit[f] (A1)	7.8 (1.4)	6.9 (2.3)	7.4 (1.9)
Hyperactivity/impulsivity[g] (A2)	5.3 (2.9)	5.7 (2.5)	5.5 (2.7)
Highest level of education, *n* (%)			
Primary school	36 (36)	33 (38)	69 (37)
Secondary school	46 (46)	28 (32)	74 (39)
University	11 (11)	13 (15)	24 (13)
Other[h]	8 (8)	14 (16)	22 (12)
Main source of income, *n* (%)			
Full- or part-time employment	32 (32)	38 (43)	70 (37)
Self-employment (full- or part-time)	9 (9)	9 (10)	18 (10)
Sickness benefit (short- or long-term)	23 (23)	19 (22)	42 (22)
Unemployment benefit	12 (12)	3 (3)	15 (8)
Other[i]	25 (25)	19 (22)	44 (23)
Type of referral, *n* (%)			
Self-initiated	27 (27)	13 (15)	40 (21)
School	1 (1)	2 (2)	3 (2)
Primary care	13 (13)	36 (41)	49 (26)
Psychiatric department	56 (55)	28 (32)	84 (44)
Other	4 (4)	7 (8)	11 (6)
Missing	0 (0)	2 (2)	2 (1)

ADHD attention-deficit/hyperactivity disorder, *DIVA 2.0* Diagnostic Interview for ADHD in Adults, second edition, *ICD-10-SE* International Statistical Classification of Diseases and Related Health Problems – 10th Revision, Swedish modification, *SD* standard deviation

[a] χ^2 test was used to compare proportions of male and female patients between the two test sites

[b] *t*-test was used to compare the mean ages of patients enrolled at the two test sites

[c] ICD-10-SE F90.0 B: ADHD, combined type

[d] ICD-10-SE F90.0 C: ADHD, predominantly inattentive type

[e] ICD-10-SE F90.0 X: ADHD, unspecified ADHD

[f] $n = 163$ (Danderyd, 91; Liljeholmen, 72)

[g] $n = 157$ (Danderyd, 86; Liljeholmen, 71)

[h] 'Other' includes occupational (7%), other (4%), and missing (1%)

[i] 'Other' includes 'studying/student loan' (7%), 'other' (13%), and 'missing' (4%)

disorders. Medications included antidepressants (67/189 [35%]), hypnotics (38/189 [20%]), anxiolytics (37/189 [20%]), and antipsychotics (5/189 [3%]; Table 3). Three patients (3/189 [2%]) had been prescribed ADHD medication (the central nervous system stimulant, osmotic-release oral system methylphenidate [OROS-MPH]) despite lacking a

Table 3 Patients' psychiatric and somatic comorbidities and prescribed psychiatric medication

Comorbidities	Danderyd (*n* = 101)	Liljeholmen (*n* = 88)	Overall (*N* = 189)
Psychiatric, *n* (%)[a]			
Any	61 (60)	31 (35)	92 (49)
None	40 (40)	57 (65)	97 (51)
Anxiety and/or depression, *n* (%)			
Anxiety	43 (43)	22 (25)	65 (34)
Anxiety only[b]	16 (16)	9 (10)	25 (13)
Depression[c]	28 (28)	9 (10)	37 (20)
Depression only[b]	7 (7)	4 (5)	11 (6)
Both anxiety and depression[d]	17 (17)	4 (5)	21 (11)
Other, *n* (%)			
Any other psychiatric diagnosis	21 (21)	14 (16)	35 (19)
Dysthymic disorder	5 (5)	4 (5)	9 (5)
Substance-related disorders	6 (6)	2 (2)	8 (4)
Antisocial personality disorder	4 (4)	3 (3)	7 (4)
Eating disorder	5 (5)	1 (1)	6 (3)
Bipolar disorder	4 (4)	1 (1)	5 (3)
Post-traumatic stress disorder	3 (3)	1 (1)	4 (2)
Somatic comorbidity, *n* (%)			
Any	86 (85)	59 (67)	145 (77)
None	15 (15)	29 (33)	44 (23)
Pain	25 (25)	11 (13)	36 (19)
Gastrointestinal disorders	23 (23)	9 (10)	32 (17)
Allergy	21 (21)	6 (7)	27 (14)
Asthma	10 (10)	9 (10)	19 (10)
Joint problems	6 (6)	6 (7)	12 (6)
Thyroid disease	8 (8)	3 (3)	11 (6)
Lactose intolerance	6 (6)	1 (1)	7 (4)
Prescribed psychiatric medication, *n* (%)			
Any	61 (60)	47 (53)	108 (57)
None	40 (40)	41 (47)	81 (43)
Antidepressants	37 (37)	30 (34)	67 (35)
Hypnotics	24 (24)	14 (16)	38 (20)
Anxiolytics	18 (18)	19 (22)	37 (20)
Antipsychotics	3 (3)	2 (2)	5 (3)
Central nervous system stimulants	3 (3)	0 (0)	3 (2)

MINI Mini International Neuropsychiatric Interview
[a]Comorbid psychiatric diagnoses were based on MINI and did not include autism. An autism diagnosis was recorded in 30/189 patients (16%)
[b]This disorder is listed as the only registered comorbidity
[c]Includes recurrent and single-episode depression
[d]MINI-identified diagnosis of recurrent or single-episode depression and MINI-identified diagnosis of anxiety

confirmed ADHD diagnosis. Following ADHD diagnosis, pharmacological ADHD treatment was recommended for 146/189 patients (77%). Most were prescribed OROS-MPH or other methylphenidate formulations (130/189 [69%]), while atomoxetine and lisdexamfetamine dimesylate were prescribed to 8/189 patients (4%) and 5/189 patients (3%), respectively.

Somatic comorbidities affected 145/189 patients (77%) at enrolment. The most frequently reported conditions were pain (36/189 [19%]), gastrointestinal disorders

(32/189 [17%]), and allergy (27/189 [14%]; Table 3). Just over one-third of patients (69/189 [37%]) had been prescribed medication for these comorbidities.

Patient-reported measures and HRQoL subgroup analyses

The mean ASRS-v.1.1 Symptom checklist score in the study population was 47.4 (SD, 13.0), indicating that the majority of patients regularly experienced multiple ADHD symptoms (Table 4). Depressive symptoms were also common, as indicated by the mean MADRS-S score of 19.8 (SD, 9.2). The mean EQ-5D index score was 0.63 (SD, 0.28), indicating poor HRQoL in the study population.

Subgroup analysis was used to identify trends associated with low EQ-5D index scores (indicating poor HRQoL) in the patient population (Fig. 1). Mean EQ-5D index scores tended to be lower in older patients than in younger patients, with the lowest mean index score recorded in patients aged 50 years or above (Fig. 1). Other variables associated with low EQ-5D index scores included patient-rated severe depressive symptoms (MADRS-S score ≥ 30), an ASRS-v.1.1 score of 60 or greater, and having multiple comorbid psychiatric disorders.

HRQoL predictor analysis

In the multivariate regression model, a high MADRS-S score (≥ 30) was the strongest predictor of low EQ-5D index scores (adjusted mean, − 0.40; $P < 0.001$, compared with scores between 1 and 11; Fig. 2). MINI-identified anxiety and depression ($P < 0.001$) and having three or more MINI-identified diagnoses ($P = 0.002$) were also strong predictors, compared with having no MINI-identified diagnoses (Fig. 2).

Adjusted mean EQ-5D index scores were significantly higher in men than in women ($P = 0.049$), in patients with secondary education than in those without ($P = 0.004$), and in patients whose main income source was full- or part-time employment, compared with those reliant on other sources ($P = 0.03$, Fig. 2). Adult ASRS-v.1.1 Symptom checklist or DIVA 2.0 scores were not significant predictors of EQ-5D index score ($P \geq 0.05$; Fig. 2).

Almost one quarter (22%) of the patient population had a WAIS-IV score of < 85 but there was no significant association between high WAIS-IV scores and HRQoL.

Discussion

Adult patients with newly diagnosed ADHD experienced a considerable disease burden and substantially impaired HRQoL in this retrospective chart review. Psychiatric comorbidities were common in the study population, and linear regression analysis identified comorbid anxiety and depression as key factors contributing to poor HRQoL. MADRS-S score was the strongest predictor of EQ-5D index score, implying an association between severe depression and poor HRQoL in adult patients with ADHD. Other variables, including low educational attainment, low levels of employment, and female sex were also associated with poor HRQoL in the study population.

Both the strengths and weaknesses of this study should be considered when interpreting the results. The study included a moderately large number of patients and integrated in-depth analyses of patients' neuropsychiatric evaluations with a variety of patient- and clinician-reported measures, including HRQoL. The variety of information extracted from the EMRs enabled the investigation of a wide range of potential factors impacting HRQoL in adult patients with ADHD. HRQoL was assessed using the EQ-5D, a validated generic HRQoL tool that provides health utility estimates and is recommended by the UK National Institute for Health and Care Excellence [22]. The use of the generic EQ-5D permits comparisons with reference populations and patients with other diseases [22].

There are, however, several limitations that should be noted. First, data for some parameters were missing for a substantial proportion of patients, which may have introduced bias. To address this, a multiple imputation

Table 4 Patient-reported measures of ADHD symptoms, depression, and HRQoL

Measure	Danderyd ($n = 101$)		Liljeholmen ($n = 88$)		Overall ($N = 189$)	
	n	Mean (SD)	n	Mean (SD)	n	Mean (SD)
ASRS-v1.1 score						
Screener	1	–	65	5.0 (1.0)	66	5.0 (1.0)
Symptom checklist	98	46.4 (13.0)	11	56.6 (8.7)	109	47.4 (13.0)
MADRS-S score[a]	93	20.3 (9.6)	72	19.1 (8.5)	165	19.8 (9.2)
EQ-5D						
Index score	95	0.64 (0.27)	67	0.61 (0.30)	162	0.63 (0.28)
VAS	91	58.1 (21.2)	66	56.4 (23.5)	157	57.4 (22.1)

ADHD attention-deficit/hyperactivity disorder, *ASRS-v1.1* Adult ADHD Self-Report Scale version 1.1, *EQ-5D* five-dimension EuroQol questionnaire, *HRQoL* health-related quality of life, *MADRS-S* Montgomery–Åsberg Depression Rating Scale – Self-reported, *PHQ-9* Patient Health Questionnaire 9, *SD* standard deviation, *VAS* visual analog scale

[a]MADRS-S scores were converted from PHQ-9 scores for 72 patients from Liljeholmen and one patient from Danderyd using a regression equation (MADRS-S = [1.206 × PHQ-9] + 4.062)

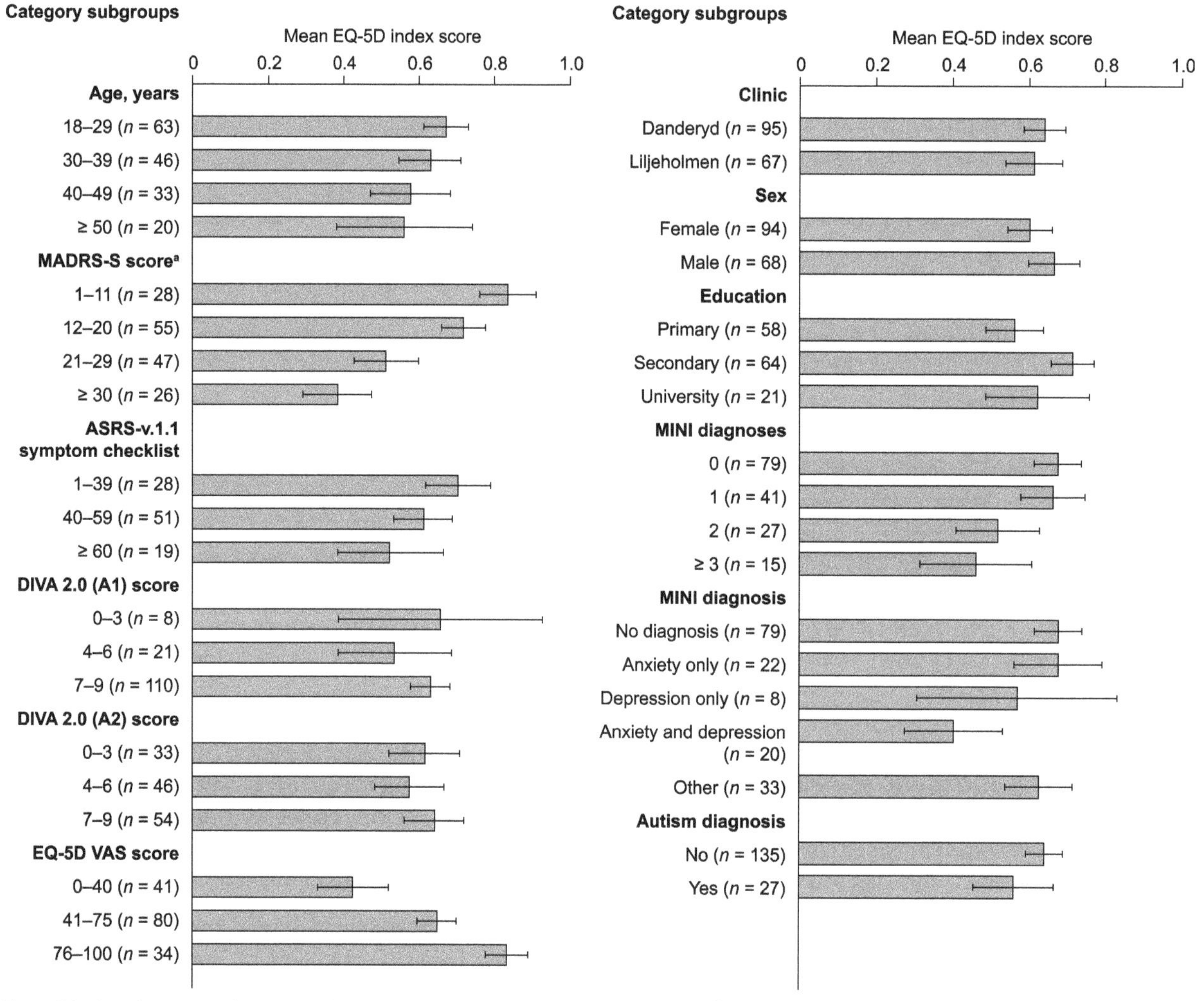

Fig. 1 EQ-5D index score subgroup analysis. Error bars show 95% confidence intervals. [a]MADRS-S derived from PHQ-9 score for patients enrolled at Liljeholmen (1.206 × PHQ-9) + 4.062. ADHD: attention-deficit/hyperactivity disorder; ASRS-v1.1: Adult ADHD Self-Report Scale version 1.1; DIVA 2.0: Diagnostic Interview for ADHD in Adults, second edition (A1: Attention deficit; A2: hyperactivity/impulsivity); EQ-5D: 5-dimension EuroQol questionnaire; MADRS-S: Montgomery–Åsberg Depression Rating Scale – Self-reported; MINI: Mini International Neuropsychiatric Interview; PHQ-9: Patient Health Questionnaire 9; VAS: visual analog scale

model was utilized to estimate missing data for the regression model. However, this method may also influence results, particularly when sample sizes are limited. Data were missing for fewer than 20% of the total patients across both sites for all imputed variables except ASRS-v.1.1 score, which was missing for 88% of Liljeholmen patients (Additional file 1: Table S1). This implies that the ASRS-v.1.1 may not be part of the routine diagnostic procedure at Liljeholmen. The high proportion of imputed data for this variable in the linear regression model precludes any reliable conclusions concerning the relationship between ASRS-v.1.1 score and HRQoL in adult patients with ADHD. Secondly, covariates for the statistical models were selected based on the data available, but other factors influencing HRQoL may not have been captured in the study. Thirdly, comorbid psychiatric diagnoses were based on the MINI for all psychiatric disorders except autism. Inclusion of autism as a separate covariate in the analyses may have led to underestimation of the impact of psychiatric comorbidities on patients' HRQoL. Other limitations to consider are the absence of a comparative control sample of EQ-5D index scores from the Swedish population and the recruitment of patients only in the city of Stockholm.

The findings of the present study strongly suggest that adult patients with ADHD experience reduced HRQoL, and support the conclusion that the manifestations of ADHD are associated with considerable disease burden. The mean EQ-5D index score in the patient population was 0.63 (SD, 0.28), which is markedly lower than published EQ-5D index scores for the healthy adult population in Sweden (range, 0.74–0.89) [23] and in the UK

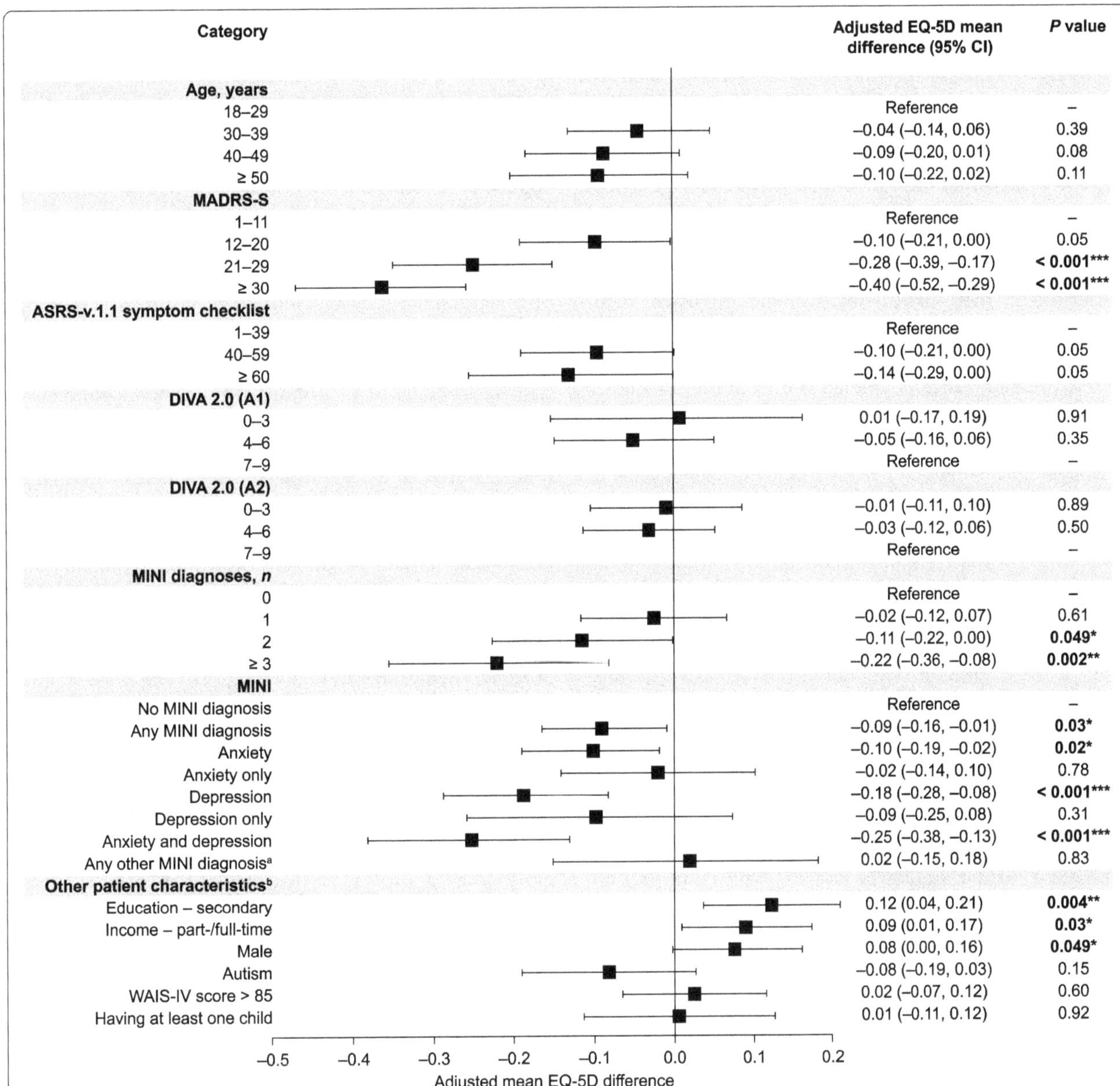

Fig. 2 EQ-5D index score linear regression model. $^{*}P < 0.05$, $^{**}P < 0.01$, $^{***}P < 0.001$. Error bars show 95% confidence intervals. [a]Any MINI diagnosis other than anxiety and depression. [b]Reference populations for binary variables (other patient characteristics): education, secondary or university vs. no secondary; main income from full- or part-time employment vs. other sources; male sex vs. female sex; autism, confirmed diagnosis vs. no diagnosis. "Reference" indicates subgroup used for statistical comparisons with other subgroups. *p* values rounded to nearest 0.01 decimal places. ADHD: attention-deficit/hyperactivity disorder; ASRS: Adult ADHD Self-Report Scale version 1.1; CI: confidence interval; DIVA 2.0: Diagnostic Interview for ADHD in Adults, second edition (A1: Attention Deficit; A2: hyperactivity/impulsivity); EQ-5D: 5-dimension EuroQol questionnaire; MADRS-S: Montgomery–Åsberg Depression Rating Scale – Self-reported; MINI: Mini International Neuropsychiatric Interview; WAIS-IV: Wechsler Adult Intelligence Scale IV

(mean, 0.86; SD, 0.28) [24]. Similarly, low EQ-5D index scores have been reported for patients with other chronic conditions including asthma, chronic obstructive pulmonary disease, diabetes, epilepsy, heart failure, and stroke (overall mean index score, 0.73) [25]. The mean EQ-5D index score in the present study is also within the range reported in a systematic review of HRQoL in adults with psoriasis (0.52–0.9) [26], but higher than that reported for people with spinal complaints (0.39) [27]. The applicability of the present study's findings to cultural/social groups outside Stockholm is uncertain, although a recent study involving seven countries concluded that the impact of ADHD on patient well-being is consistent across different socioeconomic groups [13]. Furthermore, the EQ-5D scores in the present study are similar to those reported for adult patients with ADHD in other European countries [28, 29], suggesting a broad relevance of the present findings.

To our knowledge, this is the first study to use linear regression to identify specific factors that may influence HRQoL in adult patients with ADHD. Comorbid anxiety and depression, together with patient-rated severe depressive symptoms, were identified as the strongest predictors of poor HRQoL. Given that these diagnoses are frequently comorbid with ADHD, the potential negative impact of these disorders upon patients' HRQoL should be considered in their clinical management. Adjusted mean EQ-5D index scores were also significantly higher in men than in women, who made up 57% of the patient population. A preponderance of women is uncommon in studies of ADHD, which is diagnosed more frequently in men than in women [2]. Gender is not thought to modulate the phenotypic presentation of ADHD [30], but higher rates of comorbid anxiety disorders have been reported in women than in men [31], which could contribute to the gender difference in HRQoL in the present study.

Psychiatric disorders other than depression and anxiety were common, affecting 19% of the patient population. However, only 3% of the patients in the present study were diagnosed with comorbid bipolar disorder. This is in contrast with the results of the National Comorbidity Study which reported a bipolar disorder prevalence of 19.4% among adults with ADHD [32]. It is possible that the unusually low frequency of bipolar disorder may have influenced the relationship between comorbid psychiatric disorders and HRQoL in the present study, and further studies in patients with comorbid bipolar disorder may be warranted. Over two-thirds of the patient population (77%) also reported at least one somatic comorbidity. Pain was the most frequently reported somatic comorbidity. Individuals with ADHD are more prone to accidents and injuries [33], may be more sensitive to pain [34], and may experience motor inhibition problems and heightened muscle tone [35]. Multiple studies have identified a high incidence of joint hypermobility in individuals with ADHD [36], which may also have contributed to the high prevalence of pain in the present study. Adults with ADHD are more likely to have somatic disorders, and are more likely to use non-psychiatric healthcare services, than those without ADHD [37]. In particular, somatic disorders such as obesity, sleep disorders, and asthma frequently co-occur with ADHD [38]. ADHD symptoms and functional impairment may make people with ADHD more vulnerable to somatic diseases and may affect their ability to obtain appropriate diagnosis and treatment for somatic disease. Optimum care for patients with ADHD may involve an integrated and multidisciplinary approach for identifying and treating co-occurring psychiatric and somatic disorders [39].

Other predictors of poor HRQoL included poor educational achievement and not having a main income derived from employment. In the present study, primary school was the highest level of education reached for 37% of adults with newly diagnosed ADHD, and only 13% were educated to university level. In comparison, equivalent levels in the general Stockholm population in 2014 were reported to be 16 and 45%, respectively [40]. Having an average or higher intelligence score (denoted by a WAIS-IV score of more than 85) was not significantly associated with improved HRQoL, implying that the challenges faced by patients with ADHD in school extend beyond deficits in intellectual functioning. The present results also suggest that difficulties continue into the workplace. Despite a median age of 33 years, fewer than half of the patients were able to support themselves financially through employment or self-employment, and 22% were reliant on sickness benefit as their main source of income. Thus, the present study highlights the significant impact that poor performance in school and the workplace can have on HRQoL and emphasizes the need for early diagnosis and effective clinical management of ADHD symptoms from a young age. The present study was not designed to investigate the impact of ADHD medication on HRQoL in individuals with ADHD, but a recent systematic review concluded that ADHD medication may help to reduce functional impairment and to improve HRQoL deficits [41].

European guidelines recommend an individualized, multimodal approach to treatment of ADHD in adults, including psychological treatments and medication [12]. In the present study, over two-thirds (77%) of patients were prescribed pharmacological treatment for ADHD. This figure is in line with guidance from the Swedish National Board of Health and Welfare indicating that ADHD medication is likely to be effective and appropriate in the majority of patients [42].

Conclusions

In summary, the findings of this non-interventional, retrospective study indicate that undiagnosed ADHD contributes to poor HRQoL in adults presenting with psychiatric symptoms. Furthermore, the impact of ADHD on HRQoL may be exacerbated by psychiatric comorbidities such as anxiety and depression. Adults with newly diagnosed ADHD and comorbid depression or anxiety may require particular care and resources in their management.

Abbreviations

ADHD: Attention-deficit/hyperactivity disorder; ASRS-v1.1: Adult ADHD Self-Report Scale version 1.1; DIVA 2.0: Diagnostic Interview for ADHD in Adults, second edition (A1: Attention deficit; A2: Hyperactivity/impulsivity); EQ-5D: 5-dimension EuroQol questionnaire; HRQoL: Health-related quality of life; MADRS-S: Montgomery–Åsberg Depression Rating Scale – Self-reported; MINI: Mini International Neuropsychiatric Interview; PHQ-9: Patient Health Questionnaire 9; SD: Standard deviation; VAS: Visual analogue scale; WAIS-IV: Wechsler Adult Intelligence Scale IV

Acknowledgements
The authors thank the patients and investigators involved in the study. Under the direction of the authors, Dr. M. Cottingham and Dr. K. Dodd of Oxford PharmaGenesis, Cardiff, UK, provided writing assistance for this publication. Editorial assistance in formatting, proofreading, and copyediting the manuscript, fact-checking, and coordination and collation of comments was also provided by Oxford PharmaGenesis. Shire International GmbH provided funding to Oxford PharmaGenesis for support in writing, editing, and managing this manuscript.

Funding
This study was funded by Shire Sweden AB. Shire International GmbH provided funding to Oxford PharmaGenesis for support in writing, editing, and managing this manuscript. Shire also reviewed and edited the manuscript for scientific accuracy. Although employees of Shire were involved in the design, collection, analysis, interpretation, and fact-checking of the information, the authors produced the content for this paper, interpreted the data, and decided on the submission of the manuscript for publication in *BMC Psychiatry* independently.

Authors' contributions
EA, AF, EM, JS, and YG developed the study concept and design. EA, MD, EM, JS, and YG were responsible for data acquisition, analysis, and interpretation. EA, MD, AF, EM, JS, and YG developed, reviewed, and edited the manuscript content for important intellectual content. All authors approved the final manuscript version.

Consent for publication
Not applicable.

Competing interests
Dr. Ewa Ahnemark is an employee of Shire and owns stock or stock options. The following authors have received compensation for serving as consultants or speakers for, or they or the institutions they work for have received research support or royalties from, the companies or organizations indicated: Dr. Marianne Di Schiena (Prima Child and Adult Psychiatry AB); Dr. Anne-Christine Fredman (Evolan, Lilly, Novartis, Servier, and Shire); Dr. Emma Medin (PAREXEL International); Dr. Jonas. K. Söderling (COMBINE Sweden, Novo Nordisk, and PAREXEL International); Dr. Ylva Ginsberg (Eli Lilly, HB Pharma, Janssen-Cilag, Lundbeck, and Novartis).

Author details
[1]Shire, Vasagatan 7, SE-111 20 Stockholm, Sweden. [2]Prima Child and Adult Psychiatry AB, Stockholm, Sweden. [3]PAREXEL International, Stockholm, Sweden. [4]Department of Learning, Informatics, Management and Ethics, Karolinska Institute, Stockholm, Sweden. [5]Bell Analytics, Stockholm, Sweden. [6]Department of Medical Epidemiology and Biostatistics, Karolinska Institute, Stockholm, Sweden. [7]Department of Clinical Neuroscience, Centre for Psychiatry Research, Karolinska Institute, Stockholm, Sweden. [8]Present Address: Psychiatry Centre, Stockholm County Council, Södertälje, Sweden.

References

1. Goodman DW, Mitchell S, Rhodewalt L, Surman CB. Clinical presentation, diagnosis and treatment of attention-deficit hyperactivity disorder (ADHD) in older adults: a review of the evidence and its implications for clinical care. Drugs Aging. 2016;33(1):27–36.
2. Willcutt EG. The prevalence of DSM-IV attention-deficit/hyperactivity disorder: a meta-analytic review. Neurotherapeutics. 2012;9:490–9.
3. Simon V, Czobor P, Balint S, Meszaros A, Bitter I. Prevalence and correlates of adult attention-deficit hyperactivity disorder: meta-analysis. Br J Psychiatry. 2009;194:204–11.
4. Biederman J. Advances in the neurobiology of ADHD. CNS Spectrums. 2007;12:6–7.
5. Faraone SV, Biederman J, Mick E. The age-dependent decline of attention deficit hyperactivity disorder: a meta-analysis of follow-up studies. Psychol Med. 2006;36:159–65.
6. Nylander L, Holmqvist M, Gustafson L, Gillberg C. ADHD in adult psychiatry. Minimum rates and clinical presentation in general psychiatry outpatients. Nord J Psychiatry. 2009;63:64–71.
7. Ginsberg Y, Hirvikoski T, Lindefors N. Attention deficit hyperactivity disorder (ADHD) among longer-term prison inmates is a prevalent, persistent and disabling disorder. BMC Psychiatry. 2010;10:112.
8. Agnew-Blais JC, Polanczyk GV, Danese A, Wertz J, Moffitt TE, Arseneault L. Evaluation of the persistence, remission, and emergence of attention-deficit/hyperactivity disorder in young adulthood. JAMA Psychiatry. 2016;73:713–20.
9. Caye A, Rocha T, Anselmi L, et al. Attention-deficit/hyperactivity disorder trajectories from childhood to young adulthood: evidence from a birth cohort supporting a late-onset syndrome. JAMA Psychiatry. 2016;73:705–12.
10. Giacobini M, Medin E, Ahnemark E, Russo LJ, Carlqvist P. Prevalence, patient characteristics, and pharmacological treatment of children, adolescents, and adults diagnosed with ADHD in Sweden. J Atten Disord. 2014; https://doi.org/10.1177/1087054714554617.
11. Nylander L, Holmqvist M, Gustafson L, Gillberg C. Attention-deficit/hyperactivity disorder (ADHD) and autism spectrum disorder (ASD) in adult psychiatry. A 20-year register study. Nord J Psychiatry. 2013;67:344–50.
12. Kooij SJ, Bejerot S, Blackwell A, Caci H, Casas-Brugué M, Carpentier PJ, et al. European consensus statement on diagnosis and treatment of adult ADHD: the European network adult ADHD. BMC Psychiatry. 2010;10:67.
13. Brod M, Pohlman B, Lasser R, Hodgkins P. Comparison of the burden of illness for adults with ADHD across seven countries: a qualitative study. Health Qual Life Outcomes. 2012;10:47.
14. Brod M, Schmitt E, Goodwin M, Hodgkins P, Niebler G. ADHD burden of illness in older adults: a life course perspective. Qual Life Res. 2012;21:795–9.
15. Gusi N, Olivares PR, Rajendram R. The EQ-5D health-related quality of life questionnaire. In: Preedy VR, Watson RR, editors. Handbook of disease burdens and quality of life measures. New York: Springer New York; 2010. p. 87–99.
16. World Health Organization. International statistical classification of diseases and related health problems, tenth revision. Geneva: World Health Organization; 2010.
17. Adler L, Kessler RC, Spencer T. Adult ADHD self-report scale-v1. 1 (ASRS-v1. 1) symptom checklist. New York: World Health Organization; 2003.
18. Lecrubier Y, Sheehan DV, Weiller E, Amorim P, Bonora I, Harnett Sheehan K, et al. The Mini international neuropsychiatric interview (MINI). A short diagnostic structured interview: reliability and validity according to the CIDI. Eur Psychiatry. 1997;12:224–31.
19. American Psychiatric Association. Diagnostic and statistical manual of mental disorders. 4th ed., text revision. Washington DC: American Psychiatric Association; 2000.
20. Fantino B, Moore N. The self-reported Montgomery–Åsberg depression rating scale is a useful evaluative tool in major depressive disorder. BMC Psychiatry. 2009;9:26.
21. Hawley CJ, Gale TM, Smith PS, Jain S, Farag A, Kondan R, et al. Equations for converting scores between depression scales (MADRS, SRS, PHQ-9 and BDI-II): good statistical, but weak idiographic, validity. Hum Psychopharmacol. 2013;28:544–51.
22. NICE. Guide to the methods of technology appraisal 2013. National Institute for health and care excellence; 2013. Retrieved from: http://publications.nice.org.uk/pmg9

23. Burstrom K, Johannesson M, Diderichsen F. Swedish population health-related quality of life results using the EQ-5D. Qual Life Res. 2001;10:621–35.
24. Kind P, Hardman G, Macran S. UK Population Norms for EQ-5D. University of York Centre for Health Economics Discussion Paper: 1721999.
25. Peters M, Crocker H, Jenkinson C, Doll H, Fitzpatrick R. The routine collection of patient-reported outcome measures (PROMs) for long-term conditions in primary care: a cohort survey. BMJ Open. 2014;4:e003968.
26. Moller AH, Erntoft S, Vinding GR, Jemec GB. A systematic literature review to compare quality of life in psoriasis with other chronic diseases using EQ-5D-derived utility values. Patient Relat Outcome Meas. 2015;6:167–77.
27. McDonough CM, Grove MR, Tosteson TD, Lurie JD, Hilibrand AS, Tosteson AN. Comparison of EQ-5D, HUI, and SF-36-derived societal health state values among spine patient outcomes research trial (SPORT) participants. Qual Life Res. 2005;14:1321–32.
28. Karlsdotter K, Bushe C, Hakkaart L, Sobanski E, Kan CC, Lebrec J, et al. Burden of illness and health care resource utilization in adult psychiatric outpatients with attention-deficit/hyperactivity disorder in Europe. Curr Med Res Opin. 2016;32:1547–56.
29. van Hout B, Janssen MF, Feng YS, Kohlmann T, Busschbach J, Golicki D, et al. Interim scoring for the EQ-5D-5L: mapping the EQ-5D-5L to EQ-5D-3L value sets. Value Health. 2012;15:708–15.
30. Biederman J, Faraone SV, Monuteaux MC, et al. Gender effects on attention-deficit/hyperactivity disorder in adults, revisited. Biol Psychiatry. 2004;55:692–700.
31. Wilens TE, Biederman J, Faraone SV, Martelon M, Westerberg D, Spencer TJ. Presenting ADHD symptoms, subtypes, and comorbid disorders in clinically referred adults with ADHD. J Clin Psychiatry. 2009;70:1557–62.
32. Kessler RC, Adler L, Barkley R, Biederman J, Conners CK, Demler O, Faraone SV, Greenhill LL, Howes MJ, Secnik K, et al. The prevalence and correlates of adult ADHD in the United States: results from the National Comorbidity Survey Replication. Am J Psychiatry. 2006;163:716–23.
33. Swensen A, Birnbaum HG, Ben Hamadi R, Greenberg P, Cremieux PY, Secnik K. Incidence and costs of accidents among attention-deficit/hyperactivity disorder patients. J Adolesc Health. 2004;35:346.e1–9.
34. Roi T, Elon E, Naor D, Dorit P. Alterations in pain response are partially reversed by methylphenidate (Ritalin) in adults with attention deficit hyperactivity disorder (ADHD). Pain Practice. 2015;15:4–11.
35. Stray LL, Kristensen Ø, Lomeland M, Skorstad M, Stray T, Tønnessen FE. Motor regulation problems and pain in adults diagnosed with ADHD. Behav Brain Funct. 2013;9:18.
36. Baeza-Velasco C, Grahame R, Bravo JF. A connective tissue disorder may underlie ESSENCE problems in childhood. Res Dev Disabil. 2017;60:232–42.
37. Hodgkins P, Montejano L, Sasané R, Huse D. Cost of illness and comorbidities in adults diagnosed with attention-deficit/hyperactivity disorder: a retrospective analysis. Prim Care Companion CNS Disorders. 2011;13:e1–e12.
38. Instanes JT, Klungsøyr K, Halmøy A, Fasmer OB, Haavik J. Adult ADHD and comorbid somatic disease: a systematic literature review. J Atten Disord. 2016; https://doi.org/10.1177/1087054716669589.
39. Muskens JB, Velders FP, Staal WG. Medical comorbidities in children and adolescents with autism spectrum disorders and attention deficit hyperactivity disorders: a systematic review. Eur Child Adolesc Psychiatry. 2017;26:1093–103.
40. Statistics Sweden: http://www.scb.se/. Accessed 19 May 2017.
41. Coghill DR, Banaschewski T, Soutullo C, Cottingham MG, Zuddas A. Systematic review of quality of life and functional outcomes in randomized placebo-controlled studies of medications for attention-deficit/hyperactivity disorder. Eur Child Adolesc Psychiatry. 2017;26:1283–307.
42. The National Board of Health and Welfare. Pharmacological treatment of ADHD in children and adults. Sweden; 2015.

13

Heterozygous deletion of *SCN2A* and *SCN3A* in a patient with autism spectrum disorder and Tourette syndrome

Kathrin Nickel[1*], Ludger Tebartz van Elst[1], Katharina Domschke[1], Birgitta Gläser[2], Friedrich Stock[2], Dominique Endres[1], Simon Maier[1] and Andreas Riedel[1]

Abstract

Background: Mutations in voltage-gated sodium channel (*SCN*) genes are supposed to be of importance in the etiology of psychiatric and neurological diseases, in particular in the etiology of seizures. Previous studies report a potential susceptibility region at the chromosomal locus 2q including *SCN1A*, *SCN2A* and *SCN3A* genes for autism spectrum disorder (ASD). To date, there is no previous description of a patient with comorbid ASD and Tourette syndrome showing a deletion containing *SCN2A* and *SCN3A*.

Case presentation: We present the unique complex case of a 28-year-old male patient suffering from developmental retardation and exhibiting a range of behavioral traits since birth. He received the diagnoses of ASD (in early childhood) and of Tourette syndrome (in adulthood) according to ICD-10 and DSM-5 criteria. Investigations of underlying genetic factors yielded a heterozygous microdeletion of approximately 719 kb at 2q24.3 leading to a deletion encompassing the five genes *SCN2A* (exon 1 to intron 14–15), *SCN3A*, *GRB14* (exon 1 to intron 2–3), *COBLL1* and *SCL38A11*.

Conclusions: We discuss the association of *SCN2A*, *SCN3A*, *GRB14*, *COBLL1* and *SCL38A11* deletions with ASD and Tourette syndrome and possible implications for treatment.

Keywords: Autism spectrum disorder (ASD), Tourette syndrome, *SCN2A*, *SCN3A*

Background

Mutations in neuronal voltage gated sodium channel genes such as *SCN1A*, *SCN2A* and *SCN3A* are supposed to play an important role in psychiatric disorders and neurological diseases [1]. These three sodium channel genes encoding distinct α-subunit isoforms are clustered within 600 kB on chromosome 2q24 and are highly expressed in neurons and glia throughout the central and peripheral nervous system [2, 3].

Genome-wide scan studies for autism susceptibility genes reported a potential susceptibility region at locus 2q including *SCN1A*, *SCN2A* and *SCN3A* genes [4, 5].

Dravet-Syndrome (DS) is a childhood disorder associated with mainly loss-of-function mutations in the *SCN1A* gene. It is characterized by frequent seizures and devastating effects on cognitive and behavioural development, persisting into adulthood [6]. While approximately 70–80% of DS patients show mutations in *SCN1A*, some patients have variants in other genes including *SCN2A* [7].

Mutations of the *SCN2A* gene have also been reported in patients with autism [8] as well as with benign familial infantile seizures, intractable epilepsy, infantile spasms and severe myoclonic epilepsy of infancy [9–12].

Previous investigations mainly led to case reports with deletions on chromosome 2q24 being associated with seizures complicated by neurobehavioral comorbidities such as cognitive impairment, psychiatric disorders and social problems [13–15]. To date, there are only two published cases with deletions on chromosome 2q24 displaying a phenotype with autistic features and developmental delay, but no seizures: Celle et al. [2] described the case of a 3-year old boy presenting with autistic

* Correspondence: kathrin.nickel@uniklinik-freiburg.de
[1]Section for Experimental Neuropsychiatry, Department of Psychiatry and Psychotherapy, Medical Center – University of Freiburg, Faculty of Medicine, University of Freiburg, Hauptstraße 5, D-79104 Freiburg, Germany

features, language delay, microcephaly and no history of seizures. He had an interstitial deletion of ~ 291.9 kb at band 2q24.3 with loss of the entire *SCN2A* gene and part of the *SCN3A* gene. Another case report described a 3 years and 4 months old girl with autistic features, developmental delay, mental retardation, language impairment and dysmorphic features, who carried a 2.8 Mb de novo deletion on chromosome 2q24.2 containing nine genes including *SCN2A2, SCN3A, GRB14* and *COBLL1* as well as *LOC643397, FLJ39822, LOC643405, FIGN* and *TAIP-2* [16]. Until now, there is no description of a patient with *SCN* gene mutations and autism spectrum disorder (ASD) with additional symptoms of Tourette syndrome.

Case presentation

We present the unique case of a 28-year-old male patient displaying a complex clinical picture with mental retardation and various behavioural problems since birth. Symptoms of the autism spectrum comprising difficulties in social interaction and communication are reported since childhood. Additionally, he suffers from auto-aggressive tics in terms of beating himself with objects against his head and lower jaw, head movement tics and simple vocal tics. Striking dysmorphic features are not evident.

Developmental and somatic history

Except a one-time bleeding in week 20 of gestation, pregnancy had been without any complications. No infections, medication, smoking, or intake of alcohol or drugs during pregnancy was reported. The patient was delivered in week 40 of gestation with the help of a ventouse due to irregular cardiac activity. During delivery there were minor signs of birth asphyxia. Birth weight was 2.900 g (25th percentile), birth length 51 cm (50th percentile) and head circumference 33 cm (<3rd percentile). During infancy a prominent frontal fissure was conspicuous. A premature ossification of the sagittal fissure could not be detected.

The patient showed psychomotor retardation: he walked alone only by 26 months and was not able to sit alone falling over to one side without shoring up even at the age of 2. Furthermore, tics in terms of eye blinking as well as a muscular hypotonia were described. The patient's parents reported early autistic features such as difficulties in social communication and interaction with avoiding eye contact and poor interest in social interaction. Development of speech was delayed (first words with 18 months). He refused body contact and demonstrated stereotypic patterns of behaviour such as filling bowls without showing any variations.

When examined at the age of 27 months, the patient presented some special facial features such as synophrys, epicanthus, modelled ears, a deep joined thumb and microcephaly. His weight was 10 kg (3rd percentile), his length 88 cm (25th percentile) and his head circumference 46 cm (2 cm above the 3rd percentile). The patient only spoke a few words and never a whole sentence. Mostly, he only repeated the words he had heard before in terms of an echolalia. A considerable general delay of development with severe perceptual disturbance and autistic traits was diagnosed.

Since the age of two years, the patient shows relevant aggressive symptoms such as throwing his head on the floor or biting into items. He needs extensive support concerning all activities of daily living and requires constant daily routines. During nursery school, auto-aggressive symptoms exacerbated in terms of head banging behaviour injuring his jaw and ears. At the age of 3 years, he started grinding his teeth. Later on, he presented head throwing movements against his left shoulder and banging of one row of his teeth against the other. There was a pattern of aggravation of the tic symptoms during stressful situations. He repeatedly showed refusal of meals and sleeping disturbances. At the age of 3 years, once there was a query febrile convulsion associated with an infection. Apart from that, there was no evidence for further seizures and clearly no epilepsy.

According to ICD-10 and DSM-5 classification, the clinical features of the patient are consistent with early infantile autism as well as with Tourette syndrome.

In the clinical examination, the patient presented with cauliflower-ears as a result of his head banging behaviour and subsequent repetitive ear injuries as well as various injuries of all kinds and healing stages. Dysmorphic features or additional external malformations were not noted, there was no evidence of internal abnormalities (heart, eye, inner ear) either. The patient showed a preserved ability of speech comprehension with rare speech production.

Family history

Our patient is the first son of non-consanguineous healthy German parents. His younger brother (24 years old) was diagnosed with an autism spectrum disorder (Asperger syndrome). There was no evidence of syndromal-secondary autism in the brother. He did not show intellectual impairment, dysmorphic signs or organic conditions such as a heart malformation or epilepsy. The mother's paternal grandparents were cousins. They had five healthy children. In their further progeny three mentally retarded persons were reported, one granddaughter (died at the age of approximately 27 years) and two great-grandchildren (a boy and a girl). The exact diagnosis was unknown to our patient's parents. Consanguinity of the retarded relatives' parents was denied. One of the patient's cousins (the son of his father's brother) was said to suffer from clinically apparent dyslexia and perhaps an autism spectrum disorder. A disablement of a cousin of our patient's father (son of his father's sister) could not be specified further. An assessment of the father revealed no clinical characteristics, neither with respect to striking dysmorphic features, the occurrence of tics nor with respect to autistic symptoms. Further relatives with neurodevelopmental disorders were not reported on the father's side of the family.

Cytogenetic and array-analysis

Conventional R-banded karyotyping of the patient was performed according to standard protocols with a resolution of approximately 500 bphs and revealed a structurally and numerically normal male karyotype (46,XY) in all 21 metaphases examined.

Furthermore, the genomic DNA of the patient was examined by microarray-analysis (CytoSureTM Constitutional v3 Array 180 k, OGT (Oxford Gene Technology)) according to the manufacturer's instructions. After hybridization, the array was scanned with the SureScan Microarray scanner (Agilent), the results were analyzed using CytoSure interpret software v.4.9 (OGT) against the Genome Reference Consortium human genome GRCh37 (hg19). Molecular karyotyping revealed a heterozygous deletion of approximately 719 kb (267 contiguous oligonucleotides) out of the chromosomal region 2q24.3 (karyotype according to ISCN (International System for Human Cytogenetic Nomenclature) (2016): arr[GRCh37] 2q24.3(165471418_166190427)× 1). The deletion encompasses the five genes *GRB14* (exon 1 to intron 2–3), *COBLL1*, *SLC38A11*, *SCN3A* and *SCN2A* (exon 1 to intron 14–15) listed in OMIM (Online Mendelian Inheritance in Man) (Fig. 1). With FISH (fluorescence in situ hybridization) analysis using probe RP11-150F4 (Empire Genomics) located at 2q24.3 the deletion could be confirmed. There is no evidence in literature that the microdeletion we detected is a common variant in the Caucasian population [17, 18]. "Orphanet" states a prevalence rate of a 2q24 microdeletion < 1/1000000 (worldwide) (https://www.orpha.net/data/patho/GB/uk-2q24.pdf).

The subsequently performed chromosome analysis of the parents, FISH with RP11-150F4 included, showed a normal female karyotype in the mother and a normal male karyotype in the father with no evidence of a deletion or rearrangement at 2q24.3. Therefore, it can be asserted that the deletion in the patient is a de novo mutation. The patient's younger brother (suffering from Asperger syndrome) was shown to have a normal male karyotype without a deletion or rearrangement at 2q24.3.

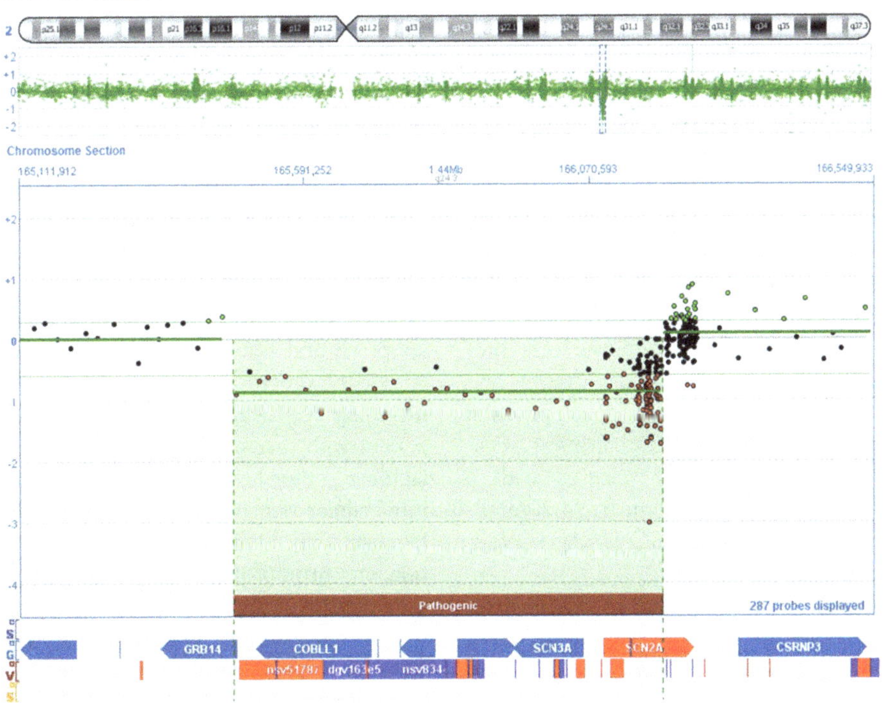

Fig. 1 Results of microarray-analysis. Molecular karyotyping revealed a deletion of approximately 719 kb out of the chromosomal region 2q24.3 encompassing the 5 genes *GRB14* (exon 1 to intron 2–3), *COBLL1*, *SLC38A11*, *SCN3A* and *SCN2A* (exon 1 to intron 14–15) listed in OMIM (Online Mendelian Inheritance in Man)

Other investigations

Magnetic resonance imaging conducted in 2014 showed no abnormalities of the patient's brain. In 1991, a detailed investigation was performed with a metabolic screening of serum, urine and cerebrospinal fluid revealing normal results. In the EEG, there was a slow baseline activity without any epilepsy suspicious potentials. A proton-spectroscopy showed no abnormalities of N-acetyl-aspartate, choline and phosphor-creatinine levels. An ophthalmologic investigation exhibited no deviations. In 1997, gastrointestinal passage was unsuspicious, and in an X-ray of the brain no stenosis of the sagittal fissure was confirmed.

Discussion and conclusions

In the present case report, we describe a 28-year-old male patient with symptoms of an early infantile autism as well as a Tourette syndrome. He carries a 719 kb deletion on chromosome 2q24.3 including the genes *SCN3A* and *SCN2A* which code for voltage-gated sodium channels. To date, no similar case has been described in the literature with respect to the phenotype of autism spectrum disorder plus Tourette syndrome but without epilepsy. The patient showed a global retardation of development (including psychomotor and language delay), various autistic traits, echolalia, severe auto-aggressive symptoms in terms of head banging, tic-specific head movements and vocal tics. There might have been one febrile convulsion at age 3; however, clearly there was no diagnosis of epilepsy. No other seizures had ever been reported. The somatic abnormalities included dysmorphic features such as synophrys, epicanthus, modelled ears, a deep joined thumb and microcephaly.

To date, there are only two case reports referring to patients with autistic features, language impairment, dysmorphic features and no history of seizures presenting a deletion of *SCN2A* and *SCN3A* genes [2, 16]. Chen et al. [16] described the most similar case to the one presented in this report. He presented a 3 years and 4 months old girl with autistic features, developmental delay, mental retardation, language impairment, dysmorphic features and no history of seizures with a 2.8 Mb de novo deletion on chromosome 2q24.2 entailing loss of nine genes including *SCN2A2*, *SCN3A*, *GRB14* and *COBLL1*.

Bartnik et al. [13] identified a de novo ~ 110 kb deletion involving exons 1–2 of *SCN2A* and non-coding exon 1a of *SCN3A* in a 25-year-old female with mental retardation, neurobehavioural and psychiatric abnormalities and a history of infantile seizures. Additionally, there are several other case reports presenting patients with a deletion on chromosome 2q24 with current seizures or a history of seizures [13–15]. In all previous case reports, no additional symptoms of Tourette syndrome have been described to date.

The presently available literature suggests that mutations in *SCN2A* can be causative for ASD, benign familial neonatal infantile seizures, intractable epilepsy, infantile spasms and severe myoclonic epilepsy of infancy [8–12].

Since sodium channels are critical for action potential generation and propagation, a causative association between seizures and sodium channel dysfunction is plausible, whereas it is more difficult to understand this link for ASD and tics [1]. It is proposed that loss of function *SCN1A* mutations associated with seizures cause reduced GABA release leading to an inappropriate inhibition in related neuronal networks [6]. Parvalbumin neurons represent inhibitory GABAergic cells that are involved in various forms of feed-forward inhibition within the striatum [19]. Postmortem studies in patients with Tourette syndrome demonstrate a consistent and profound imbalance of parvalbumin-positive neuronal distribution in the basal ganglia [20]. The selective deficit of parvalbumin-positive and cholinergic striatal interneurons in Tourette syndrome was supposed to result in an impaired cortico/thalamic control of striatal neuron firing [21]. Evidence from studies demonstrates that Na(v)1.2 (the protein encoded by *SCN2A*) is abundant in parvalbumin-positive GABAergic inhibitory interneurons, at least in the hippocampus and the temporal lobe [22].

Apart from *SCN2A* and *SCN3A* genes being affected by the presently detected deletion, *GRB14* (exon 1 to intron 2–3), *COBLL1* and *SLC38A11* were also deleted in our patient. Thus, heterozygous deletion of these genes might also play a pivotal role in conferring ASD symptoms and could even be suggested to confer symptoms of Tourette syndrome in the present case: Loss of *SLC38A11*, a putative sodium-coupled neutral amino acid transporter [23] might enhance the effects of *SCN2A* and *SCN3A* deletion. The *COBLL1* gene, encoding the Cordon-Bleu WH2 Repeat Protein Like 1 was suggested to be a negative regulator of apoptosis and associated with lower insulin resistance [24]. A deletion on chromosome 2q24.4 encompassing 47 genes including *SCN2A2*, *SCN3A* and *COBLL1* was reported in a patient with severe epilepsy [14]. *GRB14* encodes a growth factor receptor-binding protein acting as an inhibitor of intracellular signaling pathways regulating growth and metabolism [25]. One previous investigation reported a deletion on chromosome 2q comprising *GRB14* and *COBLL1* in a patient with autistic features, developmental delay, mental retardation, language impairment and dysmorphic features. In this case, additional repetitive hand movements have been described [2, 16]. Therefore, it is possible that deletions of *GRB14* and *COBLL1* may contribute to tic symptoms. An association of the above mentioned affected genes with Tourette syndrome proper, however, has not been reported in the presently available literature. From our point of view, the deletion therefore adequately explains the patient's symptomatology. Furthermore, whole genome sequencing could provide further information on whether additional mutations/variants are present in the patient's autistic brother contributing to the development of autistic symptoms in the patient.

Concerning treatment of *SCN* gene mutations, existing literature is really scarce. A causal treatment of deletions in chromosomal area 2q24.3 is not available. To date, a substitution of the missing gene products of the patient is not possible.

Promising studies reported a *SCN2A* mutation in a Chinese boy with infantile spasm responding to a modified Atkins Diet [26]. It is an "alternative" ketogenic diet with results demonstrating efficacy in the treatment of intractable seizures [27]. Evidence shows that ketones produced after a modified Atkins Diet could reduce neuron excitability by inhibiting glutamate transport and activating ATP-sensitive potassium channels [28]. Currently, there are no publications available investigating the effect of a ketogenic diet on Tic disorders or Tourette syndrome.

A review concluded that for the treatment of DS, which is often caused by loss-of-function mutations in *SCN1A*, valproate and benzodiazepines should be the first-line treatment but are often insufficient. Topiramate and levetiracetam, bromide and ketogenic diet provide efficacy as adjunctive therapy. Lamotrigine and carbamazepine should be avoided as they are supposed to lead to an increased occurrence of seizures [29]. Another promising drug is stiripentol showing efficacy in a combination with valproate and clobazam [29, 30]. Among patients with DS, a treatment with cannabidiol resulted in a reduction in seizure frequency compared to placebo, nevertheless higher rates of adverse events have been reported [31].

For the future, further research into targeted treatment options for *SCN2A* and *SCN3A* deletions is warranted. Previous studies primarily focused on patients with seizures and reported about medication with antiepileptic drugs or Atkins diets. In our case, the patient presented additional symptoms of Tourette syndrome, but no epilepsy. It remains to be elucidated whether the heterozygous loss of *SCN2A* and *SCN3A* or *GRB14*, *COBLL1* and *SLC38A11*, respectively, might also contribute to the development of tics, which remains subject to investigation in large hypothesis-driven association studies.

Abbreviations

ASD: autism spectrum disorder; ATP: adenosine triphosphate; COBL: Cordon-Bleu; DS: Dravet-Syndrome; DSM: Diagnostic and Statistical Manual of Mental Disorders; EEG: electroencephalography; FISH: fluorescence in situ hybridization; GABA: gamma-aminobutyric acid; GRB: growth factor receptor-bound protein; ICD: International Statistical Classification of Diseases; ISCN: International System for Human Cytogenetic Nomenclature; OGT: Oxford Gene Technology; OMIM: Online Mendelian Inheritance in Man; SCN: sodium voltage-gated channel; SLC: solute carrier

Acknowledgements

Not applicable.

Funding

There is no funding to report.

Authors' contributions

KN, LTvE, KD, DE, SM and AR discussed, analysed and interpreted the patient data regarding clinical presentation, cytogenetic aspects and treatment options. KN, LTvE, KD, DE, SM and AR contributed to the manuscript. BG performed the CGH analysis, interpreted the data with respect to the cytogenetic aspects and created the fig. FS investigated and depicted the family history. KN and AR wrote the manuscript. All authors read and approved the final version of the manuscript.

Authors' information

Not applicable.

Consent for publication

Written informed consent was obtained from the parents of the patient for publication of the case report.

Competing interests

Kathrin Nickel: no conflict of interest. Ludger Tebartz van Elst has received advisory boards, lectures, or travel grants within the last 3 years: Eli Lilly, Janssen-Cilag, Novartis, Shire, UCB, GSK, Servier, Janssen, and Cyberonics. Katharina Domschke: no conflict of interest. Birgitta Gläser: no conflict of interest. Friedrich Stock: no conflict of interest. Dominique Endres: no conflict of interest. Simon Maier: no conflict of interest. Andreas Riedel: no conflict of interest.

Author details

[1]Section for Experimental Neuropsychiatry, Department of Psychiatry and Psychotherapy, Medical Center – University of Freiburg, Faculty of Medicine, University of Freiburg, Hauptstraße 5, D-79104 Freiburg, Germany. [2]Institute of Human Genetics, Medical Center – University of Freiburg, Faculty of Medicine, University of Freiburg, Breisacher Straße 33, D-79106 Freiburg, Germany.

References

1. Imbrici P, Camerino DC, Tricarico D. Major channels involved in neuropsychiatric disorders and therapeutic perspectives. Front Genet. 2013;4:76.
2. Celle ME, Cuoco C, Porta S, Gimelli G, Tassano E. Interstitial 2q24.3 deletion including SCN2A and SCN3A genes in a patient with autistic features, psychomotor delay, microcephaly and no history of seizures. Gene. 2013; 532:294–6.
3. Meisler MH, O'Brien JE, Sharkey LM. Sodium channel gene family: epilepsy mutations, gene interactions and modifier effects. J Physiol. 2010;588(Pt 11): 1841–8.
4. Philippe A, Martinez M, Guilloud-Bataille M, Gillberg C, Råstam M, Sponheim E, et al. Genome-wide scan for autism susceptibility genes. Paris autism research international Sibpair study. Hum Mol Genet. 1999;8:805–12.

5. Weiss LA, Escayg A, Kearney JA, Trudeau M, MacDonald BT, Mori M, et al. Sodium channels SCN1A, SCN2A and SCN3A in familial autism. Mol Psychiatry. 2003;8:186–94.
6. Bender AC, Morse RP, Scott RC, Holmes GL, Lenck-Santini P-P. SCN1A mutations in Dravet syndrome: impact of interneuron dysfunction on neural networks and cognitive outcome. Epilepsy Behav EB. 2012;23:177–86.
7. Le SV, Le PHT, Le TKV, Kieu Huynh TT, Hang Do TT. A mutation in GABRB3 associated with Dravet syndrome. Am J Med Genet A. 2017;173:2126–31.
8. Sanders SJ, Murtha MT, Gupta AR, Murdoch JD, Raubeson MJ, Willsey AJ, et al. De novo mutations revealed by whole-exome sequencing are strongly associated with autism. Nature. 2012;485:237–41.
9. Berkovic SF, Heron SE, Giordano L, Marini C, Guerrini R, Kaplan RE, et al. Benign familial neonatal-infantile seizures: characterization of a new sodium channelopathy. Ann Neurol. 2004;55:550–7.
10. Kamiya K, Kaneda M, Sugawara T, Mazaki E, Okamura N, Montal M, et al. A nonsense mutation of the sodium channel gene SCN2A in a patient with intractable epilepsy and mental decline. J Neurosci. 2004;24:2690–8.
11. Liao Y, Anttonen A-K, Liukkonen E, Gaily E, Maljevic S, Schubert S, et al. SCN2A mutation associated with neonatal epilepsy, late-onset episodic ataxia, myoclonus, and pain. Neurology. 2010;75:1454–8.
12. Ogiwara I, Ito K, Sawaishi Y, Osaka H, Mazaki E, Inoue I, et al. De novo mutations of voltage-gated sodium channel alphaII gene SCN2A in intractable epilepsies. Neurology. 2009;73:1046–53.
13. Bartnik M, Chun-Hui Tsai A, Xia Z, Cheung SW, Stankiewicz P. Disruption of the SCN2A and SCN3A genes in a patient with mental retardation, neurobehavioral and psychiatric abnormalities, and a history of infantile seizures. Clin Genet. 2011;80:191–5.
14. Davidsson J, Collin A, Olsson ME, Lundgren J, Soller M. Deletion of the SCN gene cluster on 2q24.4 is associated with severe epilepsy: an array-based genotype-phenotype correlation and a comprehensive review of previously published cases. Epilepsy Res. 2008;81:69–79.
15. Holland KD, Kearney JA, Glauser TA, Buck G, Keddache M, Blankston JR, et al. Mutation of sodium channel SCN3A in a patient with cryptogenic pediatric partial epilepsy. Neurosci Lett. 2008;433:65–70.
16. Chen C-P, Lin S-P, Chern S-R, Chen Y-J, Tsai F-J, Wu P-C, et al. Array-CGH detection of a de novo 2.8 Mb deletion in 2q24.2-->q24.3 in a girl with autistic features and developmental delay. Eur J Med Genet. 2010;53:217–20.
17. Uddin LQ, Dajani DR, Voorhies W, Bednarz H, Kana RK. Progress and roadblocks in the search for brain-based biomarkers of autism and attention-deficit/hyperactivity disorder. Transl Psychiatry. 2017;7:e1218.
18. Cooper GM, Coe BP, Girirajan S, Rosenfeld JA, Vu TH, Baker C, et al. A copy number variation morbidity map of developmental delay. Nat Genet. 2011; 43:838–46.
19. Gurney K, Prescott TJ, Wickens JR, Redgrave P. Computational models of the basal ganglia: from robots to membranes. Trends Neurosci. 2004;27:453–9.
20. Kalanithi PSA, Zheng W, Kataoka Y, DiFiglia M, Grantz H, Saper CB, et al. Altered parvalbumin-positive neuron distribution in basal ganglia of individuals with Tourette syndrome. Proc Natl Acad Sci U S A. 2005;102:13307–12.
21. Kataoka Y, Kalanithi PSA, Grantz H, Schwartz ML, Saper C, Leckman JF, et al. Decreased number of parvalbumin and cholinergic interneurons in the striatum of individuals with Tourette syndrome. J Comp Neurol. 2010;518:277–91.
22. Wang W, Takashima S, Segawa Y, Itoh M, Shi X, Hwang S-K, et al. The developmental changes of Na(v)1.1 and Na(v)1.2 expression in the human hippocampus and temporal lobe. Brain Res. 2011;1389:61–70.
23. Mackenzie B, Erickson JD. Sodium-coupled neutral amino acid (system N/a) transporters of the SLC38 gene family. Pflugers Arch. 2004;447:784–95.
24. Han SH, Kim S-H, Kim H-J, Lee Y, Choi S-Y, Park G, et al. Cobll1 is linked to drug resistance and blastic transformation in chronic myeloid leukemia. Leukemia. 2017;31:1532–9.
25. Holt LJ, Siddle K. Grb10 and Grb14: enigmatic regulators of insulin action--and more? Biochem J. 2005;388(Pt 2):393–406.
26. Wong VCN, Fung CW, Kwong AKY. SCN2A mutation in a Chinese boy with infantile spasm - response to modified Atkins diet. Brain and Development. 2015;37:729–32.
27. Kossoff EH, Cervenka MC, Henry BJ, Haney CA, Turner Z. A decade of the modified Atkins diet (2003–2013): results, insights, and future directions. Epilepsy Behav EB. 2013;29:437–42.
28. Lutas A, Yellen G. The ketogenic diet: metabolic influences on brain excitability and epilepsy. Trends Neurosci. 2013;36:32–40.
29. Chiron C. Current therapeutic procedures in Dravet syndrome. Dev Med Child Neurol. 2011;53(Suppl 2):16–8.
30. Chiron C, Marchand MC, Tran A, Rey E, d'Athis P, Vincent J, et al. Stiripentol in severe myoclonic epilepsy in infancy: a randomised placebo-controlled syndrome-dedicated trial. STICLO study group. Lancet Lond Engl. 2000;356:1638–42.
31. Devinsky O, Cross JH, Laux L, Marsh E, Miller I, Nabbout R, et al. Trial of Cannabidiol for drug-resistant seizures in the Dravet syndrome. N Engl J Med. 2017;376:2011–20.

Identification and treatment of offenders with attention-deficit/hyperactivity disorder in the prison population: a practical approach based upon expert consensus

Susan Young[1*], Gisli Gudjonsson[2], Prathiba Chitsabesan[3], Bill Colley[4], Emad Farrag[5], Andrew Forrester[6], Jack Hollingdale[7], Keira Kim[8], Alexandra Lewis[9,10], Sarah Maginn[11], Peter Mason[12], Sarah Ryan[13], Jade Smith[14], Emma Woodhouse[15,16] and Philip Asherson[17]

Abstract

Background: Around 25% of prisoners meet diagnostic criteria for attention-deficit/hyperactivity disorder (ADHD). Because ADHD is associated with increased recidivism and other functional and behavioural problems, appropriate diagnosis and treatment can be a critical intervention to improve outcomes. While ADHD is a treatable condition, best managed by a combination of medication and psychological treatments, among individuals in the criminal justice system ADHD remains both mis- and under-diagnosed and consequently inadequately treated. We aimed to identify barriers within the prison system that prevent appropriate intervention, and provide a practical approach to identify and treat incarcerated offenders with ADHD.

Methods: The United Kingdom ADHD Partnership hosted a consensus meeting to discuss practical interventions for youth (< 18 years) and adult (≥18 years) offenders with ADHD. Experts at the meeting addressed prisoners' needs for effective identification, treatment, and multiagency liaison, and considered the requirement of different approaches based on age or gender.

Results: The authors developed a consensus statement that offers practical advice to anyone working with prison populations. We identified specific barriers within the prison and criminal justice system such as the lack of adequate: staff and offender awareness of ADHD symptoms and treatments; trained mental health staff; use of appropriate screening and diagnostic tools; appropriate multimodal interventions; care management; supportive services; multiagency liaison; and preparation for prison release. Through discussion, a consensus was reached regarding prisoners' needs, effective identification, treatment and multiagency liaison and considered how this may differ for age and gender.

Conclusions: This practical approach based upon expert consensus will inform effective identification and treatment of offenders with ADHD. Appropriate intervention is expected to have a positive impact on the offender and society and lead to increased productivity, decreased resource utilization, and most importantly reduced rates of re-offending. Research is still needed, however, to identify optimal clinical operating models and to monitor their implementation and measure their success. Furthermore, government support will likely be required to effect change in criminal justice and mental health service policies.

Keywords: Attention-deficit/hyperactivity disorder (ADHD), Prison population, Identification, Treatment, Interventions, Consensus, UKAP

* Correspondence: suzyyoung@aol.com
[1]Psychology Services Limited, Croydon, UK
Full list of author information is available at the end of the article

Background

Effective identification and treatment of offenders with attention-deficit/hyperactivity disorder (ADHD) in the prison population is likely to have a positive impact on the offender and society. ADHD is associated with early age criminality [1], a high rate of recidivism [2], and a two to three-fold increased risk of later arrest, conviction, and imprisonment [1]. While ADHD is a treatable condition best managed by a combination of appropriate medication and psychological treatments [3], among individuals in the criminal justice system ADHD remains both mis- and under-diagnosed [4–6] and consequently inadequately treated.

ADHD is characterized by symptoms of pervasive and impairing inattention and/or hyperactivity and impulsivity [7] that starts during childhood or early adolescence and persists in around half of individuals into adulthood [8], where it is associated with significant personal, social, and occupational problems [9]. Compared with inmates without ADHD, inmates with ADHD symptoms demonstrate a high frequency and severity of functional impairment that worsen in proportion to the severity of their ADHD symptoms [4, 5].

Worldwide prevalence rates estimate that 5.3% of children and 2.5% of adults meet diagnotic criteria for ADHD [10, 11]. Meta-analyses of 42 prisons, based on international data derived from symptom-based clinical diagnostic interviews, indicated that 25.5% of the prison population overall met diagnostic criteria for ADHD [12]. Compared with the worldwide prevalance of ADHD, this is a five-fold increase among youth prisoners (< 18 years) and a ten-fold increase among adult prisoners (≥18 years) [12].

Among incarcerated adults with ADHD, there is an increased risk of associated coexisting psychopathology [13] that often confounds and influences treatment options. Given the high risk of co-morbid mood disorders among youth and adult offenders with ADHD [5], paired with their high risk of self-harm or suicide in the first weeks of prison reception [14], it is imperative to identify prisoners at risk of aggression, violence, self-harm, and suicide who might benefit from treatment for ADHD. It is also important to identify prisoners with ADHD with co-morbid substance use disorders, so that they may undergo detoxification treatment in prison before receiving treatment for ADHD. Adults with undiagnosed ADHD treated for other mental health disorders such as major depression, anxiety, bipolar, and/or personality disorders, have poor clinical and functional outcomes if ADHD goes untreated [5]. When appropriately diagnosed and treated for ADHD, there is likely improved ADHD symptom control, emotional lability, and overall functioning. Furthermore, outcome studies indicate reduced rates of transport accidents, criminality, and suicidal behaviour during periods of treatment for ADHD [5, 15–17].

Although there is a large evidence base for ADHD treatments for individuals in the community, similar evidence is limited for those in the prison population. A literature review of non-offender populations with ADHD reported that the combination of pharmacological and non-pharmacological treatment was most consistently associated with improved long-term outcomes and large effect sizes [3]. An Icelandic study of non-offender adults with ADHD reported that those who received the multi-modal treatment of ADHD medication plus the ADHD version of Reasoning and Rehabilitation 2 for Youths and Adults (R&R2ADHD) [18], experienced a significant reduction in ADHD and co-morbid symptoms and demonstrated improved functional outcomes [19–21]. A Swedish national database study of released prisoners reported that rates of violent reoffending were reduced by 42% during periods when they were receiving antipsychotics, psychostimulants, and/or drugs for addictive disorders, compared to periods in which they were not receiving medication [22]. Another Swedish database study reported that among those treated for ADHD, criminal conviction rates were reduced by 32% in men and 41% in women over a 3 year period [23].

As of October 2015 the World Prison Population List conservatively estimated that up to 11 million people were held in penal institutions throughout the world [24]. With around a quarter of prisoners worldwide meeting diagnostic criteria for ADHD, we estimate that 2.8 million prisoners have ADHD.

Given the large population of prisoners with ADHD combined with their increased risk of recidivism, appropriate intervention is crucial. By expanding upon the consensus of the United Kingdom Adult ADHD network (UKAAN) on the identification and management of offenders with ADHD [6], we aimed to identify existing barriers within the prison system that prevent appropriate intervention, and provide a practical approach to effectively identify and treat incarcerated offenders with ADHD.

Methods

The United Kingdom ADHD Partnership (UKAP; www.UKADHD.com) hosted a meeting in November 2016, where researchers, prison staff, clinicians, and patient representatives with expertise in offender mental health and ADHD, convened to discuss identification and treatment of youth and adult offenders with ADHD in the prison population. Each author attended the meeting. The authors represent a multidisciplinary group including both prescribing and non-prescribing clinical and academic experts, with extensive experience working with individuals with ADHD, including prisoners (for further details see Authors' Information subsection of the Declarations section). The meeting included presentations with electronic slides, discussions, and group work. Presentations and discussions were recorded and later transcribed.

The meeting commenced with four presentations:

- The Facts: What We Know from Empirical Data
- Needs, Problems, and Obstacles when Assessing and Treating ADHD in a Young Offender Institution
- Needs, Problems, and Obstacles when Assessing and Treating ADHD in an Adult Prison
- Beyond the Gates: Needs, Multiagency Liaison, and the Care Pathway

Following the presentations, all attendees separated into three small groups. Each group was tasked with providing practical solutions relevant to their assigned topic. The methodological orientation that underpinned the focus of the discussion groups was phenomenological, using the empirical research base and their clinical experience. Group leaders facilitated the small-group discussions while scribes took notes and summarized their groups' answers to the following topical questions:

1. Identification and Assessment
   - How do we identify ADHD among youth offenders? Among adult offenders? What are the screening tools?
   - What should trigger additional assessments and referrals? And to whom?
   - What should these assessments involve for youth offenders? For adult offenders?
   - Are there significant gender differences to take into account?
2. Interventions and Treatment
   - What are the appropriate pharmacological treatments for youth offenders? For adult offenders?
   - What are the appropriate non-pharmacological treatments for youth offenders? For adult offenders?
   - What is the evidence base for these treatments?
   - Are there significant gender differences to take into account?
3. Care Management and Multiagency Liaison
   - What agencies need to be involved in developing a care plan for youth offenders? For adult offenders?
   - What might trigger multiagency liaison?
   - What should be considered when providing support to families and carers?
   - What kind of educational, behavioural, and/or socialization support should be established to meet the needs of this population?
   - Are there significant gender differences to take into account?

Following the small-group work, all attendees re-assembled together. The leaders then presented their findings in a feedback session to all the attendees for another round of discussion and debate, until a final consensus was reached. The medical writer consolidated the meeting transcription, electronic slide presentations, and small-group notes into the manuscript. Lastly, the meeting transcription and manuscript were circulated to all authors for review to ensure agreement. The consensus reported here reflects the views of the authors based on their experience and is supported by published research; and aimed to provide practical guidance to health care professionals working with prisoners with ADHD.

Results

The authors successfully came to a consensus on a practical approach to identify and treat prisoners with ADHD. While our approach draws primarily from our experiences in the UK, we believe it can be easily adapted for use in other countries.

Identification and assessment

The identification and accurate diagnosis (including confirmation of a previous diagnosis) of ADHD among prisoners is a process reliant on the availability of medical records, mental health clinicians trained to conduct interview assessments for ADHD, prison staff trained to recognise potential patients with ADHD, and suitable screening and diagnostic instruments. It will be necessary to use identification and assessment tools that are specific to youth or adult offenders. According to best practice all new prisoners should receive an initial reception screen for mental health problems, including ADHD, followed by a comprehensive second screen shortly after their reception screen [25, 26].

Identifying prisoners with ADHD

While some prisoners present with a history of ADHD diagnosed during childhood, others present with no history of ADHD, or alternative diagnoses such as specific learning difficulties (dyslexia, dyspraxia) or conduct problems. It is therefore important to review the medical history and confirm the presence of other common mental health and neurodevelopmental disorders that may overlap with ADHD — highlighting the need for a careful diagnostic assessment. In our experience, many offenders who had a prior diagnosis of ADHD were untreated or failed to adhere to their treatment programme. In making a new diagnosis, there are specific indicators among the prison population that, in our experience, suggest the presence of ADHD and are as follows:

- Symptoms of inattention, which are often missed among offenders of both genders

- Symptoms of impulsivity, emotional dysregulation, and poor self-control, which are especially important to recognize as the prisoner may be at risk of aggression and violence towards others, or self-harm and suicide
- A history of educational failure, school expulsion, inability to work, driving offences, and impulsive aggression, and/or
- A history of chronic mental health problems or a history of failed treatment programmes for conditions such as mood disorders, anxiety, depression, post-traumatic stress disorder, emotional instability, self-harm, and/or borderline personality disorder.

We have observed that assessors commonly view hyperactivity as a 'male' ADHD symptom and inattention as a 'female' ADHD symptom. This bias may interfere with making an accurate diagnosis of ADHD in males who lack overt hyperactivity and in females who display hyperactive behaviour. Diagnosing ADHD in offenders can be additionally challenging because it is often complicated by the high frequency of co-occurring conditions. In addition to common disorders seen in the prison population such as anxiety, depression, post-traumatic stress disorders, substance abuse and self-harm, borderline personality disorders are commonly found among female offenders [27, 28], and conduct and antisocial personality disorder among males; all potentially masking the diagnosis of ADHD. Consequently, further training is often required to support the accurate identification of ADHD symptoms and distinguish these from other disorders.

Prison staff ADHD awareness training

Currently there is very limited training about ADHD for prison staff. Raising awareness of ADHD was however considered to be essential by the consensus group. ADHD awareness training is likely to reshape misconceptions or stereotypes of ADHD and may improve the outcomes of offenders with ADHD within the criminal justice system. It is important to understand that although ADHD is a pervasive condition that persists into adulthood in around half of cases, it is treatable at all ages. Prison officers, clinicians, educators, therapists, and mentors therefore should be trained to recognize the signs and symptoms of ADHD and further educated on available treatments and expected outcomes.

ADHD awareness training should ideally raise the visibility of the disorder. Increased understanding and recognition of ADHD will likely help prison staff to better manage offenders with ADHD presenting with difficult behaviours that were previously unattributed to the disorder [2]. While any member of prison staff can refer a prisoner for a mental health assessment at any time, referrals are dependent on their vigilance and ability to make appropriate observations.

Delivery of ADHD awareness training (alongside training for mental health more generally) in the prison setting may have logistical challenges, such as lockdown requirements to allow staff to attend workshops. However, training in mental health issues, including ADHD, is essential for this high-risk population and needs to be addressed at each institution.

Screening for youth offenders

Primary screen

As is the case for many prisons, all youth offenders are subject to a reception screen upon admission. Screening preferences and practices vary greatly between institutions world-wide, and while no evident gold standard method exists, healthcare standards offer guidance for best practices for youth in secure settings [29]. Nurses with mental health experience usually administer the primary screen to assess the overall physical and mental health of the offenders.

The National Health Service England (NHSE) mandates using the comprehensive health assessment tool (CHAT) in youth offender institutions throughout England and Wales. Because of the NHSE requirements, we recommend using the CHAT as the primary screen in all youth offender institutions. The CHAT is a validated semi-structured interview designed to screen for health issues among all young offenders admitted to a secure facility [30]. CHAT is divided into four sections covering: physical health, mental health, substance abuse, and neurodisability. It is available in electronic format; however, the mental health section takes approximately one hour to complete.

Questions pertaining to ADHD symptoms are included in the mental health section of the CHAT, but because they focus on externalizing rather than internalizing symptoms the assessors will need to take extra care in considering all symptoms, including the inattention symptoms of ADHD. While we acknowledge the poor specificity of CHAT, it is a sensitive tool for detecting mental health problems that include ADHD. It is therefore important to emphasize that the CHAT should be used as a primary screen to flag potential mental health issues before going on to more detailed assessments.

If any chronic or serious mental health issue is suspected, then the offender should be referred for a secondary screen involving a more comprehensive assessment by a multidisciplinary mental health team including nurses, psychologists, and psychiatrists who are specially trained to recognize ADHD as well as other mental health conditions commonly seen in young offenders.

Secondary screen and clinical diagnosis

At the time of clinical assessment, we recommend that a trained clinician administer a standard validated rating scale such as the Swanson, Nolan, and Pelham teacher and parent rating scale (SNAP-IV) [31] and/or the Conners' comprehensive behaviour rating scale (Conners' CBRS) [32] to assist in making the diagnosis and to gather necessary collateral information. A diagnosis of ADHD usually requires supporting evidence from teacher, therapist, employer, or parent reports. In cases where screens indicate a possible ADHD diagnosis, we recommend that clinicians always conduct a full diagnostic interview for ADHD, as well as carefully assess for commonly occurring co-morbid conditions such as drug abuse, personality disorders, emotional problems, and learning difficulties. The ADHD Child Evaluation (ACE) [33] is one such tool used for assessing ADHD symptoms, possible co-morbid problems, and associated impairments. The ACE is a semi-structured diagnostic interview providing either DSM-5 or ICD-10 [7] criteria and is available in 19 languages free of charge in paper form. Those who are symptomatic on screening, but have a confirmed pre-existing diagnosis of ADHD may not require a diagnostic interview. This will largely depend on how long ago the diagnosis was made and is a matter of clinical judgment.

Screening for adult offenders

Primary screen

In adult prisons offenders are subject to a reception screen upon admission, to review their overall physical and mental health. In most institutions, however, the mental health section of the primary screen for adult offenders does not include questions pertaining to ADHD symptoms. For example, the screening tool Health & Wellbeing Needs Assessment Toolkit (HWBNA) published by the Public Health England Health & Justice Team, to be used in all 118 adult English Prisons, has no mention of ADHD. Screening preferences and practices vary greatly between adult institutions world-wide and while no evident gold standard method exists, several valid tools are available [25].

Some prisons have adopted the short screening version of the Adult ADHD Self Rating Scale (ASRS), [34] yet in our experience, because of the wording of the questions, this is less suitable for prison populations. We identify this as problematic and therefore suggest using the brief version of the Barkley Adult ADHD rating scale (B-BAARS) as part of the primary mental health screen. The B-BAARS is a short, six-item screen with excellent specificity and sensitivity for predicting a diagnosis of ADHD in the offender population, and is available free of charge [33, 35].

Ideally, nurses with mental health experience should administer the primary screen in adult institutions as this increases the validity of the screens by ensuring questions are understood and properly rated by the offenders [36]; however, this is usually not the case. Nurses in adult prisons and police stations tend to be physical health nurses without mental health experience. This may cause difficulties with identifying ADHD symptoms, as well as other mental health disorders, in the primary screen and may prevent triggering a secondary screen among adult offenders. Because of this, we recommend employing nurses with mental health experience throughout the criminal justice system offender pathway to adequately assess the overall physical and mental health of adult offenders.

If any co-morbid mental health disorder is suspected, then the offender should be referred for a secondary screen involving a more comprehensive assessment by a multidisciplinary mental health team including nurses, psychologists, and psychiatrists who are specially trained to recognize ADHD as well as other adult mental health conditions.

Secondary screen and clinical diagnosis

In cases where a B-BAARS score or results from another screen indicate a likely ADHD diagnosis, we recommend a clinician trained in the assessment of ADHD conduct a full diagnostic interview. This may include the full 18-item version of the BAARS to ascertain the severity of ADHD. Whenever possible, the interview should be supported by collateral reports (e.g., parent, therapist, and previous medical history) to gain a comprehensive description of their symptoms and impairments across the lifespan. While informant reports are not always required, they can be particularly useful as offenders with ADHD often have very poor recollections of their childhood behaviour and tend to minimise impairments arising from ADHD. Extra care is needed when evaluating all of the offenders' symptoms to avoid focusing only on externalising behaviours.

We have identified three comprehensive semi-structured diagnostic interview tools that are suitable for adult prison populations: the Conners' Adult ADHD Diagnostic Interview for DSM-IV (CAADID) [37], the Diagnostic Interview for ADHD in adults (DIVA-2) [38, 39], and the ACE+ (ACE for adults) [40]. While the CAADID and DIVA-2 are the more established methods, the ACE+ has an advantage because it includes a section that considers coexisting conditions and whether they are co-morbid or reflect a differential diagnosis. For this reason, the ACE+ may be preferred when establishing the diagnosis of ADHD in the presence of co-morbid disorders. The DIVA-2 is widely used throughout Europe and should be used in conjunction with a systematic assessment of co-morbidity because it does not include a prompt to evaluate the presence of common co-morbid conditions. Both the ACE+ and DIVA-2 are available in many languages other than English and are free of charge in paper form.

Each of these interviews provides age-appropriate examples of each of the ADHD symptoms that can be applied when evaluating adults. Relevant descriptions of adult ADHD symptoms include: internal restlessness; excessive mind wandering that interferes with tasks such as reading, writing and listening to TV or conversations; getting bored quickly then losing ability to focus; and feelings of irritability and impatience when waiting in queues. Clinicians also need to be aware that symptoms of emotional dysregulation such as frequent inappropriate levels of irritability, frustration, and anger (while not part of the formal diagnostic criteria) can be used to support the diagnosis [7].

While continuous performance tests (CPT) perform reasonably well at discriminating between people with ADHD from non-psychiatric controls, and may contribute to the diagnostic assessment, they are far less able to discriminate ADHD from other common psychiatric disorders seen in prison populations [38]. Given these validity issues and the logistical problems of bringing information technology equipment into prisons, we cannot recommend their use in prison populations.

Interventions and treatment

Providing appropriate pharmacological and non-pharmacological interventions in prison populations is a process reliant on prison staff and offender self-awareness of ADHD symptoms and treatments, the availability of trained mental health clinicians, and the administration of specifically targeted multimodal treatments. Although female offenders often present with a more complex profile due to pregnancy, motherhood, and high levels of co-morbidity [13], all pharmacological and non-pharmacological treatments can be administered irrespective of age and gender. During pregnancy, ADHD pharmacological treatments can be used, but should be restricted to cases where treatment is required to reduce significant distress and behavioural problems, where the potential risks of no treatment outweigh risks of treatment [41].

It will be necessary to educate offenders on the efficacy of multimodal treatments and expected outcomes and to obtain informed consent for permission to treat. Following a new or confirmed previous diagnosis of ADHD and a careful evaluation of possible co-morbid conditions, we recommended the following multi-modal treatment for incarcerated offenders, as summarized in Fig. 1.

We have observed that staff support in pharmacological treatment and involvement in psychological treatment programmes has a positive and direct impact on offender adherence to and engagement in the prescribed treatment plan. Staff lack of knowledge about ADHD can interfere with medication administration and offender engagement in psychological treatment programmes. Conversely, staff awareness of ADHD symptoms, and observation of positive treatment effects, usually increases engagement with and support for the treatment process, and makes it much more likely they become involved in the delivery of offenders' psychological treatments.

According to principle and law, punishment for criminal offence is the loss of liberty, and prisoners' human rights are fully protected unless restrictions are unavoidably and demonstrably 'necessitated by the fact of incarceration' [42]. The Mandela Rules expressly state the fundamental prohibitions on torture and inhumane treatment, and emphasize that imprisonment is itself the punishment and should not carry additional 'pains' [42]. Solitary confinement is arguably considered to be an additional 'pain', with especially significant adverse effects for people with serious mental illness; it has negative psychological consequences and restricts the inmates access to mental health services [43, 44]. Although ADHD is often un-recognized as a serious mental illness, we contend that severe cases should be recognized as such, and particularly when ADHD related behaviours are severe enough to lead to isolation of sentenced prisoners. We have observed that solitary confinement exacerbates prisoners' ADHD symptoms [45], and recommend increasing efforts to ensure that offenders with ADHD are prevented from receiving this punishment. The same argument can be applied to severe cases of other mental health disorders, so it not unique to ADHD. This may require prisons to reduce the use of solitary confinement for all prisoners and to ensure that it is only used as a last resort, for short periods of time to manage acute situations, and never as a punishment.

Given the high prevalence of neurodevelopmental disorders (traumatic brain injury, communication disorders, dyslexia, learning disabilities, autistic spectrum disorder, and ADHD) among young offenders [46], it is especially important to staff the prisons appropriately with educational psychologists and speech/language therapists to meet their needs adequately. Currently, prisoners with these needs are either inadequately supported or receive these necessary services only upon release.

Pharmacological treatments for offenders

Treatment with ADHD medication is effective in reducing symptoms of inattention, hyperactivity, and impulsiveness [47] and is also reported to be associated with a significant reduction in violent reoffending (around 42%) on release from prison [22] and similarly in criminal convictions [23]. By reducing their ADHD symptoms, the offender is likely better equipped to engage in and benefit from psychological, educational, and occupational interventions. It is important for offenders and prison staff to understand that, although ADHD medication reduces ADHD

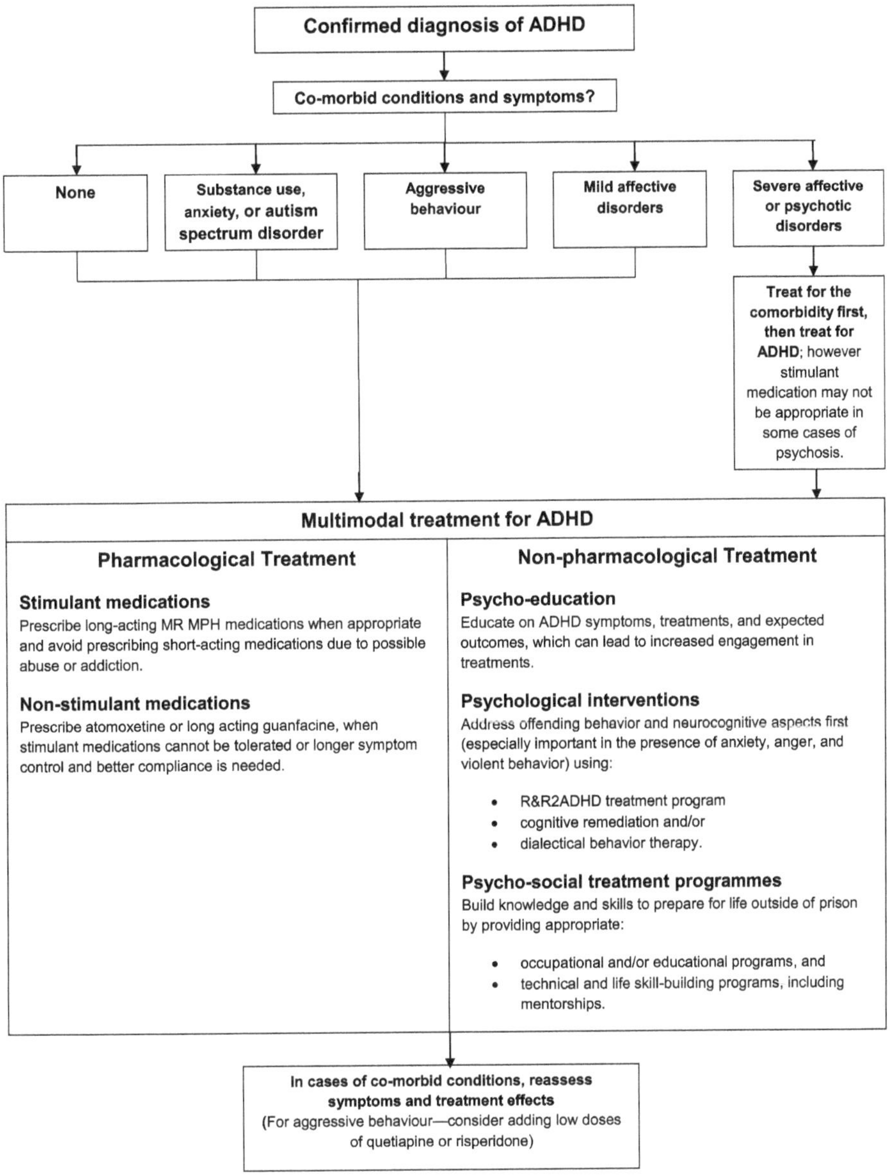

Fig. 1 Multimodal Treatment for Incarcerated Offenders with ADHD

symptoms, it does not cure the disorder, and concomitant non-pharmacological treatments are nearly always necessary to help the offender manage ADHD related problems and improve their behaviour.

Given the lack of sufficient high quality evidence from randomized-control trials for treatment among prisoners, it is important to emphasize that clinicians trained in the diagnosis and treatment of ADHD should administer ADHD medications, to carefully asses for risks of abuse potential and possible risks of exacerbating other co-morbid conditions. Medication can be administered to all offenders irrespective of age and gender, but type and dosage should be made on an individual basis, especially in the case of pregnancy.

With respect to psychoeducation, the offender needs to be educated on the benefits and side effects of pharmacological treatment and the implications of remaining untreated or discontinuing treatment. This education is not only necessary in obtaining informed consent to treat, but is important in engaging them in their own treatment. Such engagement will encourage offenders to take an active role in their treatment and can cause them to perceive some control over their situation, which can have an empowering effect. Offenders need to be given adequate opportunities to provide feedback on the medication's effect and to titrate for therapeutic doses. Support during the early stage of treatment is critical in helping offenders take full advantage of the reductions in ADHD symptoms and in helping manage the medication's side effects.

We recommend prescribing stimulant medications first line because these have a quicker response than non-stimulants and a greater average effect size. Drugs with a high risk of abuse, such as immediate release preparations of methylphenidate (MPH) and dexamfetamine (DEX), should be avoided in prison populations due to the potential for abuse. Injected or insufflated (snorted) MPH and DEX cause a rapid release of dopamine that can give the user a 'high'. This does not occur, however, when these medications are taken orally. The oral administration of therapeutic doses of MPH or DEX is therefore essential in reducing the abuse potential of stimulant medications [48].

We recommend prescribing long acting or modified release preparations of methylphenidate (MR MPH) that are difficult to take in any other way than by mouth (e.g. Concerta XL). Lisdexamfetamine (Elvanse) is a long acting preparation that has a unique advantage, because even if injected, the active drug is released slowly at a similar rate in to the brain as when taken by mouth. These extended release formulations are usually taken in the morning and give active control of symptoms for 8–14 h in most cases.

MR MPH, lisdexamfetamine, along with all other stimulants, are controlled substances and thus subject to strict dispensary logistics that often interfere with treatment compliance and efficacy. Restrictions on movements within the prison can limit the regular and timely administration of stimulant (and other) medications. In some cases, staff are needed to escort prisoners to the healthcare unit to receive medication, although in most cases prisoners can take themselves to a dispensary, or receive medication from a wheeled cart. Escorting not only over burdens the staff, but stigmatizes the offender and further complicates adherence. Although stimulants are controlled substances, they can usually be dispensed in the same manner as other non-stimulant medications that are not kept in possession, which improves adherence. The practice of dispensing drugs varies by prison, but non-stimulants are easier to dispense as there are less procedures for nursing staff to follow.

Preliminary results of a pilot study of Concerta XL in adult offenders with ADHD (CIAO) indicated a significant reduction in total critical incidents (assaults, fights, property damage, self-harm, drug use, and acts of disobedience) among prisoners in the UK who were treated for 12 weeks. In relation to dose, over half of the prisoners took 18-36 mg and only 4% took the maximum dose of 90 mg, indicating a lack of drug seeking behaviour with regard to Concerta XL in this population. This was in line with our clinical experience that suggests greater abuse potential for sedative antidepressants and antipsychotics than stimulants within the prison population. The findings from this study were successfully used to secure further funding the National Institute of Health Research (NIHR) for an ongoing randomised controlled trial in 200 young adult offenders following a similar study design. We anticipate that the reports from these studies will inform optimal medical treatment of ADHD in prisons and raise public awareness for the need for effective treatment of offenders with ADHD (unpublished report for pilot study available from PA).

In alignment with national guidelines [49], we recommend prescribing non-stimulants, such as atomoxetine in adolescents under 18 and adults, and/or long-acting guanfacine in adolescents under 18: when stimulants do not adequately treat symptoms or cause adverse effects, when a sustained 24-h effect is required, or there is clear drug seeking behaviour for stimulant medications (a rare event in our experience). In adults there is no data for the use of guanfacine, so atomoxetine is the non-stimulant of choice. Non-stimulants are easy to administer as they are not a controlled substance and would therefore bypass dispensary logistics and potentially improve treatment compliance. Although atomoxetine and long-acting guanfacine take several weeks to reach optimal effect, they have a significantly longer effect on symptom control over a 24-h period and can maintain their effect when individual doses are missed. They are particularly useful for patients who have a rapid return of severe ADHD symptoms once stimulant effects wear off during the day. Additionally, non-stimulants are the medication of choice for patients with a previous history of stimulant abuse.

Pharmacological treatments for offenders with co-morbid conditions

In the presence of co-morbid anxiety, autism spectrum disorder (ASD), aggressive behaviour, or mild affective symptoms, ADHD should usually be treated first, followed by a careful evaluation of the medication's effect on the co-morbid symptoms. While adults with ADHD are reported to misuse drugs [50, 51], detoxification is provided by prison mental health services, and despite reports in the media about drug abuse in prison, there is no longer regular access to major drugs of abuse. Substance abuse is stabilised and under control in most cases in prison settings, so that diagnostic assessments and treatment for ADHD can proceed.

Symptoms commonly shared between ADHD and co-morbid disorders may be better managed with pharmacological treatments for ADHD rather than with pharmacological treatments for the co-morbid disorders themselves. For example, irritability and low mood symptoms secondary to ADHD are alleviated more effectively by ADHD medication than with antidepressants or antipsychotics. Similarly, we have observed that conditions such as post-traumatic stress disorder and borderline personality disorder sometimes improve following treatment of concurrent ADHD. Subsequent treatments for co-morbid disorders may be required and can be added one at a time to discriminate their effects. Conversely, in the presence of psychosis, bipolar disorder, and/or a clear depressive episode, ADHD should not be treated first. Care should be taken, however, to avoid mistaking the ADHD symptoms of emotional instability for the episodic mood changes of bipolar disorder or the chronic symptoms of a personality disorder.

In the case of co-morbid anxiety disorder, pharmacological treatment for the anxiety can be added if the stimulant exacerbates the anxiety. Alternatively, the stimulant can be discontinued and replaced by atomoxetine. In the case of co-morbid symptoms of aggressive behaviours, a low dose of quetiapine or risperidone may be added if the symptoms are not adequately treated by stimulants or atomoxetine. While high doses of quetiapine are sedative and are used to treat psychosis, low doses have a mildly sedative effect that can help reduce irritability and emotional liability associated with ADHD.

Unfortunately, there are insufficient studies of the treatment of ADHD in co-morbid cases, and offenders presenting with complex mix of co-morbidities. Our recommendations are therefore based on the experience of the authors, which are aligned with recommendations from guideline groups such as NICE [49]. In our experience, while a significant proportion of offenders with co-morbid conditions respond positively to the treatment of ADHD, there are cases that show limited or no response. Severe adverse effects on co-morbid conditions, including risk of psychosis, however appear to be extremely rare. The most common complaint is appetite loss. Overall, we conclude that while further work is needed to identify the predictors of good and poor response among patients with co-morbid conditions, the potential benefits of treatment outweigh the potential risks. The risks are minimised by careful monitoring of treatment effects during the titration phase of drug administration. In accordance with published guidelines [49], when titrating stimulants we recommend weekly assessments for 4–5 weeks, and less often for non-stimulants .

Non-pharmacological treatments for offenders

Non-pharmacological treatments in the prison setting consist of psychological, educational, and occupational treatment programmes. These interventions should aim to: facilitate changes in life-long patterns of poor behavioural control, increase life satisfaction, build useful skills, and help the offender plan for civilian life after release. Mentorship programmes embedded in the treatment plan are likely to be additionally beneficial. Pharmacological treatment of ADHD symptoms will enable offenders who respond to such treatments to better engage in and benefit from non-pharmacological interventions in this setting. It is important to emphasize that, although ADHD medication can improve symptoms, concomitant non-pharmacological treatments are nearly always necessary to help the offender manage ADHD related problems and improve their behaviour.

Offender psychoeducation

There is a need to change common misconceptions and stereotypes about ADHD symptoms and treatments. Young people and adults find it helpful to understand that ADHD is a neurobiological disorder evident early in life and distinct from other behavioural problems. It is especially important for offenders to understand that although ADHD is pervasive, treatment may help improve self-control and level of function. In our experience prisoners value improvements in attention span and reduced levels of physical restlessness and emotional impulsivity that would enable them to benefit from education. Mental health professionals working with prisoners with ADHD should provide a clear explanation of ADHD symptoms, treatments, and expected outcomes, and educate the offender on the potential risks of remaining untreated or discontinuing treatment. Additionally, we recommend giving offenders an easy-to-read pamphlet that briefly highlights some facts about ADHD.

Offender psychoeducation is an integral part of intervention that should be initiated during imprisonment to increase its efficacy and to avoid overwhelming the offender upon release. We commonly observe that offenders are not adequately educated about their condition and take a passive role in their treatment plan. Furthermore, we have observed that an offender's increased understanding of their condition helps them to engage in their pharmacologic and psychological treatment programmes and increase their sense of self-empowerment.

Psychological treatment programmes

Many UK prisons implement offending behaviour programmes that focus on addressing the risk of future offending behaviour, but these do not provide treatment for clinical conditions for offenders with ADHD. We recommend implementing a neurocognitive intervention that addresses offending behaviour and ADHD related and other behavioural co-morbid executive function deficits such as: difficulty with time-keeping, organizing, planning, and self-regulating emotions and behaviour.

Given the logistical limitations inherent in correctional institutions (e.g. restrictions on movement and variations in sentencing), it is important that treatment programmes are suitable and feasible for the prison environment. Appropriate programmes include those that can be: completed in a relatively short amount of time (less than

4 months), delivered in a small group setting with about 10 to 12 inmates once or twice per week, and administered to all offenders irrespective of age and gender.

To augment and fortify interventions we recommend providing the offender with personal support from a mentor (i.e. coach or champion). Prison staff, officers, substance abuse staff, primary and secondary care clinicians, educators, volunteers, and when appropriate even fellow prisoners, can be trained to provide one-on-one skill-building sessions. These one-on-one sessions emphasize a personal approach and can help the offender bridge lessons from the therapy room to daily life.

To the best of our knowledge the only psychological treatment programme developed to address antisocial behaviour and executive functioning deficits is Reasoning and Rehabilitation 2 ADHD (R&R2ADHD). R&R2ADHD is a treatment programme based on cognitive behaviour therapy designed to build pro-social competence [18] and may be used in non-offender and prison populations. It can be administered to all offenders irrespective of age and gender and completed in approximately 2 months. The programme's short duration, comprised of 15 treatment sessions deliverable up to 2 times per week, makes it favourable to ensure completion. R&R2ADHD has an additional advantage of being suitable for both youth and adult offenders. Furthermore, mentorship is embedded within the programme — whereof an assigned coach or mentor meets one-on-one with the offender between sessions to help them consolidate and apply newly learned skills in their daily life.

While the evidence for R&R2ADHD efficacy is predominantly community based with a majority of male samples [19–21], results from a pilot trial at Her Majesty's Prison Youth Offender Institution (HMP/ YOI) Feltham (a level 3 youth offender institution in the UK) indicated high rates of completion and universally positive feedback from enrolled youth offenders. We observed that the positive impact of R&R2ADHD on the youth offenders with ADHD at HMP/YOI Feltham was even more significant when prison staff were involved in the treatment programme. Oftentimes prison staff and officers have an established rapport with offenders, and involving them seems to improve offender engagement in the treatment programme. According to the 2013 London Mayor's Office for Policing and Crime (MOPAC) report, R&R2ADHD was mentioned as an example of good practice and has received the full support of London prison governors and lead staff [52].

Other psychological approaches that may be helpful include cognitive remediation therapy (CRT) [53] and dialectical behavioural therapy (DBT) [54]. CRT applies techniques historically used to treat individuals with traumatic brain injury (e.g. deficits in planning, time management, and attention, impulse control). DBT was developed for the treatment of borderline personality disorder. Ideally, psychological interventions should take an eclectic approach drawing on these paradigms as well as cognitive behaviour therapy (CBT). The Young-Bramham Programme, is one such CBT intervention that can be used for adolescents and adults with ADHD [55].

Educational and occupational treatment programmes

Children with ADHD are at an increased risk of academic underachievement [56] and repeating an academic year [57], therefore all prisoners should have numeracy and literacy assessments to identify academic impairments. An appropriate individualized education plan based upon academic assessments developed by the prison education department can be additionally informed by mental health screen results, and previous mental health and school records, pending prisoner consent to information sharing between departments. The CHAT screening tool assesses for learning difficulties in young people (in the neurodisability section, part 5). These results should be used in developing a young offender's education plan, and will consequently inform overall holistic care.

It is important that the education plan addresses gaps in the offenders' academic core skills, focuses on strengths, includes ADHD support strategies, and is appropriate for those disengaged from the education system. Education support workers and volunteers from outside private organizations can be helpful with implementing the education plan. While education services have information pertinent to learning difficulties, they do not automatically liaise with mental health services. We have observed that problems with information sharing are primary barriers that need to be to overcome. Therefore, we recommend an ad hoc liaison between mental health and education services to ensure effective intervention.

Prison rules most often require that offenders complete an academic course (related to reading and writing) before participating in technical skill-building workshops. Because symptoms of inattention, hyperactivity, and behavioural difficulties can prevent the offender from meaningful participation in academic courses, this requirement is inherently biased against them. Imposing this requirement upon offenders with ADHD who are at risk of disengaging from and failing the academic course may result in extended prison time. For example, in England and Wales, if an offender fails the Imprisonment for Public Protection (IPP) course they are subject to an increased prison sentence.

We recommend waiving the requirement to complete an academic course and directing offenders towards educational and occupational programmes that suit their strengths (e.g. creative, technical, and/or athletic skills). Focusing on their strengths may not only reduce the occurrence of extended sentencing, but also the rate of offenders with ADHD in solitary confinement. In cases where solitary confinement has not been averted, we recommend shortening the period(s) of isolation and giving the offender an activity to occupy them while confined.

Participation in technical skill-building workshops can provide hands on experience and the opportunity to learn occupational and technical skills useful for life during and after prison. In our experience, maintenance jobs throughout the prison (e.g., housekeeping, kitchen, and garden work) that provide the opportunity to be physically active and occupied, are highly sought after by ADHD offenders.

In addition to acquiring technical skills, it is important that offenders are taught necessary personal life skills to equip them to successfully navigate civilian life after prison and not re-offend. Given the likelihood of executive function deficits, offenders with ADHD most often need help planning how to attain their goals. Long-term desires and goals (e.g., health, wealth, and happiness) need to be broken down into realistic achievable short-term plans and goals (e.g., self-care and employment). R&R2ADHD [18] notably includes a module that focuses on offender needs of this nature.

Care management and multiagency liaison

As for people with mental health problems or related complex needs, offenders with ADHD require assistance from a wide variety of supportive services and agencies. It is important that these services are accessed and coordinated during imprisonment, not only to infer maximal benefit, but to ensure continuity of care once the prisoner is released. Supportive services and agencies, although distinct and separate entities, will need to liaise with each other to exchange information and help ensure comprehensive care. For example, education services should automatically be contacted when an offender with mental health issues is identified.

Care plan and care coordination

In England people having complex needs are often eligible to receive a Care Programme Approach (CPA). A CPA is a structured multidisciplinary care management format designed to support people with severe and enduring mental health problems. Service users are allocated a care plan coordinator (e.g., community psychiatric nurse, social worker, psychologist or psychiatrist) who is responsible to review, access, and coordinate multiple available services on their behalf [58]. The structure of a CPA requires that issues are clearly addressed according to distinct domains of need (e.g., mental health, medication, accommodation, education, financial) and consequently clearly identifies which agencies are responsible to fulfil those needs. While the care plan coordinator is central to a CPA, it is important for them to encourage the service user to take an active role in their care plan as much as possible.

A CPA is routinely implemented for high risk patients in inpatient settings, yet less commonly in community mental health settings. Although the National Institute for Health and Clinical Excellence 2018 (NICE) guidelines [59] recommend that individuals with ADHD aged 16 and over receive a CPA, many offenders with ADHD are not adequately identified and subsequently do not receive an appropriate care management plan. In our experience, continual failure to properly identify offenders with ADHD and meet their needs can lead to some individuals to persist in offending behaviours and 'fall through the gap'.

We recommend offenders with ADHD receive a CPA or similar care management plan and are assigned a care plan coordinator to oversee the plan. We also recommend implementing a medication management plan, which should be a core component of the care plan. A medication management plan addresses the need for regular built-in reviews by a suitably trained psychiatrist, and the need for monitoring medication adherence, which should be a key task of the care coordinator. When transitioning from youth to adult or between different institutions or out of prison, it is vital to maintain robust care coordination, continuity of care, and uninterrupted treatment with ADHD medication; using the CPA format can be effective in mitigating problems with service discontinuity that can arise during transitions. A sample CPA based on numerous 'real life' cases is provided in the supplementary material, see Additional file 1.

Supportive services and agencies

The following people, services, and agencies may need to be accessed and coordinated according to the offenders' individual needs:

- Parents and carers — adults responsible to provide general support at home and, where appropriate, give consent to treat
- Care plan coordinators — trained workers designated as the main point of contact responsible to develop a care plan and review, access, and coordinate appropriate available services
- Criminal justice services including diversion services — police, court, prison, and offender management unit staff responsible to move offenders through the offender pathway while safeguarding rights; an intermediary may be required
- Mental health services, including forensic mental health services — trained physicians, psychiatrists,

psychologists, nurses, and therapists responsible to provide appropriate evaluations and treatments
- Primary and secondary care physicians — paediatricians, general practitioners, psychiatrists, and specialist physicians responsible to provide appropriate evaluations and treatments
- Social services — social workers responsible to access available financial support for appropriate healthcare, housing, and child care needs
- Educational services — teachers, therapists, nurses, and trained volunteers, responsible to provide appropriate evaluations and develop and implement individualized educational plans
- Mentorship programmes — trained coaches or champions responsible to provide one-on-one treatment or skill-building sessions
- Addiction services — trained clinicians, officers, or workers responsible to provide appropriate interventions and recovery support services
- Adoption and foster care agencies — trained workers responsible to access appropriate placements for youth offenders or children of offenders
- Probation services — trained officers responsible to supervise offenders and provide appropriate interventions
- Occupational, rehabilitation, and therapeutic services — trained workers, therapists, job coaches, and volunteers responsible to provide and/or access appropriate skill-building courses and employment opportunities to help the offender regain independence
- Immigration services — trained workers responsible to administrate and adjudicate cases of foreign offenders

Support for female offenders

Despite women's inclination to seek help, female offenders with ADHD may be less likely to be identified [12] and consequently less likely to receive effective support. As mentioned previously, pregnancy, responsibilities of parenting, and the risk of commonly prevalent co-morbid disorders complicate intervention and additionally cause female offenders to require varied and unique services. The immediate access of social and foster care services is crucial when an offender is pregnant and/or has child custody issues.

Support for youth offenders

In developing a care plan for youth offenders it is important to involve parents or carers, whenever appropriate or possible. They can be helpful in supporting the youth once released, especially when it comes to medication compliance. Additionally, parents or carers may be required to give consent for treatment when the youth is under 18 years old, however, obtaining consent may be problematic in some cases. When the family is a part of the offenders' problems or a family member is the victim, careful consideration is required before contacting and involving them. In addition to providing psychoeducation for the offender, families need to be educated on the facts about ADHD symptoms, treatments, and expected outcomes. The care plan coordinator should direct families to parent groups or other supportive organizations and resources to help them meet their child's complex needs. The CHAT screening tool includes a care plan summary that highlights the young person's needs. This information should be communicated to all professionals working with the young person in secure care, and to parents, carers, and care plan coordinators following release to ensure good continuity of care.

Support for adult offenders

In developing a care plan for adult offenders it is important to encourage them to take an active role in their care management. When adults have been in the prison system for many years, it can be difficult to motivate them to engage in intervention and supportive services. We have observed that youth offender services and pathways are generally more developed and effective than those for adult offenders. Therefore, we recommend adult prisons adopt many of the same models and tools, such as mentorship programmes and comprehensive screens like the CHAT, which are used in youth offending institutions.

Support upon prison release

Prison release and the transition into civilian life is a period of increased vulnerability requiring offenders with ADHD to receive specific timely support. There is a need for further research on ways to best support offenders with ADHD who are released from prison; meanwhile we recommend implementing a critical time intervention approach [60], in which a designated person meets with the offender just before and immediately after release from prison to help implement their care plan and ensure subsequent engagement in healthcare. Appropriate support would include: connecting the offender with their care plan coordinator, ensuring registration with a primary care physician, and helping them understand the implications of discontinuing treatment. Because uninterrupted treatment with ADHD medication is vitally important, we further emphasize the need to implement a medication management plan.

Discussion

There is strong evidence of a high prevalence of offenders (both youth and adults, males and females) with ADHD in prison and who have increased risk of associated coexisting conditions and higher rates of recidivism. Paired with the evidence that treatment improves symptoms and outcomes, accurate identification and comprehensive treatment is warranted. Effective intervention is expected to have a positive impact on the offender and society and lead to increased productivity, decreased resource utilization, and most importantly reduced rates of re-offending.

The United Kingdom ADHD Partnership therefore hosted a meeting of experts on the topic who reviewed the literature and shared personal experiences. It was concluded that there were specific barriers within the prison that hindered the recognition of offenders within the system with ADHD. These include inadequate staff and offender awareness of ADHD symptoms and treatments; lack of training for mental health staff; inappropriate use of screening and diagnostic tools; inappropriate multimodal interventions, care management, supportive services, and multiagency liaison; and a lack of preparation for prison release to address the ongoing needs and care of prisoners with ADHD.

We successfully came to a consensus on practical ways to address these problems and it was clear that the work needs to commence with recognition and identification, and this will involve training. To appropriately care for the individual needs of each offender we recognize that a separate pathway for each mental health disorder (including ADHD) would need to be created. Realizing this may be a problem, we therefore aim to influence criminal justice systems to create a unifying mental health approach with different interventions that address each disorder. We envision a fully integrated intervention pathway—in which the information gathered from screenings and assessments is automatically shared with appropriate service departments for the immediate and coordinated implementation of necessary interventions.

The increased use of the CHAT screening tool, the launch of healthcare standards and commissioning guidance, and the development and implementation of the SECURE STAIRS (an integrated framework of care funded by the NHSE) together are supporting a unifying mental health approach within the secure estate for children and young people in England. Additionally, the NHSE's report The Five Year Forward View for Mental Health [61] outlines general recommendations to support all offenders in the criminal justice system who are experiencing mental health problems. The report recommends expanding liaison and diversion schemes nationally and urges the establishment of comprehensive pathways and quality standards. We advise increasing the use of the B-BAARS [33, 35] as a screening tool to support the identification of adult offenders with ADHD. Our approach based upon expert consensus is directly aligned with these current efforts and offers practical solutions to address the un-met needs of offenders with ADHD.

Table 1 Recommendations

Identification and Assessment

1. Prison staff training to develop awareness of ADHD symptoms and co-morbid conditions (including how these may differ by age and gender), treatments, expected outcomes and the potential impact of prison regime on the offender with ADHD (e.g. greater risk of suicide, impact of segregation). This should include recognition that many offender mental health issues are secondary to ADHD.
2. For youths, adoption of a suitable primary screen (e.g. CHAT) and a clinical diagnostic interview (e.g. ACE). If a rating scale is given (e.g. SNAP-IV, CBRS) this should be sensitive to both inattention and hyperactivity/impulsivity symptoms.
3. For adults, adoption of a suitable primary screen (e.g. B-BAARS) and a clinical diagnostic interview (e.g. ACE+, CAADID, DIVA-2). If a rating scale is given (e.g. BAARS) this should be sensitive to both inattention and hyperactivity/impulsivity symptoms.

Interventions and Treatment

4. All treatments should include psychoeducation about ADHD, including symptoms, co-morbidity, pharmacological and non-pharmacological treatments, side-effects of treatment and expected outcomes.
5. Adoption of appropriate pharmacological and non-pharmacological treatments (see Fig. 1).
6. Adoption of appropriate educational and occupational programmes designed to increase engagement (see Fig. 1).
7. Educational and occupational programmes should be prioritised that advance vocational, creative, technical, and/or athletic skills.

Care Management and Multiagency Liaison

8. There should be close liaison between education and mental health services within the criminal justice system
9. A care plan coordinator should be assigned to the offender while in prison.
10. A comprehensive care plan should be established, including a medication management plan, for the offender while in prison (see Additional file 1, online supplementary material).
11. The care plan should also plan to prepare the offender with ADHD for release from prison (e.g. effecting a seamless transition to ensure continuity of care and uninterrupted treatment with ADHD medication; arranging appropriate links with supportive services and agencies).
12. A critical time intervention approach should be established for a designated person to support the offender through the release process, support implementation of the care plan and ensure engagement in healthcare.

The outcome of the review and consensus is detailed above and the key conclusions and recommendations that arose from it are briefly summarised in Table 1.

While a practical approach to effectively identify and treat offenders with ADHD was achieved at the meeting, it was clear that future research is needed to identify optimal clinical operating models and monitor their implementation and measure their success. It will be valuable to investigate the impact of accurate identification and specifically targeted multimodal treatments on offender health, behaviour, and offence related outcomes. Further research on the needs of female offenders is needed.

A recent study investigating the economic consequences of ADHD in prison has conservatively estimated that the financial burdon of medical and behaviour-related prison care is £11.7 million per annum [62] and future research should evaluate the financial benefits to society of effectively treating offenders with ADHD (compared with not-treating) using functional related outcomes. It will be essential to demonstrate the cost effectiveness of intervention using health economic modelling techniques to garner governmental support and effect change in criminal justice and mental health service policies.

Conclusion

This consensus will inform effective identification and treatment of offenders with ADHD. Appropriate intervention is expected to have a positive impact on the offender and society and may lead to increased productivity, decreased resource utilization, and most importantly reduced rates of re-offending.

Acknowledgements

We acknowledge the assistance of Luke Aldridge-Waddon, Emma-Louise Bush, and Alexander Nolan who attended the consensus meeting and took notes during the small group sessions. We also want to thank Dr. Jennifer Kahle for attending the meeting and for assisting the note takers.

Funding

The meeting was funded by the UK ADHD partnership (UKAP). UKAP has been supported with unrestricted donations from Shire. SY, BC, EF, JH, EW, and GG are consultants with UKAP. None of the authors received funds for attending the meeting or writing the manuscript, aside from KK who received funds for developing the consensus statement.

Authors' contributions

SY and GG led the planning and scientific input of this consensus statement. All authors attended the consensus meeting. KK interpreted the meeting results and wrote the first draft with input from SY and GG, subsequent drafts with input from PA, and the final draft with input from all authors. All authors have read and approved the final manuscript.

Authors' information

Authors have the following expertise - Participation in UK Department of Health initiatives (e.g. NICE Guidelines, NHS England Clinical Reference Group for Offenders): SY, GG, AF, AL, PA. Past or current employment in ADHD specialist clinical or educational services: SY, BC, EW, PA. Past or current employment in general clinical services but with a special interest in ADHD: GG, PC, EF, AF, JH, AL, SM, PM, SR, JS. Past or current service provision in criminal justice services: SY, GG, PC, AF, JH, AL, SM, PM, EW, PA. ADHD committee membership (e.g. UK Adult ADHD Network, ADHD Foundation, ADHD Europe, European Network of Adult ADHD): SY, GG, BC, EF, JH, PM, JS, EW, PA. Criminal justice committee membership (e.g. National Appropriate Adult Network; expert evidence to a public account committee at the House of Lords/House of Commons): GG, AF. Participation in Position Papers on mental health and/or the criminal justice service for professional bodies (e.g. British Psychological Society, Royal College of Psychiatry, World Psychiatric Association Taskforce): SY, GG, AF, SM. KK is a medical writer who worked with this group on a previous ADHD consensus statement.

Consent for publication

Not applicable.

Competing interests

SY has received honoraria for consultancy, sponsorship for attendance at scientific meetings, educational talks, and/or research awards from Janssen, Lilly, HB Pharma, and/or Shire. PM has received honoraria for consultancy and lectures from Lilly, Shire, and Flynn Pharma. AL has received honoraria for consultancy from Lilly. The remaining authors have no disclosures.

Author details

[1]Psychology Services Limited, Croydon, UK. [2]Institute of Psychiatry, Psychology and Neuroscience, Department of Psychology, King's College London, London, UK. [3]Offender Health Research Network, Division of Psychology and Mental Health and Division of Medicine and Health, University of Manchester, Manchester, UK. [4]CLC Consultancy, Dunkeld, Scotland, UK. [5]Sussex Partnership NHS Foundation Trust, Children & Young People's Service, Tunbridge Wells Kent, UK. [6]Forensic Psychiatry and Offender Health Research Network, Division of Psychology and Mental Health and Division of Medicine and Health, University of Manchester, Manchester, UK. [7]Division of Psychology and Language Science, University College London, London, UK. [8]Independent Medical Writer, San Diego, California, USA. [9]Barnet Enfield & Haringey Mental Health NHS Trust, HMP/YOI Feltham, Feltham, UK. [10]Health & Justice Central Team, NHS, London, UK. [11]Kent Prisons, Oxleas NHS Foundation Trust, Dartford, UK. [12]Cheshire & Wirral Partnership NHS Foundation Trust, The Stein Centre, St Catherine's Hospital, Birkenhead, UK. [13]Tees, Esk & Wear Valley NHS Foundation Trust, HMP Frankland, Durham, UK. [14]Humber NHS Foundation Trust, East Yorkshire, London, UK. [15]Institute of Psychiatry, Psychology, and Neuroscience, Department of Forensic and Neurodevelopmental Sciences, King's College London, London, UK. [16]South London & Maudsley NHS Foundation Trust, National Adult Outpatient Neurodevelopmental Clinic, and National Autism Unit, London, UK. [17]Institute of Psychiatry, Psychology, and Neuroscience, King's College London, London, UK.

References

1. Mohr-Jensen C, Steinhausen HC. A meta-analysis and systematic review of the risks associated with childhood attention-deficit hyperactivity disorder on long-term outcome of arrests, convictions, and incarcerations. Clin Psychol Rev. 2016;48:32–42.
2. Young S, Wells J, Gudjonsson GH. Predictors of offending among prisoners: the role of attention-deficit hyperactivity disorder and substance use. J Psychopharmacol. 2011;25(11):1524–32.
3. Arnold LE, Hodgkins P, Caci H, Kahle J, Young S. Effect of treatment modality on long-term outcomes in attention-deficit/hyperactivity disorder: a systematic review. PLoS One. 2015;10(2):e0116407.
4. Young S, Gudjonsson GH, Goodwin EJ, Jotangia A, Farooq R, Haddrick D, Adamou M. Beyond the gates: identifying and managing offenders with attention deficit hyperactivity disorder in community probation services. AIMS Public Health. 2014;1(1):33–42.
5. Ginsberg Y, Quintero J, Anand E, Casillas M, Upadhyaya HP. Underdiagnosis of attention-deficit/hyperactivity disorder in adult patients: a review of the literature. Prim Care Companion CNS Disord. 2014;16(3):PCC.13r01600.
6. Young S, Adamou M, Bolea B, Gudjonsson GH, Müller U, Pitts M, Thome J, Asherson P. The identification and management of ADHD offenders within the criminal justice system: a consensus statement from the UK adult ADHD network and criminal justice agencies. BMC Psychiatry. 2011;11(1):32.

7. American Psychiatric Association. The diagnostic and statistical manual of mental disorders. 5th ed. Arlington: VA; 2013.
8. Faraone SV, Biederman J, Mick E. The age-dependent decline of attention deficit hyperactivity disorder: a meta-analysis of follow-up studies. Psychol Med. 2006;36(2):159–65.
9. Shaw M, Hodgkins P, Caci H, Young S, Kahle J, Woods AG, Arnold LE. A systematic review and analysis of long-term outcomes in attention deficit hyperactivity disorder: effects of treatment and non-treatment. BMC Med. 2012;10:99.
10. Polanczyk G, de Lima MS, Horta BL, Biederman J, Rohde LA. The worldwide prevalence of ADHD: a systematic review and metaregression analysis. Am J Psychiatr. 2007;164(6):942–8.
11. Simon V, Czobor P, Balint S, Meszaros A, Bitter I. Prevalence and correlates of adult attention-deficit hyperactivity disorder: meta-analysis. Br J Psychiatry. 2009;194(3):204–11.
12. Young S, Moss D, Sedgwick O, Fridman M, Hodgkins P. A meta-analysis of the prevalence of attention deficit hyperactivity disorder in incarcerated populations. Psychol Med. 2015;45(2):247–58.
13. Young S, Sedgwick O, Fridman M, Gudjonsson G, Hodgkins P, Lantigua M, González RA. Co-morbid psychiatric disorders among incarcerated ADHD populations: a meta-analysis. Psychol Med. 2015;45(12):2499–510.
14. Shaw J, Baker D, Hunt IM, Moloney A, Appleby L. Suicide by prisoners. Natl Clin Surv. 2004;184(3):263–7.
15. Chang Z, Lichtenstein P, D'Onofrio BM, Sjolander A, Larsson H. Serious transport accidents in adults with attention-deficit/hyperactivity disorder and the effect of medication: a population-based study. JAMA Psychiatry. 2014;71(3):319–25.
16. Lichtenstein P, Larsson H. Medication for attention deficit-hyperactivity disorder and criminality. N Engl J Med. 2013;368(8):776.
17. Chen Q, Sjolander A, Runeson B, D'Onofrio BM, Lichtenstein P, Larsson H. Drug treatment for attention-deficit/hyperactivity disorder and suicidal behaviour: register based study. BMJ. 2014;348:g3769.
18. Young S, Ross RR. R&R2 for ADHD youths and adults: A prosocial competence training Program. Ottawa: Congitive Centre of Canada; 2007.
19. Young S, Emilsson B, Sigurdsson JF, Khondoker M, Philipp-Wiegmann F, Baldursson G, Olafsdottir H, Gudjonsson GH. A randomized controlled trial reporting functional outcomes of cognitive-behavioural therapy in medication-treated adults with ADHD and comorbid psychopathology. Eur Arch Psychiatry Clin Neurosci. 2017;267(3):267-76.
20. Young S, Khondoker M, Emilsson B, Sigurdsson JF, Philipp-Wiegmann F, Baldursson G, Olafsdottir H, Gudjonsson GH. Cognitive–behavioural therapy in medication-treated adults with attention-deficit/hyperactivity disorder and co-morbid psychopathology: a randomized controlled trial using multi-level analysis. Psychol Med. 2015;45(13):2793–804.
21. Emilsson B, Gudjonsson GH, Sigurdsson JF, Baldursson G, Einarsson E, Olafsdottir H, Young S. Cognitive behaviour therapy in medication-treated adults with ADHD and persistent symptoms: a randomized controlled trial. BMC Psychiatry. 2011;11:116.
22. Chang Z, Lichtenstein P, Langstrom N, Larsson H, Fazel S. Association between prescription of major psychotropic medications and violent reoffending after prison release. Jama. 2016;316(17):1798–807.
23. Lichtenstein P, Halldner L, Zetterqvist J, Sjolander A, Serlachius E, Fazel S, Langstrom N, Larsson H. Medication for attention deficit-hyperactivity disorder and criminality. N Engl J Med. 2012;367(21):2006–14.
24. Walmsley R: World prison population list., 11th edn: world prison brief; 2015.
25. Martin MS, Colman I, Simpson AI, McKenzie K. Mental health screening tools in correctional institutions: a systematic review. BMC Psychiatry. 2013;13:275.
26. Senior J, Birmingham L, Harty MA, Hassan L, Hayes AJ, Kendall K, King C, Lathlean J, Lowthian C, Mills A, et al. Identification and management of prisoners with severe psychiatric illness by specialist mental health services. Psychol Med. 2013;43(7):1511–20.
27. Konstenius M, Larsson H, Lundholm L, Philips B, van de Glind G, Jayaram-Lindström N, Franck J. An epidemiological study of ADHD, substance use, and comorbid problems in incarcerated women in Sweden. J Atten Disord. 2012;19(1):44–52.
28. Hollingdale J, Woodhouse E, Asherson P, Gudjonsson GH, Young S. A pilot study examining ADHD and Behavioural disturbance in female mentally disordered offenders. AIMS Public Health. 2014;1(2):100–8.
29. Royal College of Paediatrics and Child Health. Healthcare standards for children and young people in secure settings. London: Royal Collect of Paediatrics and Child Health; 2013. https://www.rcpch.ac.uk/cypss. Accessed 29 Aug 2018.
30. Chitsabesan P, Lennox C, Theodosiou L, Law H, Bailey S, Shaw J. The development of the comprehensive health assessment tool for young offenders within the secure estate. J Forensic Psychiatry Psychol. 2014;25(1):1–25.
31. Bussing R, Fernandez M, Harwood M, Hou W, Garvan CW, Eyberg SM, Swanson JM. Parent and teacher SNAP-IV ratings of attention deficit hyperactivity disorder symptoms. Assessment. 2008;15(3):317–28.
32. Conners CK, Pitkanen J, Rzepa SR. Conners comprehensive behavior rating scale. In: Kreutzer JS, DeLuca J, Caplan B, editors. Encyclopedia of Clinical Neuropsychology. Edn. New York: Springer; 2011. p. 678–80.
33. ADHD Child Evaluation (ACE) [https://www.psychology-services.uk.com/resources.htm]. Accessed 29 Aug 2018.
34. Kessler RC, Adler LA, Gruber MJ, Sarawate CA, Spencer T, Van Brunt DL. Validity of the World Health Organization adult ADHD self-report scale (ASRS) screener in a representative sample of health plan members. Int J Methods Psychiatr Res. 2007;16(2):52–65.
35. Young S, González RA, Mutch L, Mallet-Lambert I, O'Rourke L, Hickey N, Asherson P, Gudjonsson GH. Diagnostic accuracy of a brief screening tool for attention deficit hyperactivity disorder in UK prison inmates. Psychol Med. 2016;46(7):1449–58.
36. Brown K, Cullen A, Kooyman I, Forrester A. Mental health expertise at prison reception. J Forensic Psychiatry Psychol. 2015;26(1):107–15.
37. Epstein JN, Johnson DE, Conners CK: CAADID: Conners adult ADHD Diagnstic interview for DSM-IV: multi health systems (MHS); 2001.
38. Diagnosing ADHD in Adults: an examination of the discriminative validity of neuropsychological tests and diagnostic assessment instruments. J Atten Disord. 2018;22(11):1019-31.
39. Ramos-Quiroga JA, Nasillo V, Richarte V, Corrales M, Palma F, Ibáñez P, Michelsen M, Van de Glind G, Casas M, Kooij JJS. Criteria and concurrent validity of DIVA 2.0. J Atten Disord. 2016:1-10. https://doi.org/10.1177/1087054716646451.
40. ACE+ [https://www.psychology-services.uk.com/resources.htm]. Accessed 29 Aug 2018.
41. UK Adult ADHD. Network: handbook for attention deficit hyperactivity disorder in adults. London: UK: springer science & business media; 2013.
42. Naylor B. Human rights and their application in prisons , Monash University Faculty of Law Legal Studies Research Paper No. Prison Serv J 2016. 2016; 9(227):17–22.
43. Forrester A, Piper, M, World psychiatric association: prison public health position statement. 2017.
44. Metzner JL, Fellner J. Solitary confinement and mental illness in U.S. prisons: a Challengefor medical ethics. J Am Acad Psychiatry Law. 2010;38(1):104–8.
45. Young S, Gudjonsson G, O'Rourke L, Woodhouse E, Ashwood K, Murphy D, Asherson P. Attention-deficit-hyperactivity disorder and associated functional impairments in mentally disordered offenders. Psychiatry Res. 2015;230(2):387–93.
46. Hughes N, Williams H, Chitsabesan P, Davies R, Mounce L. Nobody made the connection: the prevalence of neurodisability in young people who offend. London: The Office of the Children's Commissioner; 2012.
47. Ginsberg Y, Lindefors N. Methylphenidate treatment of adult male prison inmates with attention-deficit hyperactivity disorder: randomised double-blind placebo-controlled trial with open-label extension. Br J Psychiatry. 2012;200(1):68–73.
48. Volkow ND, Swanson JM. Variables that affect the clinical use and abuse of methylphenidate in the treatment of ADHD. Am J Psychiatr. 2003;160(11):1909–18.
49. Attention deficit hyperactivity disorder Diagnosis and management of ADHD in children, young people and adults. NICE Clinical Guideline 72; 2009.
50. Young S, González R, Wolff K, Xenitidis K, Mutch L, Mallet-Lambert I, Gudjonsson GH. Transitions and motivations for substance misuse in prison inmates with ADHD and conduct disorder: validation of a new instrument. J Dual Diagn. (in press)
51. Young S, González R, Wolff K, Xenitidis K, Mutch LM-LI, Gudjonsson GH. Substance and alcohol misuse, drug pathways and offending behaviours in association with ADHD in prison inmates. J Atten Disord. (in press)
52. King S, Gieve M. Evaluation of a pilot to deliver forensic mental health interventions to young people at risk of violent offending. Commissioned by MOPAC. London: The Tavistock Institute; 2013.
53. Solanto MV, Marks DJ, Wasserstein J, Mitchell K, Abikoff H, Alvir JM, Kofman MD. Efficacy of meta-cognitive therapy for adult ADHD. Am J Psychiatr. 2010;167(8):958–68.
54. Philipsen A, Graf E, Jans T, Matthies S, Borel P, Colla M, Gentschow L, Langner D, Jacob C, Gross-Lesch S, et al. A randomized controlled multicenter trial on the multimodal treatment of adult attention-deficit hyperactivity disorder: enrollment and characteristics of the study sample. Atten Deficit Hyperact disord. 2014;6(1):35–47.

55. Young S, Bramham J. Cognitive-behavioural therapy for ADHD in adolescents and adults: A Psychological Guide to Practice. 2nd ed. Chichester: Wiley.; 2012.
56. Barry TD, Lyman RD, Klinger LG. Academic underachievement and attention-deficit/hyperactivity disorder: the negative impact of symptom severity on school performance. J Sch Psychol. 2002;40(3):259–83.
57. Biederman J, Faraone S, Milberger S, Guite J, Mick E, Chen L, Mennin D, Marrs A, Ouellette C, Moore P, et al. A prospective 4-year follow-up study of attention-deficit hyperactivity and related disorders. Arch Gen Psychiatry. 1996;53(5):437–46.
58. Care Programme Approach [http://www.nhs.uk/Conditions/social-care-and-support-guide/Pages/care-programme-approach.aspx]. Accessed 29 Aug 2018.
59. Attention deficit hyperactivity disorder: Diagnosis and management: NICE guideline [NG87]. 2018. https://www.nice.org.uk/guidance/ng87. Accessed 29 Aug 2018.
60. Jarrett M, Thornicroft G, Forrester A, Harty M, Senior J, King C, Huckle S, Parrott J, Dunn G, Shaw J. Continuity of care for recently released prisoners with mental illness: a pilot randomised controlled trial testing the feasibility of a critical time intervention. Epidemiol Psychiatr Sci. 2012;21(2):187–93.
61. National Health Service England. The five year forward view for mental health. Mental Health Taskforce Strategy. 2016:1–81. https://www.england.nhs.uk/mental-health/taskforce/. Accessed 29 Aug 2018.
62. Young S, Gonzalez R, Fridman M, Hodgkins P, Kim K, Gudjonsson G. The economic consequences of ADHD in the Scottish prison system. BMC Psychiatry. 18:210. https://doi.org/10.1186/s12888-018-1792-x.

15

FADS1-FADS2 and *ELOVL2* gene polymorphisms in susceptibility to autism spectrum disorders in Chinese children

Caihong Sun[1†], Mingyang Zou[1†], Xuelai Wang[1], Wei Xia[1], Yongjuan Ma[1], Shuang Liang[1], Yanqiu Hao[2], Lijie Wu[1*] and Songbin Fu[3*]

Abstract

Backgroud: Autism spectrum disorders (ASD) are a complex group of neurodevelopmental disorders with a genetic basis. The role of long-chain polyunsaturated fatty acids (LC-PUFAs) and the occurrence of autism has been the focus of many recent studies. The present study investigates whether genetic variants of the *fatty acid desaturase* (*FADS*) 1/2 and *elongation of very long-chain fatty acids protein* (*ELOVL*) 2 genes, which are involved in LC-PUFA metabolism, are associated with ASD risk.

Methods: A cohort of 243 ASD patients and 243 unrelated healthy controls were enrolled in this case control study. Sixteen tag single nucleotide polymorphisms from the *FADS1–2* and *ELOVL2* genes were genotyped using the Sequenom Mass Array.

Results: There were significant differences in allelic distribution of *FADS2 rs526126* (OR = 0.55, 95% CI = 0.42–0.72, $p_{FDR} < 0.05$) between autistic children and controls. *FADS2 rs526126* and *ELOVL2 rs10498676* were associated with decreased ASD risk in recessive model (OR = 0.07, 95% CI = 0.02–0.22, $p_{FDR} < 0.01$; OR = 0.56, 95% CI = 0.35–0.89, $p_{FDR} = 0.042$), while *ELOVL2 rs17606561*, *rs3756963*, and *rs9468304* were associated with increased ASD risk in overdominant model (OR = 1.63, 95% CI = 1.12–2.36, $p_{FDR} = 0.036$; OR = 1.64, 95% CI = 1.14–2.37, $p_{FDR} = 0.039$; OR = 1.75, 95% CI = 1.22–2.50, $p_{FDR} = 0.017$). The A/A genotype of *rs10498676* was correlated with a decline in the Autism Diagnostic Interview-Revised communication (verbal and nonverbal) domain.

Conclusions: These findings provide evidence of an association between *FADS2* and *ELOVL2* polymorphisms and ASD susceptibility in Chinese children.

Keywords: Autism spectrum disorders, *FADS1–2; ELOVL2*, Long-chain polyunsaturated fatty acids, Single nucleotide polymorphisms

Background

Autism spectrum disorders (ASD) are a heterogeneous group of neurodevelopmental disorders characterized by abnormal social interaction, impaired language and communication, and repetitive stereotypic behaviors or a narrow range of interests [1]. ASD likely result from complex interactions between multiple genes and environmental factors, with some studies suggesting that genetics play a role in the majority of autism cases [2]. Genomic analyses have revealed that single nucleotide polymorphisms (SNPs) in specific genes are associated with predisposition to ASD and may explain the phenotypic variability observed in patients [3].

Polyunsaturated fatty acid (PUFAs) are classified as omega-3 (n-3) or omega-6 (n-6) depending on the location of the last double bond relative to the terminal methyl group in the carbon chain [4]. The essential PUFA precursors linoleic acid (LA, 18:2n-6) and alpha-linolenic acid (ALA, 18:3n-3) are metabolized by elongation and desaturation into long-chain (> 20 C atoms) (LC-) PUFAs, such as

* Correspondence: wulijiehyd@126.com; fusb@ems.hrbmu.edu.cn
†Caihong Sun and Mingyang Zou contributed equally to this work.
[1]Department of Children's and Adolescent Health, Public Health College, Harbin Medical University, Harbin 150081, China
[3]Laboratory of Medical Genetics, Harbin Medical University, Harbin 150081, China

arachidonic acid (AA, 20:4n-6), eicosapentaenoic acid (EPA, 20:5n-3), and docosahexaenoic acid (DHA, 22:6n-3). The two types of PUFA share and compete for the same enzymes in their biosynthesis (Fig. 1). Rate-limiting LC-PUFA biosynthetic enzymes in humans include delta-5 and -6 desaturase, and elongases 2 encoded by *fatty acid desaturase* (*FADS*)*1*, *FADS2*, and *elongation of very long-chain fatty acids protein* (*ELOVL*)*2*, respectively. Independent of dietary effects, polymorphisms in these genes have been shown to affect LC-PUFA status in different ethnic groups [5–9]. LC-PUFAs are indispensible components of neuronal membranes and modulate the integrity, fluidity, and function of transmembrane proteins. They also act as second messengers in intracellular signaling pathways or regulate gene transcription and expression, neurogenesis, neuroprotection, and neurotransmission, and serve as precursors for the synthesis of eicosanoids and docosanoids, which are potent regulators of immune and inflammatory processes in the brain [4, 10]. In particular, DHA and AA, the principal LC-PUFAs in the brain, that mediate many physiological effects. Numerous epidemiological and experimental studies have reported a link between LC-PUFA content in blood and certain tissues and mental health as well as cognitive and motor development [7, 11–13]. As such, there is great interest in investigating the potential connection between LC-PUFA levels and the occurrence of autism.

Although there is evidence to suggest that autistic patients have abnormal LC-PUFA metabolism that manifests as a reduction in their levels [14–17], few studies have explored the relationship between genes involved in LC-PUFA metabolism and risk of ASD. *FADS1/2* and *ELOVL2* gene polymorphisms may be the primary determinants not only of LC-PUFA status, but also of the biological effects exerted by LC-PUFAs [9]. We previously reported that serum LC-PUFA levels and delta-6 and -5 desaturase and elongase 2 were downregulated in a rat model of ASD relative to control rats under the same dietary conditions [18]. These findings indicate that mutations in the *FADS1/2* and *ELOVL2* genes resulting in abnormal expression of delta-6 and -5 desaturase and elongase 2, possibly due to perturbed LC-PUFA status during critical stages of neural development that increases susceptibility to ASD. To clarify the etiology of ASD, the present study investigated the relationship between *FADS1/2* and *ELOVL2* gene polymorphisms and ASD risk as well as clinical features of ASD in a Chinese Han population.

Methods

Subjects

A total of 243 consecutive patients with ASD were recruited from the Child Development and Behavior

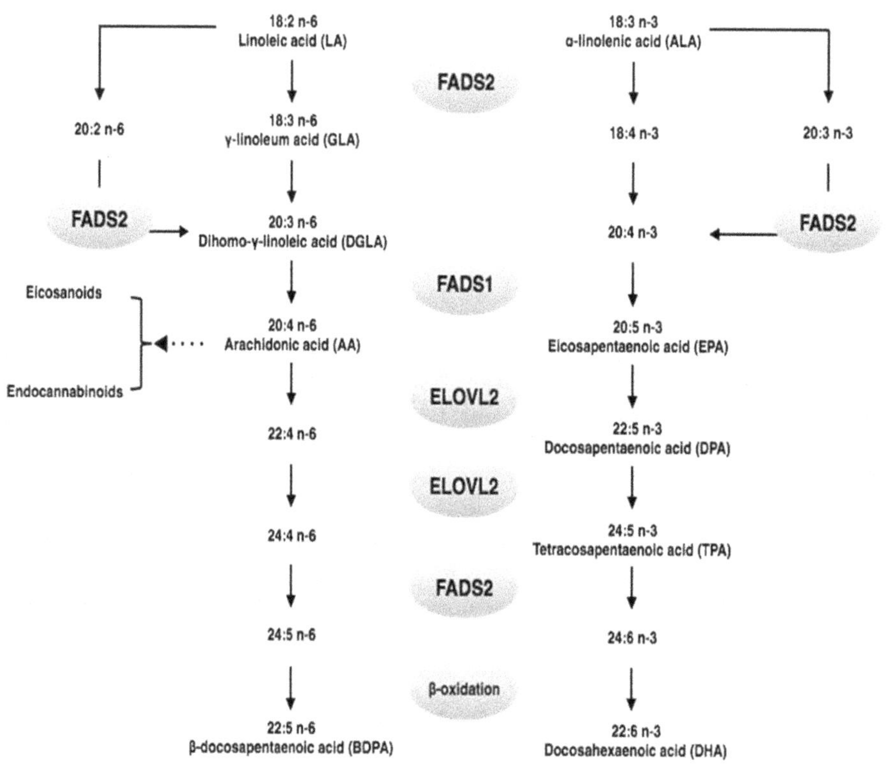

Fig. 1 Metabolic pathways for endogenous n-6 and n-3 polyunsaturated fatty acids

Research Center of Harbin Medical University, Harbin, China, from May 2013 to March 2016. Inclusion criteria were a diagnosis of ASD, which was made by a specialist clinician according to Diagnostic and Statistical Manual of Mental Disorders, Fifth Edition (DSM-V) criteria. One of the following methods was used as an aid to diagnose: Childhood Autism Rating Scales, Autism Behavior Checklist, Autism Diagnostic Observation Schedule (ADOS), Autism Diagnostic Interview-Revised (ADI-R). Exclusion criteria were children with significant sensory and motor impairment, known genetic disorders, seizures at the time of enrollment, and any other neurological conditions suspected to be associated with autism. Unrelated healthy children ($n = 243$) without history of developmental delay or other neurological disorders were randomly selected from normal kindergartens in Harbin, China as the controls. All study subjects were of Chinese Han ethnicity.

Clinical assessment

Autism-specific behaviors and symptoms were evaluated according to ADOS and ADI-R, which were administered during interviews with patients or their guardians and scored by a clinical psychologist or trainee who met standard requirements for research reliability. Due to applicability, cooperativity and compliance from patients and their guardians, some cases did not complete above two examinations. Only 184 of 243 ASD cases completed the ADOS and/or ADI-R. The ADOS was available for 174 assessments (71.6% of sample), the ADI-R for 176 assessments (72.4%). Nine participants were excluded due to missing data. Sample characteristics are provided in Additional file 1: Table S1.

ADOS is a semi-structured standardized observational assessment that is organized into four modules according to developmental and expressive language level. The calibrated severity score (CSS), which is a standardized score of the relative severity of autism-specific behaviors, is less influenced by participant demographics than by raw scores [19]. The ADOS CSS algorithm encompasses social affect (SA) and restricted repetitive behavior (RRB) domains, which are consistent with DSM-V [20]; these allow comparisons of assessments across modules and times. Procedures for deriving the ADOS-CSS, SA-CSS and RRB-CSS are detailed in the original study [19, 21].

ADI-R is a semi-structured parent interview that assesses autism symptoms across three domains: social, communication, and repetitive behavior. Although the algorithm scores were originally designed to provide categorical diagnostic information, taking language level and age at the time of interview into account, ADI-R domain and total scores can be used as estimates of the severity of core ASD symptoms [22]. Higher adjusted ADI-R scores indicate greater impairment. Before similar strategies used in ADOS can be applied to ADI-R, ADI-R scores must be statistically adjusted for language level indicated by the ADOS module, intelligence quotients (IQ), sex and age. The IQ scores were derived from the Wechsler Preschool and Primary Scales of Intelligence, Wechsler Intelligence Scale for Children or the Peabody Picture Vocabulary Test.

SNP selection and genotyping

We used genotyping data from the Chinese Han in Beijing (CHB) panel of the HapMap Project Phase II to select tag SNPs in *FADS1/2* and *ELOVL2* genes using the Tagger program incorporated with Haploview v.4.2 software (Broad Institute of Massachusetts Institute of Technology and Harvard, Cambridge, MA, USA) according to the following criteria: pairwise tagging ($r^2 \geq 0.8$) and minor allele frequency ≥ 0.05, leading to the identification of 16 tag SNPs (one in *FADS1* and seven in *FADS2* that captured more than 34 initially identified SNPs; and eight in *ELOVL2* that captured more than 45 initially identified SNPs). Detailed information for tag SNPs are showed in Additional file 1: Table S2.

Blood samples were obtained from each participant in an EDTA-containing tube. Genomic DNA was extracted using the Qiagen QIAamp DNA Mini kit (Qiagen, Hilden, Germany) according to the manufacturer's instructions. DNA quality was confirmed on a 1% agarose gel, and DNA concentrations were determined by measuring the absorbance at 260 nm using a NanoDrop 2000 spectrophotometer (Thermo Fisher Scientific, Waltham, MA, USA). SNPs were genotyped using the MassArray platform (Sequenom, San Diego, CA, USA) with the primers showed in Additional file 1: Table S3. For genotyping, investigators were blinded to case/control status, and 30 random samples were tested in duplicate for all 16 tag SNPs for quality control, with a reproducibility of 100%.

Statistical analyses

Haploview v.4.2 software was used to evaluate deviations from Hardy–Weinberg equilibrium (HWE) among controls, as well as for analysis of linkage disequilibrium (LD) and haplotype construction. SNPstats software (http://bioinfo.iconcologia.net/SNPstats) was used to calculate the odds ratios (ORs) and 95% confidence intervals (CIs) in different genetic models. SNP associated analyses were estimated under the following genetic models: codominant, dominant, recessive, overdominant and log-additive model. When the values of Akaike' information criterion (AIC) and Bayesian information criterion (BIC) are the lowest, the genetic model is the optimal model for the SNP. Benjamini-Hochberg approach based on false discovery rate (FDR) criterion was applied to avoid the type I error in multiple comparisons. Potential relationships between genetic and phenotypic characteristics were evaluated by one-way analysis of variance with adjustment for language level, IQ, sex and age at the time of assessment, and the *Bonferroni* correction was applied in multiple testing. Data were analyzed using SPSS v.17.0 software (SPSS Inc., Chicago, IL, USA). All reported p values were two-tailed, and statistical significance was defined at the $\alpha = 0.05$ level.

Results

Clinical characteristics

The 243 cases included 204 boys and 39 girls with a mean age of 5.19 ± 1.96 years. The 243 controls included 192 boys and 51 girls with a mean age of 4.96 ± 0.97 years. There were no differences in terms of age and gender between cases and controls ($p = 0.101$ and $p = 0.161$, respectively).

Association between the SNPs and ASD risk

Call rates for the 16 tag SNPs exceeded 95%. These differences in genotyping efficiency were attributable to different sample sizes for each SNP measured. The *rs2845573* was excluded from statistical analyses because the corresponding genotypes in the control group deviated from HWE ($p < 0.05$). The genotype distributions of the remaining SNPs were in agreement with HWE in the control group ($p > 0.05$; Table 1).

Table 2 summarized the allele frequencies of the SNPs in ASD patients and controls. Allele frequencies for *FADS2 rs526126* and *ELOVL2 rs9468304* differed significantly between cases and controls ($p < 0.05$). The *rs526126* G allele (OR = 0.55, 95% CI = 0.42–0.72, $p < 0.001$) was associated with a lower risk of ASD, whereas the *rs9468304* G allele (OR = 1.37, 95% CI = 1.05–1.79, $p = 0.035$) was associated with a higher risk of ASD. The allele distributions of other tag SNPs were non-significant. However, the positive result of *rs9468304* presented no statistical significance after FDR-based correction.

We analyzed the association of the SNPs with ASD risk in five genetic models (Additional file 1: Table S4). As shown in Table 3, there were significant differences in genotype frequencies of *rs526126, rs17606561, rs3756963, rs10498676*, and *rs9468304* between the patient and control groups ($p < 0.05$). After the p values were adjusted by FDR-based correction, *FADS2 rs526126* (OR = 0.07, 95% CI = 0.02–0.22, $p_{FDR} < 0.01$), and *ELOVL2 rs10498676* (OR = 0.56, 95% CI = 0.35–0.89, $p_{FDR} = 0.042$) were associated with a reduced risk of ASD in the recessive model. Whereas *ELOVL2 rs17606561* (OR = 1.63; 95% CI = 1.12–2.36, $p_{FDR} = 0.036$), *rs3756963* (OR = 1.64, 95% CI = 1.14–2.37, $p_{FDR} = 0.039$) and *rs9468304* (OR = 1.75, 95% CI = 1.22–2.50, $p_{FDR} = 0.017$) were associated with an increased risk of ASD in the overdominant model. There were no associations for the remaining SNPs under any kind of genetic model.

Haplotype analysis

In the *FADS1/2* gene cluster, LD analysis of seven SNPs identified one haplotype block consisting of two SNPs (*rs174585* and *rs174593*) that produced two haplotypes with frequencies > 1% (Fig. 2a and Table 4). There were no differences in the frequencies of these haplotypes between ASD patients and controls.

Table 1 Characteristics of *FADS1–2* and *ELOVL2* tag SNPs

SNP ID	Gene	Genomic position (bp)	Genic position	Reference allele [a]	Call rate %	MAF [b]	HWE [b] (p)
rs174546	*FADS1*	61,802,358	3'UTR	C	98.6	0.322	0.958
rs2845573	*FADS2*	61,834,436	intron	A	98.8	0.071	**< 0.001***
rs174585	*FADS2*	61,844,222	intron	G	99.8	0.091	0.786
rs174593	*FADS2*	61,851,359	intron	T	100.0	0.095	1.000
rs174602	*FADS2*	61,856,942	intron	T	98.3	0.241	0.455
rs498793	*FADS2*	61,857,233	intron	T	99.0	0.075	0.266
rs526126	*FADS2*	61,857,413	intron	C	96.7	0.428	0.175
rs174616	*FADS2*	61,861,650	intron	G	99.8	0.152	0.994
rs17606561	*ELOVL2*	10,982,126	3'UTR	G	99.8	0.215	0.580
rs2236212	*ELOVL2*	10,994,782	intron	C	98.1	0.332	1.000
rs3798712	*ELOVL2*	11,007,869	intron	A	98.8	0.233	0.912
rs953413	*ELOVL2*	11,012,626	intron	A	97.9	0.095	0.186
rs3756963	*ELOVL2*	11,021,921	intron	T	99.7	0.229	0.492
rs10498676	*ELOVL2*	11,026,766	intron	G	98.1	0.450	0.100
rs6936315	*ELOVL2*	11,035,739	intron	T	98.8	0.288	1.000
rs9468304	*ELOVL2*	11,041,932	intron	A	99.8	0.320	0.408

MAF minor allele frequency, *HWE* Hardy-Weinberg equilibrium, * $p < 0.05$
[a] determined by most frequent allele among controls
[b] among controls ($n = 243$)

Table 2 Distribution of allelic frequencies of SNPs in cases and controls (n, %)

SNPs	Allele (major:minor)	Control (243)		Case (243)		OR(95%CI)	p	p_{FDR}
		major	minor	major	minor			
rs174546	C:T	324(67.8)	154(32.2)	328(68.3)	152(31.7)	0.98(0.75–1.29)	0.855	0.916
rs174585	G:A	440(90.9)	44(9.1)	452(93.0)	34(7.0)	0.75(0.47–1.20)	0.230	0.493
rs498793	C:T	444(92.5)	36(7.5)	444(92.1)	38(7.9)	1.07(0.66–1.72)	0.823	1.029
rs174602	T:C	360(75.9)	114(24.1)	375(77.5)	109(22.5)	0.94(0.70–1.28)	0.575	0.958
rs174593	T:C	440(90.5)	46(9.5)	451(92.8)	35(7.2)	0.73(0.46–1.16)	0.202	0.505
rs526126	C:G	275(56.6)	211(43.4)	315(69.4)	139(30.6)	0.55(0.42–0.72)	**< 0.001**	**< 0.05***
rs174616	G:A	412(84.8)	74(15.2)	414(85.5)	70(14.5)	0.93(0.65–1.33)	0.738	1.107
rs17606561	G:A	380(78.5)	104(21.5)	360(74.1)	126(25.9)	1.31(0.97–1.77)	0.104	0.390
rs2236212	C:G	318(66.8)	158(33.2)	317(66.3)	161(33.7)	1.01(0.77–1.32)	0.873	0.873
rs3798712	A:G	365(76.7)	111(23.3)	374(77.3)	110(22.7)	0.94(0.69–1.27)	0.828	0.955
rs953413	A:G	436(90.5)	46(9.5)	415(88.3)	55(11.7)	1.28(0.84–1.93)	0.280	0.525
rs3756963	T:C	373(77.1)	111(22.9)	354(72.8)	132(27.2)	1.28(0.96–1.72)	0.129	0.387
rs10498676	G:A	263(55.0)	215(45.0)	289(60.7)	187(39.3)	0.79(0.61–1.02)	0.075	0.375
rs6936315	T:C	339(71.2)	137(28.8)	349(72.1)	135(27.9)	0.92(0.70–1.23)	0.760	1.036
rs9468304	A:G	329(68.0)	155(32.0)	299(61.5)	187(38.5)	1.37(1.05–1.79)	**0.035**	0.263

Major major allele, *minor* minor allele, *OR* Odds ratio, *CI* confidence interval, *FDR* false discovery rate, p_{FDR} FDR corrected p value, $^{*}p < 0.05$

In the *ELOVL2* gene, LD analysis of eight SNPs identified one haplotype block consisting of six SNPs (*rs17606561, rs2236212, rs3798712, rs953413, rs3756963,* and *rs10498676*) that produced five haplotypes with frequencies > 1 (Fig. 2b and Table 4). There were no differences in the frequencies of these haplotypes between ASD patients and controls.

Association between genotype and ASD symptoms

According to above positive results, only 5 SNPs (*rs526126, rs17606561, rs3756963, rs10498676, rs9468304*) were selected in analyses of the relationships between gene polymorphisms and a series of ASD-specific features, including ADI-R and ADOS domains. Analysis of variance revealed that the A/A genotype of *rs10498676* had lower scores for ADI-R social, ADI-R verbal and nonverbal communication (Comm-V and -NV, respectively) than the G/G and A/G genotypes after adjusting for language level, IQ, sex and age. However, the positive result of ADI-R social presented no statistical significance after *Bonferroni* correction (Table 5). There were no associations for the remaining 4 SNPs (Additional file 1: Table S5).

Discussion

In this population-based case-control study, we aimed to investigate the effect of gene variations involved in LC-PUFA pathways and metabolism on the risk of ASD using allele, genotype, and haplotype analyses. We also investigated associations between gene polymorphisms and clinical features of ASD. This is the first study to investigate the association between *FADS1/2* and *ELOVL2* gene polymorphisms and ASD risk.

Our team previously found that significantly lower serum levels of AA, DHA and docosapentaenoic acid (DPA, 22:5n-3) in autistic children than in controls [14]. Then, the following animal experiments, we strictly controlled dietary conditions in both groups in order to reduce the effects of dietary factors, and we still found that serum n-3 and n-6 PUFA levels were lower in ASD model rats relative to controls. Moreover, we observed that the expression of rate-limiting PUFA metabolic enzymes was downregulated in the ASD group [18]. However, genetic mutations were not taken into consideration in our previous work. Investigating the role of genes involved in LC-PUFA metabolism may provide valuable insight into genetic susceptibility to ASD.

The *FADS1* and *FADS2* genes are seated head-to-head in a cluster on chromosome 11 (11q12–q13) and expressed in most human tissues, particularly in the liver, heart, and brain. An Avon longitudinal study in over 4000 pregnant women and their children indicated that *FADS* polymorphisms influenced maternal erythrocyte the concentrations of n-3 DHA, which disrupted the baby's DHA supply in utero [23]. Animal studies have shown that irreversible and persistent changes in hypothalamic phospholipid composition resulted from abnormally high n-6:n-3 ratio early in life, the same as a dysfunction or down-regulation of the conversion of ALA to DHA by the delta-6 desaturase enzyme [24]. These two findings suggest that *FADS* polymorphisms may lead to irreversible structural and functional changes in neurons. In CHIANTI study reported that polymorphisms in the *FADS1/2* gene cluster accounted for as much as 18.6 of the variance in plasma and erythrocyte

Table 3 SNPs in significant genetic models associated with ASD risk

SNPs	Model	genotype	Control (243)	Case (243)	OR (95% CI)	p	p_{FDR}
rs174546	overdominant	C/C-T/T	133 (55.6)	136 (56.7)	1.00	0.82	0.82
		T/C	106 (44.4)	104 (43.3)	0.96 (0.67–1.38)		
rs174585	dominant	G/G	199 (82.2)	210 (86.4)	1.00	0.2	0.375
		A/G-A/A	43 (17.8)	33 (13.6)	0.73 (0.44–1.19)		
rs498793	overdominant	C/C-T/T	210 (87.5%)	207 (85.9%)	1.00	0.6	0.75
		T/C	30 (12.5%)	34 (14.1%)	1.15 (0.68–1.95)		
rs174602	overdominant	T/T-C/C	145 (61.2)	157 (64.9)	1.00	0.4	0.667
		C/T	92 (38.8)	85 (35.1)	0.85 (0.59–1.24)		
rs174593	recessive	T/T-C/T	241 (99.2)	243 (100)	1.00	0.095	0.204
		C/C	2 (0.8)	0 (0)	NA		
rs526126	recessive	C/C-G/C	203 (83.5)	224 (98.7)	1.00	**< 0.0001**	**< 0.01***
		G/G	40 (16.5)	3 (1.3)	**0.07 (0.02–0.22)**		
rs174616	overdominant	G/G-A/A	181 (74.5)	188 (77.7)	1.00	0.41	0.615
		A/G	62 (25.5)	54 (22.3)	0.84 (0.55–1.27)		
rs17606561	overdominant	G/G-A/A	164 (67.8)	137 (56.4)	1.00	**0.0096**	**0.036***
		A/G	78 (32.2)	106 (43.6)	**1.63 (1.12–2.36)**		
rs2236212	recessive	C/C-G/C	212 (89.1)	210 (87.9)	1.00	0.68	0.729
		G/G	26 (10.9)	29 (12.1)	1.13 (0.64–1.98)		
rs3798712	overdominant	A/A-G/G	151 (63.5)	160 (66.1)	1.00	0.54	0.736
		G/A	87 (36.5)	82 (33.9)	0.89 (0.61–1.29)		
rs953413	recessive	A/A-G/A	241 (100)	232 (98.7)	1.00	0.039	0.098
		G/G	0 (0)	3 (1.3)	NA		
rs3756963	overdominant	T/T-C/C	161 (66.5)	133 (54.7)	1.00	**0.0078**	**0.039***
		C/T	81 (33.5)	110 (45.3)	**1.64 (1.14–2.37)**		
rs10498676	recessive	G/G-A/G	184 (77)	204 (85.7)	1.00	**0.014**	**0.042***
		A/A	55 (23)	34 (14.3)	**0.56 (0.35–0.89)**		
rs6936315	overdominant	T/T-C/C	141 (59.2)	149 (61.6)	1.00	0.6	0.692
		C/T	97 (40.8)	93 (38.4)	0.91 (0.63–1.31)		
rs9468304	overdominant	A/A-G/G	143 (59.1)	110 (45.3)	1.00	**0.0023**	**0.017***
		G/A	99 (40.9)	133 (54.7)	**1.75 (1.22–2.50)**		

OR Odds ratio, *CI* confidence interval, p_{FDR} FDR corrected p value,* $p < 0.05$, *NA* is not applicable

PUFA concentrations [25], and up to 28.5 of the variance in serum LC-PUFA content [9]. Moreover, the *FADS1/2* gene cluster is mainly involved in regulating the levels of pro- and anti-inflammatory eicosanoids synthesized from LC-PUFAs [26]. In our results, the frequencies of the minor allele G and genotype G/G of *rs526126* were lower in ASD cases than in controls, suggesting that individuals with the G allele have a lower risk of ASD. In other studies of this locus, *rs526126* G allele carriers had lower AA levels as well as reduced desaturase activity, as indicated by AA/dihomo-γ-linoleic acid (DGLA, 20:3n-6), γ-linoleic acid (GLA,18:3n-6)/LA, and AA/LA ratios [27]. The AA/DGLA, GLA/LA, and AA/LA product-to-precursor ratios are used to estimate FADS1, FADS2, and aggregate FADS1/2 desaturase indices, respectively. Moran et al. also found that the G allele of *rs526126* was nominally also related to lower levels of AA and lower FADS1 index, and the maternal G/G genotype was associated with higher child cognition scores, although this was not statistically significant [28]. In addition to the n-6 pathway, the minor allele G was positively associated with levels of desaturase subtrates (ALA) and negatively associated with levels of desaturase products (EPA and DHA) as well as ratios of n-3 (EPA/ALA) pathway components [23]. There are two possible explanations for the protective effects of allele G of *rs526126*. Firstly, eicosanoids, as the strongly pro-inflammatory factors, such as prostaglandins, thromboxanes, leukotrienes, and lipoxins that are transformed from AA via the cyclooxygenase and lipoxygenase pathways, are related to increased neuroinflammation, which is thought to damage nervous

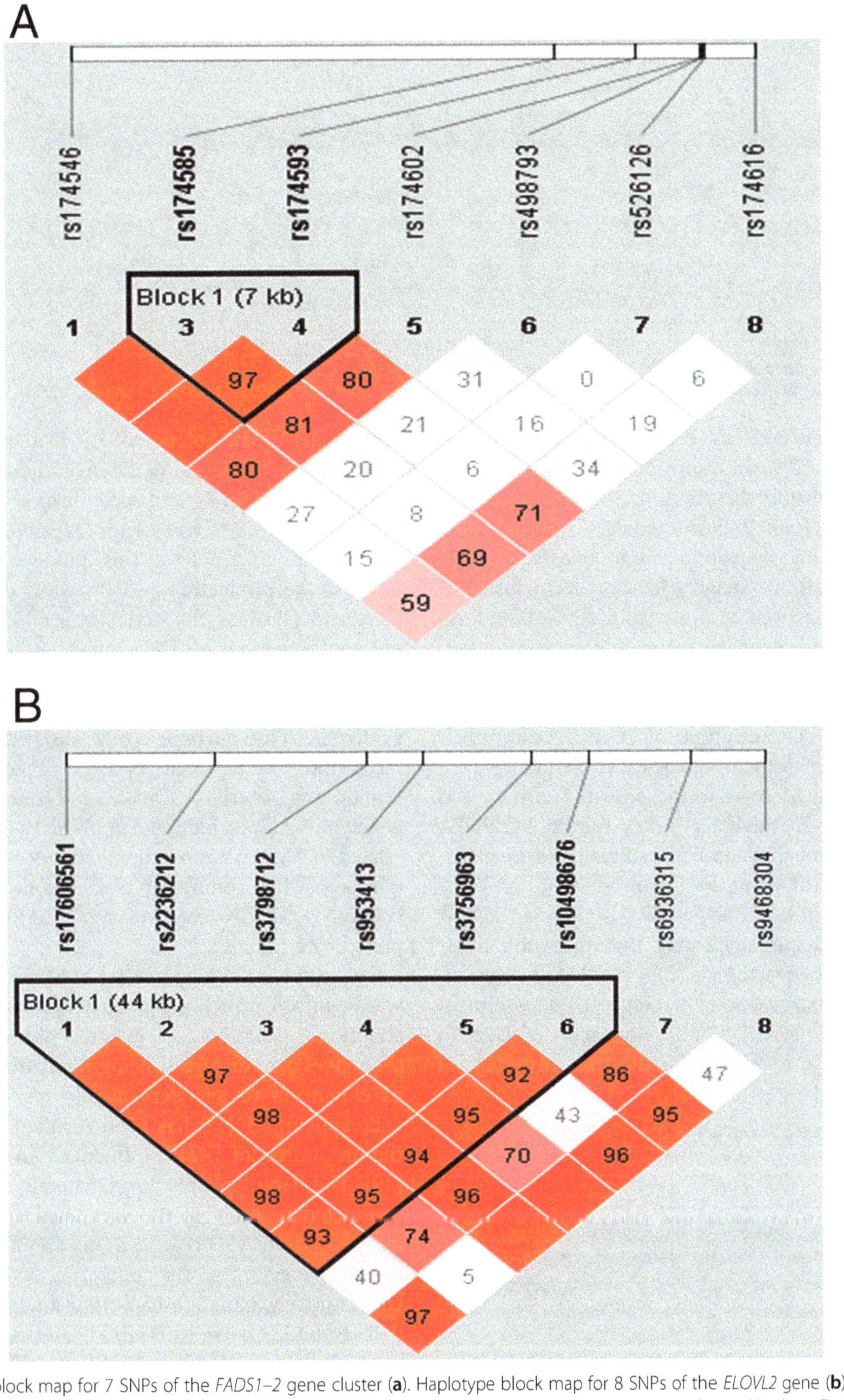

Fig. 2 Haplotype block map for 7 SNPs of the *FADS1–2* gene cluster (**a**). Haplotype block map for 8 SNPs of the *ELOVL2* gene (**b**). The haplotypes were constructed based on the prevalence of individual SNPs and LD between them. Numbers in squares indicate D′ values. Explanation of color scheme: if D′ < 1 and LOD (log of the likelihood odds ratio) < 2, the cell is white; if D′ = 1 and LOD < 2, the cell color is blue; if D′ < 1 and LOD ≥ 2, the cell color is shades of pink or red; if D′ = 1 and LOD ≥ 2, the cell color is bright red

Table 4 Distribution of *FADS1–2* and *ELOVL2* haplotypes in cases and controls (frequency more than 1%)

No.	Haplotype	Case ratio (243)	Control ratio (243)	*p*	OR (95 CI)
FADS1–2					
1	GT [a]	0.926	0.903	0.207	1.00
2	AC [a]	0.068	0.089	0.232	0.74(0.45–1.20)
ELOVL2					
1	GCAATA [b]	0.380	0.439	0.057	1.00
2	ACAACG [b]	0.253	0.203	0.066	1.46(1.04–2.05)
3	GGGATG [b]	0.216	0.230	0.640	1.10(0.80–1.52)
4	GGAGTG [b]	0.116	0.087	0.161	1.57(0.99–2.47)
5	GCAACG [b]	0.010	0.017	0.404	0.72(0.23–2.25)

[a] The order of SNPs in estimated analysis of haplotypes frequency: *rs174585* and *rs174593*
[b] The order of SNPs in estimated analysis of haplotypes frequency: *rs17606561*, *rs2236212*, *rs3798712*, *rs953413*, *rs3756963* and *rs10498676*

system development and has been associated with ASD [29]. Additionally, EPA can also produce eicosanoids, the lightly pro-inflammatory factors [26]. Secondly, endocannabinoids derived from PUFAs modulate synaptic function by suppressing neurotransmitter release, thereby acting as retrograde messengers in short-term forms of synaptic plasticity as well as presynaptically in long-term potentiation at both excitatory and inhibitory synapses [4, 11, 13, 30]. Genetic variant in *FADS2* (*rs526126*) may reduce desaturase activity, functionality, or expression, resulting in lower concentrations of LC-PUFAs and their derivatives, with downstream biological consequences.

ELOVL2 is located on chromosome 6 (6p24.2) and encodes elongase 2, which has a key role in LC-PUFA biosynthesis. Although delta-6 desaturase has been accepted as a control point in the production of DHA from ALA, when dietary ALA or EPA is abundant, DHA levels do not increase, suggesting that there are other control points in the reactions of EPA to DHA. In particular, in the sequential reactions of EPA → DPA → tetracosapentaenoic acid (TPA, 24:5n-3), elongation of DPA to TPA by *ELOVL2* is a key step in the transformation of EPA to DHA [31]. Ablation of *Elovl2* in mice caused severe reduction in the levels of DHA and β-docosapentaenoic acid (BDPA, 22:5n-6), and accumulation of EPA, DPA and 22:4n-6 in both liver and serum [32]. SNPs in *ELOVL2* that reduce the efficiency of this process are expected to increase the production of DPA while decreasing that of TPA and DHA as the end product [31, 33]. Given the essential function of DHA in brain development and cognition-enhancing [4, 10], we speculated that SNPs in *ELOVL2* influence ASD susceptibility by modulating DHA synthesis. The current study showed that the allele distributions of tag SNPs in *ELOVL2* gene did not differ significantly between ASD cases and controls. However, the genotype analyses indicated four SNPs were significantly related to ASD risk in overdominate/recessive model. Given our somewhat conflicting observations, the relationship between *ELOVL2* gene and risk of ASD must be interpreted with cautious.

Table 5 The genotype association of the *rs10498676* with ASD specific features in the recessive model

Items	n	G/G-A/G	A/A	*F*	*p*
ADI-R social	163	23.04±4.61	21.56±5.66	4.601	0.033
ADI-R comm-V	117	17.82±3.29	15.58±3.91	**9.221**	**0.003***
ADI-R comm-NV	163	11.36±2.61	9.96±3.52	**8.814**	**0.003***
ADI-R RR	163	5.43±2.77	6.04±2.89	0.335	0.564
ADOS-CSS	160	6.82±1.44	6.92±1.41	0.110	0.740
SA-CSS	160	7.16±1.57	7.27±1.49	0.113	0.737
RRB-CSS	160	6.39±1.88	6.38±1.77	0.000	0.993

ADI-R Autism Diagnostic Interview-Revised, *ADI-R comm-V* ADI-R communication for verbal, *ADI-R comm-NV* ADI-R communication for nonverbal, *ADI-R RR* ADI-R restricted repetitive behaviors, *ADOS* Autism Diagnostic Observation Schedule, *CSS* calibrated severity scores, *SA* social affect, *RRB* restricted repetitive behaviors, *F* statistic values from analysis of variance, * $p < p_{\text{Bonferroni}} = 0.05/7$

Except for rs17606561, most of SNPs in this study lied within intron, which performed vital roles in gene transcription. Mutations in introns, although non-coding sequences, can disturb splicing regulatory elements, such as enhancers or silencers, finally resulting in aberrant gene splicing [34]. It has been certified that the SNPs in the first intron of *FADS2* influenced *FADS1/2* expression [35]. The haplotyple block, as generally genetic unit, was conducted to evaluate the combined effect of the polymorphisms on ASD risk, and was an effective way of improving detection power comparing with single markers. Unfortunately, although haploview analyses demonstrated that strong LD between *rs174585* and *rs174593* in *FADS2* gene, and *rs17606561, rs2236212, rs3798712, rs953413, rs3756963* and *rs10498676* in *ELOVL2* gene (D' = 0.97, mean D' = 0.98, respectively), there were no marked association between the two reconstruction haplotype blocks of these tag SNPs in this study and ASD, which may have been a function of small size.

Estimating the severity of core autism features is critical for comparing samples across studies, tracking the course of the disorder over time, and quantifying treatment effects. However, the established measures for rating autism severity including the Childhood Autism Rating Scales, Autism Behavior Checklist, and raw ADOS scores yield variable results. This is may be attributable in part to differences in phenotypic characteristics such as IQ, language level, and chronological age, which affect the behavioral phenotypes of ASD and potentially masking the actual severity of core ASD symptoms. Gotham et al. addressed this heterogeneity by creating CSS based on raw total scores [19]. The CSS is relatively irrespective of the effect of phenotypic characteristics than the raw scores and allows scores to be compared across time, age, and modules. The use of ADOS and domain CSS has proven useful in characterizing samples for genetic and neurobiological studies [36, 37]. However, in the current literature we failed to uncover the relationship between *FADS2* and *ELOVL2* SNPs and ADOS and domain CSS. Our analysis revealed that *ELOVL2 rs10498676* is correlated with ADI-R comm-V and -NV after adjusting for age and language level. Compared with G/G and A/G genotypes, individuals with the A/A genotype had lower comm-V and -NV scores, which was in accordance with our previous finding that the minor A allele of *rs10498676* protected individuals against ASD. However, a caveat is that corrected ADI-R diagnostic scores may not represent the severity of ASD core symptoms.

The results of this study should be interpreted in light of several important limitations. Firstly, there were no data available regarding the LC-PUFA levels of the study subjects, and the relatively limited sample size decreased the power of the study. Secondly, both AIC and BIC can be derived from a model's likelihood and resulting maximum likelihood estimate in the context of regression. Although AIC and BIC as the more general estimators can be used for model selection, this strategy could increase type I error due to their parsimony principle. To further verity or choose the optimally genetic model, diverse model selection strategies are worthy being performed. Finally, we did not include a replication cohort. Additional studies with larger samples and/or family-based association testing are needed to verify the precise contribution of gene polymorphisms to ASD.

Conclusions

LC-PUFA metabolism is an important area of ASD research, given their roles in brain development and in the modulation of inflammatory response in the brain. Our results demonstrate that *FADS2* and *ELOVL2* SNPs differed between ASD cases and controls and suggest that these genes contribute to genetic susceptibility to ASD in a Chinese Han population. These findings provide new evidence for the contribution of genetic susceptibility to the etiology of ASD.

Abbreviations

AA: Arachidonic acid; ADI-R comm-NV: ADI-R communication for nonverbal; ADI-R comm-V: ADI-R communication for verbal; ADI-R RR: ADI-R restricted repetitive behaviors; ADI-R: Autism Diagnostic Interview-Revised; ADOS: Autism Diagnostic Observation Schedule; AIC: Akaike' information criterion; ALA: Alpha-linolenic acid; ASD: Autism Spectrum Disorders; BDPA: β-docosapentaenoic acid; BIC: Bayesian information criterion; CHB: Chinese Han in Beijing; CI: Confidence interval; CSS: Calibrated severity scores; DGLA: Dihomo-γ-linolenicacid; DHA: Docosahexanoic acid; DPA: Docosapentaenoic acid; DSM-V: Diagnostic and Statistical Manual of Mental Disorders, Fifth Edition; ELOVL2: Elongation of very long chain fatty acids 2/elongase 2; EPA: Eicosapentaenoic acid; FADS1: Fatty acid desaturase 1/delta-5-desaturase; FADS2: Fatty acid desaturase 2/ delta-6-desaturase; GLA: γ-linolenicacid; HWE: Hardy-Weinberg equilibrium; IQ: Intelligence quotient; LA: Linoleic acid; LD: Linkage disequilibrium; MAF: Minor Allele Frequency; OR: Odd ratio; PUFA: Polyunsaturated fatty acid; RRB: Restricted repetitive behaviors; SA: Social affect; SNP: Single nucleotide polymorphism; TPA: Tetracosapentaenoic acid

Acknowledgements

We thank all patients and their parents for their support and participation.

Funding

The design of this study, collection, analysis and writing the manuscript were supported by the National Nature Science Foundation of China (No.81302443), and experiments were supported by the National key research and development program (2016YFC1000504).

Authors' contributions

LW and WX conceived and designed the research; XW and MZ performed the experiments; MZ analyzed the data; CS and SF contributed reagents/materials/analysis tools; CS, SL, YH and YM performed clinical assessment; MZ wrote the paper. All authors read and approved the final manuscript.

Consent for publication

Not applicable

Competing interests

The authors declare that they have no competing interests.

Author details

[1]Department of Children's and Adolescent Health, Public Health College, Harbin Medical University, Harbin 150081, China. [2]Department of Pediatric, The Second Affiliated Hospital, Harbin Medical University, Harbin 150081, China. [3]Laboratory of Medical Genetics, Harbin Medical University, Harbin 150081, China.

References

1. American Psychiatric Association. The Diagnostic and Statistical Manual of Mental Disorders. 5th ed. Washington; 2013.
2. Gadad BS, Hewitson L, Young KA, German DC. Neuropathology and animal models of autism: genetic and environmental factors. Autism Res Treat. 2013;2013:731935. https://doi.org/10.1155/2013/731935.
3. Mefford HC, Batshaw ML, Hoffman EP. Genomics, intellectual disability, and autism. N Engl J Med. 2012;366(8):733–43. https://doi.org/10.1056/NEJMra1114194.
4. Bazinet RP, Laye S. Polyunsaturated fatty acids and their metabolites in brain function and disease. Nat Rev Neurosci. 2014;15(12):771–85. https://doi.org/10.1038/nrn3820.

5. Hartwig FP, Davies NM, Horta BL, Victora CG, Davey SG. Effect modification of FADS2 polymorphisms on the association between breastfeeding and intelligence: protocol for a collaborative meta-analysis. BMJ Open. 2016;6(6): e010067. https://doi.org/10.1136/bmjopen-2015-010067.
6. Yeates AJ, Love TM, Engstrom K, Mulhern MS, McSorley EM, Grzesik K, Alhamdow A, Wahlberg K, Thurston SW, Davidson PW, et al. Genetic variation in FADS genes is associated with maternal long-chain PUFA status but not with cognitive development of infants in a high fish-eating observational study. Prostaglandins Leukot Essent Fatty Acids. 2015;102–103: 13–20. https://doi.org/10.1016/j.plefa.2015.08.004.
7. Schuchardt JP, Kobe T, Witte V, Willers J, Gingrich A, Tesky V, Pantel J, Rujescu D, Illig T, Floel A, et al. Genetic variants of the FADS gene cluster are associated with erythrocyte membrane LC PUFA levels in patients with mild cognitive impairment. J Nutr Health Aging. 2016;20(6):611–20. https://doi.org/10.1007/s12603-016-0720-3.
8. Tintle NL, Pottala JV, Lacey S, Ramachandran V, Westra J, Rogers A, Clark J, Olthoff B, Larson M, Harris W, et al. A genome-wide association study of saturated, mono- and polyunsaturated red blood cell fatty acids in the Framingham heart offspring study. Prostaglandins Leukot Essent Fatty Acids. 2015;94:65–72. https://doi.org/10.1016/j.plefa.2014.11.007.
9. Glaser C, Lattka E, Rzehak P, Steer C, Koletzko B. Genetic variation in polyunsaturated fatty acid metabolism and its potential relevance for human development and health. Matern Child Nutr. 2011;7:27–40. https://doi.org/10.1111/j.1740-8709.2011.00319.x.
10. Weiser MJ, Butt CM, Mohajeri MH. Docosahexaenoic acid and cognition throughout the lifespan. Nutrients. 2016;8(2):99. https://doi.org/10.3390/nu8020099.
11. Thomazeau A, Bosch-Bouju C, Manzoni O, Laye S. Nutritional n-3 PUFA deficiency abolishes endocannabinoid gating of hippocampal long-term potentiation. Cereb Cortex. 2017;27(4):2571–9. https://doi.org/10.1093/cercor/bhw052.
12. Joffre C, Nadjar A, Lebbadi M, Calon F, Laye S. N-3 LCPUFA improves cognition: the young, the old and the sick. Prostaglandins Leukot Essent Fatty Acids. 2014;91(1–2):1–20. https://doi.org/10.1016/j.plefa.2014.05.001.
13. Lafourcade M, Larrieu T, Mato S, Duffaud A, Sepers M, Matias I, De Smedt-Peyrusse V, Labrousse VF, Bretillon L, Matute C, et al. Nutritional omega-3 deficiency abolishes endocannabinoid-mediated neuronal functions. Nat Neurosci. 2011;14(3):345–50. https://doi.org/10.1038/nn.2736.
14. Wang H, Liang S, Wang M, Gao J, Sun C, Wang J, Xia W, Wu S, Sumner SJ, Zhang F, et al. Potential serum biomarkers from a metabolomics study of autism. J Psychiatry Neurosci. 2016;41(1):27–37. https://doi.org/10.1503/jpn.140009.
15. Al-Farsi YM, Waly MI, Deth RC, Al-Sharbati MM, Al-Shafaee M, Al-Farsi O, Al-Khaduri MM, Al-Adawi S, Hodgson NW, Gupta I, et al. Impact of nutrition on serum levels of docosahexaenoic acid among Omani children with autism. Nutrition. 2013;29(9):1142–6. https://doi.org/10.1016/j.nut.2013.03.009.
16. Parletta N, Niyonsenga T, Duff J. Omega-3 and Omega-6 polyunsaturated fatty acid levels and correlations with symptoms in children with attention deficit hyperactivity disorder, autistic Spectrum disorder and typically developing controls. PLoS One. 2016;11(5):e0156432. https://doi.org/10.1371/journal.pone.0156432.
17. Brigandi SA, Shao H, Qian SY, Shen Y, Wu BL, Kang JX. Autistic children exhibit decreased levels of essential fatty acids in red blood cells. Int J Mol Sci. 2015;16(5):10061–76. https://doi.org/10.3390/ijms160510061.
18. Zhao G, Gao J, Liang S, Wang X, Sun C, Xia W, Hao Y, Li X, Cao Y, Wu L. Study of the serum levels of polyunsaturated fatty acids and the expression of related liver metabolic enzymes in a rat valproate-induced autism model. Int J Dev Neurosci. 2015;44:14–21. https://doi.org/10.1016/j.ijdevneu.2015.04.350.
19. Gotham K, Pickles A, Lord C. Standardizing ADOS scores for a measure of severity in autism spectrum disorders. J Autism Dev Disord. 2009;39(5):693–705. https://doi.org/10.1007/s10803-008-0674-3.
20. Gotham K, Risi S, Pickles A, Lord C. The autism diagnostic observation schedule: revised algorithms for improved diagnostic validity. J Autism Dev Disord. 2007;37(4):613–27. https://doi.org/10.1007/s10803-006-0280-1.
21. Hus V, Gotham K, Lord C. Standardizing ADOS domain scores: separating severity of social affect and restricted and repetitive behaviors. J Autism Dev Disord. 2014;44(10):2400–12. https://doi.org/10.1007/s10803-012-1719-1.
22. Hus V, Lord C. Effects of child characteristics on the autism diagnostic interview-revised: implications for use of scores as a measure of ASD severity. J Autism Dev Disord. 2013;43(2):371–81. https://doi.org/10.1007/s10803-012-1576-y.
23. Koletzko B, Lattka E, Zeilinger S, Illig T, Steer C. Genetic variants of the fatty acid desaturase gene cluster predict amounts of red blood cell docosahexaenoic and other polyunsaturated fatty acids in pregnant women: findings from the Avon longitudinal study of parents and children. Am J Clin Nutr. 2011;93(1):211–9. https://doi.org/10.3945/ajcn.110.006189.
24. Li D, Weisinger HS, Weisinger RS, Mathai M, Armitage JA, Vingrys AJ, Sinclair AJ. Omega 6 to omega 3 fatty acid imbalance early in life leads to persistent reductions in DHA levels in glycerophospholipids in rat hypothalamus even after long-term omega 3 fatty acid repletion. Prostaglandins Leukot Essent Fatty Acids. 2006;74(6):391–9. https://doi.org/10.1016/j.plefa.2006.03.010.
25. Tanaka T, Shen J, Abecasis GR, Kisialiou A, Ordovas JM, Guralnik JM, Singleton A, Bandinelli S, Cherubini A, Arnett D, et al. Genome-wide association study of plasma polyunsaturated fatty acids in the InCHIANTI study. PLoS Genet. 2009;5(1):e1000338. https://doi.org/10.1371/journal.pgen.1000338.
26. Tosi F, Sartori F, Guarini P, Olivieri O, Martinelli N. Delta-5 and delta-6 desaturases: crucial enzymes in polyunsaturated fatty acid-related pathways with pleiotropic influences in health and disease. Adv Exp Med Biol. 2014; 824:61–81. https://doi.org/10.1007/978-3-319-07320-0_7.
27. Roke K, Ralston JC, Abdelmagid S, Nielsen DE, Badawi A, El-Sohemy A, Ma DW, Mutch DM. Variation in the FADS1/2 gene cluster alters plasma n-6 PUFA and is weakly associated with hsCRP levels in healthy young adults. Prostaglandins Leukot Essent Fatty Acids. 2013;89(4):257–63. https://doi.org/10.1016/j.plefa.2013.06.003.
28. Moran M, Morales E, Bustamante M, Gonzalez JR, Guxens M, Torrent M, Mendez M, Garcia-Esteban R, Julvez J, Forns J, et al. Genetic variants of the FADS gene cluster and ELOVL gene family, Colostrums LC-PUFA levels, breastfeeding, and child cognition. PLoS One. 2011;6(2):e17181. https://doi.org/10.1371/journal.pone.0017181.
29. Young AM, Chakrabarti B, Roberts D, Lai MC, Suckling J, Baron-Cohen S. From molecules to neural morphology: understanding neuroinflammation in autism spectrum condition. Mol Autism. 2016;7:9. https://doi.org/10.1186/s13229-016-0068-x.
30. Drumond A, Madeira N, Fonseca R. Endocannabinoid signaling and memory dynamics: a synaptic perspective. Neurobiol Learn Mem. 2016; https://doi.org/10.1016/j.nlm.2016.07.031.
31. Gregory MK, Gibson RA, Cook-Johnson RJ, Cleland LG, James MJ. Elongase reactions as control points in long-chain polyunsaturated fatty acid synthesis. PLoS One. 2011;6(12):e29662. https://doi.org/10.1371/journal.pone.0029662.
32. Pauter AM, Olsson P, Asadi A, Herslof B, Csikasz RI, Zadravec D, Jacobsson A. Elovl2 ablation demonstrates that systemic DHA is endogenously produced and is essential for lipid homeostasis in mice. J Lipid Res. 2014;55(4):718–28. https://doi.org/10.1194/jlr.M046151.
33. Lemaitre RN, Tanaka T, Tang W, Manichaikul A, Foy M, Kabagambe EK, Nettleton JA, King IB, Weng LC, Bhattacharya S, et al. Genetic loci associated with plasma phospholipid n-3 fatty acids: a meta-analysis of genome-wide association studies from the CHARGE consortium. PLoS Genet. 2011;7(7): e1002193. https://doi.org/10.1371/journal.pgen.1002193.
34. Baralle D, Baralle M. Splicing in action: assessing disease causing sequence changes. J Med Genet. 2005;42(10):737–48. https://doi.org/10.1136/jmg.2004.029538.
35. Reardon HT, Zhang J, Kothapalli KS, Kim AJ, Park WJ, Brenna JT. Insertion-deletions in a FADS2 intron 1 conserved regulatory locus control expression of fatty acid desaturases 1 and 2 and modulate response to simvastatin. Prostaglandins Leukot Essent Fatty Acids. 2012;87(1):25–33. https://doi.org/10.1016/j.plefa.2012.04.011.
36. Hus Bal V, Lord C. Replication of standardized ADOS domain scores in the Simons simplex collection. Autism Res. 2015;8(5):583–92. https://doi.org/10.1002/aur.1474.
37. Shumway S, Farmer C, Thurm A, Joseph L, Black D, Golden C. The ADOS calibrated severity score: relationship to phenotypic variables and stability over time. Autism Res. 2012;5(4):267–76. https://doi.org/10.1002/aur.1238.

16

Health care and societal costs of the management of children and adolescents with attention-deficit/hyperactivity disorder in Spain

Javier Quintero[1], Josep A. Ramos-Quiroga[2], Javier San Sebastián[3], Francisco Montañés[4], Alberto Fernández-Jaén[5], José Martínez-Raga[6], Marta García Giral[7], Montserrat Graell[8], María J. Mardomingo[9], César Soutullo[10], Jesús Eiris[11], Montserrat Téllez[12], Montserrat Pamias[13], Javier Correas[14], Juncal Sabaté[15], Laura García-Orti[15] and José A. Alda[16*]

Abstract

Background: Attention-deficit/hyperactivity disorder (ADHD) is a common neurodevelopmental condition in childhood (5.3% to 7.1% worldwide prevalence), with substantial overall financial burden to children/adolescents, their families, and society. The aims of this study were to describe the clinical characteristics of children and adolescents with ADHD in Spain, estimate the associated direct/indirect costs of the disorder, and assess whether the characteristics and financial costs differed between children/adolescents adequately responding to currently available pharmacotherapies compared with children/adolescents for whom pharmacotherapies failed.

Methods: This was a multicenter, cross-sectional, descriptive analysis conducted in 15 health units representative of the overall Spanish population. Data on demographic characteristics, socio-occupational status, social relationships, clinical variables of the disease, and pharmacological and non-pharmacological treatments received were collected in 321 children and adolescents with ADHD. Direct and indirect costs were estimated over one year from both a health care system and a societal perspective.

Results: The estimated average cost of ADHD per year per child/adolescent was €5733 in 2012 prices; direct costs accounted for 60.2% of the total costs (€3450). Support from a psychologist/educational psychologist represented 45.2% of direct costs and 27.2% of total costs. Pharmacotherapy accounted for 25.8% of direct costs and 15.5% of total costs. Among indirect costs (€2283), 65.2% was due to caregiver expenses. The total annual costs were significantly higher for children/adolescents who responded poorly to pharmacological treatment (€7654 versus €5517; $P = 0.024$), the difference being mainly due to significantly higher direct costs, particularly with larger expenses for non-pharmacological treatment ($P = 0.012$).

Conclusions: ADHD has a significant personal, familial, and financial impact on the Spanish health system and society. Successful pharmacological intervention was associated with lower overall expenses in the management of the disorder.

Keywords: ADHD, Adolescence, School children, Economic evaluation

* Correspondence: jalda@sjdhospitalbarcelona.org
[16]Child and Adolescent Psychiatry and Psychology Department, Hospital Sant Joan de Déu, Esplugues de Llobregat, 08950 Barcelona, Spain
Full list of author information is available at the end of the article

Background

Attention-deficit/hyperactivity disorder (ADHD) is a common neurodevelopmental condition in childhood, with an estimated worldwide prevalence in children/adolescents ranging from 5.3% to 7.1%, with little variation across countries and regions [1–3]. ADHD is characterized by developmentally inappropriate levels of inattention, hyperactivity, or impulsivity that have a significant impact on different aspects of the child/adolescent's everyday life, including social, academic, or occupational activities. The severity of ADHD and presence of particular symptoms is highly heterogeneous, and the Diagnostic and Statistical Manual of Mental Disorders Fifth Edition (DSM-5) distinguishes clinical current presentations as predominantly inattentive, predominantly hyperactive/impulsive, or combined when symptoms of inattention or hyperactivity/impulsivity coexist [4]. In addition to the core symptoms, children/adolescents with ADHD have increased rates of comorbidities, including conduct disorder, learning disabilities, oppositional defiant disorder, or depressive disorders, that have further impact on the child/adolescent's everyday life [5].

ADHD significantly impairs psychosocial functioning and adjustment, and children/adolescents usually have difficulties in interpersonal relationships with peers/family [6, 7]. Furthermore, poor academic performance is more common in children/adolescents with ADHD than in those without ADHD [8]. Consequently, compared with non-ADHD children/adolescents, children/adolescents with ADHD have low self-perception and self-esteem, and impaired quality of life [9–11]. Children/adolescents with ADHD have an increased risk of mortality, and school-age children with ADHD are also more likely to require emergency treatment or be admitted to hospital due to accidental injuries, whereas adolescents with ADHD have higher rates of early and more severe substance use, and of serious delinquent behaviors than their non-ADHD peers [12–15].

Health-economics literature has consistently shown that the overall financial burden of ADHD to children/adolescents, their families, and society is substantial [11, 16–18]. A study on costs of brain disorders in 30 European countries estimated that the direct annual costs of ADHD in 2010 were €781 per person, representing a total of €2546 million. These figures are lower than for autism (total of €15,109 million) and slightly lower than for conduct disorder (total of €3671 million) [19]. Moreover, ADHD annual health care costs per child/adolescent vary substantially across European countries (from €716 in Germany to €2134 in the Netherlands), and are of a similar order of magnitude in the US ($621 to $2720) [11]. However, comparisons are difficult regarding other types of costs; for instance, special educational support may be provided within mainstream schools in some countries (e.g. the UK), but are completely external in others (e.g., Spain).

Systematic reviews of the literature have shown that the pharmacological treatment of ADHD is associated with a substantial benefit in outcomes in the short term, and is cost-effective compared with placebo, no treatment, or behavioral therapy only [20, 21]. Analyses on the effect of treatment on long-term outcomes are scarce, but it has also been reported that untreated individuals experience worse outcomes overall than those receiving any treatment [10, 22, 23]. Therefore, individuals who are untreated or inappropriately treated, or who do not respond adequately to treatment, may experience and/or contribute to a significant increase in the short- and long-term financial burden of the disease as a result of additional expenses that can be attributed to the health, social, educational, and justice systems. There are few studies on the economic impact of ADHD in Europe to date, and those available are not directly comparable with studies published in the US because of putative underlying variations in treatment approaches or public health policies [5].

The objective of this multicenter, cross-sectional study was to estimate the associated direct and indirect costs from both a health care system and a societal perspective over a 1-year time period in Spanish children/adolescents with ADHD. In addition, we assessed whether the characteristics and financial costs differed between children/adolescents responding well (good responders) versus those who responded poorly (poor responders) to currently available pharmacotherapies.

Participants and methods

Study design

This was a multicenter, cross-sectional, descriptive study in a sample of children/adolescents with ADHD in the context of the Spanish research project "Plan of Action in ADHD (PANDAH)". A total of 321 children/adolescents were recruited between 1 December 2012 and 30 April 2013 from 15 health care centers (7 privately and 8 publicly funded) representative of the overall Spanish population.

Study population

The study included children/adolescents with DSM-IV Text Revision (DSM-IV-TR) diagnostic criteria for ADHD, aged ≤18 years, and without intellectual disability (i.e. intelligence quotient ≥70), as estimated by the treating physician. Children/adolescents were excluded if they had one of the following conditions: a severe medical disease other than asthma (e.g. neoplasm, diabetes mellitus, Crohn's disease), neurological disorders (e.g. epilepsy), severe psychiatric disorders (including psychosis, bipolar disorder, and pervasive developmental disorders), symptoms of major depression before the onset of ADHD, or ADHD symptoms during episodes of depression.

To minimize selection bias, child/adolescent psychiatry or pediatric neurology units initially recruited the first child/adolescent who attended on a given day who fulfilled study inclusion criteria. When additional children/adolescents attended on the same day, only those consecutive to the first one were enrolled.

Sample size calculation

To detect a mean cost difference of €2000 between good responders and poor responders, and assuming a standard deviation (SD) of €5000 and €7000, respectively, we calculated that the total sample size needed was 350 children/adolescents ($\alpha = 0.05$; $\beta = 0.2$). As the study was conducted in 15 different health care centers, each one should recruit between 20 and 30 children/adolescents.

Ethical considerations

The central Ethics Committee that approved the study was the Niño Jesús Hospital Committee (Madrid), and all children/adolescents or their legal representatives signed a written informed consent form prior to participation in the study.

Data collection

A case report form (CRF) to be completed by the investigators was specifically designed for the study. First, a pilot study was conducted at 3 of the participating centers and data entered for 2 children/adolescents; this served to detect possible misleading questions, or other problems encountered by the investigators when completing the questionnaires. Second, all participating investigators were trained in the usage of the final CRF through a conference call. The CRFs were collected each week from all participating centers to build a common database.

Study variables

At the time of recruitment, the following data were collected and recorded by the investigators during the interview: a) current demographic characteristics of children/adolescents; b) socio-occupational status; c) social relationships; d) date of diagnosis, ADHD subtype, and psychiatric comorbidities based on DSM-IV-TR criteria [24]; e) ADHD symptom severity for the last 6 months (baseline or current severity) using ADHD rating scale-IV (ADHD-RS-IV) [25]; f) severity of the disease at the time of recruitment evaluated using the Clinical Global Impression questionnaire [26]; g) general current functioning of the child/adolescent using the Children's Global Assessment Scale (CGAS) [27]; h) the lowest known CGAS score during the previous year; and i) pharmacological and non-pharmacological ADHD-related treatments received in the previous 12 months. Available drugs for ADHD treatment in Spain at the time of the study included methylphenidate (MPH) OROS, MPH pellets, MPH immediate release (IR), and atomoxetine. Finally, the parents/caregivers were asked to provide data on utilization of health care services by the child/adolescent for the prior 12 months and their own work productivity, assessed using the Work Productivity and Activity Impairment questionnaire [28].

Data analyses and statistics

Descriptive analysis

Descriptive analyses were summarized by means (SDs) or medians and interquartile ranges for continuous variables, and absolute numbers and percentages for categorical variables.

Cost analysis

The study was performed using a health care system and a societal perspective to estimate both direct and indirect costs, and adopted a 1-year time period.

All costs are expressed in 2012 Euros. Direct medical costs were defined as the cost of resources consumed to detect and treat the disorder, including costs of diagnostic tests, blood tests, emergency/outpatient visits, hospital admissions, and medication use. Direct medical costs were estimated by multiplying the amount of consumed resources by unit costs. These were obtained from the individual official reimbursed process in each particular region because, in Spain, health care is a competence of each autonomous community. Transport to treatment center was classified as a non-medical direct cost, and estimated based on public transport or taxi tickets given to the child/adolescent and parent/caregiver. Total direct costs were the sum of medical and non-medical costs. Indirect costs were those faced because of ADHD symptoms, and defined as the costs of the child/adolescent's parents or caregivers, and the cost of lost productivity – as a consequence of hours spent in medical visits or missing workdays due to sick leave – applied to parents or caregivers. The cost of lost productivity was calculated by multiplying the estimated number of lost working hours by the average wage per working-hour [29]. More intangible costs, such as grade repetition, school drop-out, and time spent attending psychologist/educational psychologist visits, were described as proportions or means (SDs) (e.g. mean [SD] number of visits per year).

Comparison between good responders and poor responders

Good responders were defined as children/adolescents treated pharmacologically for at least 9 months who had an ADHD-RS-IV total score ≤ 18 (i.e. never, rarely, or sometimes ill) for at least the 3 previous months [30, 31]. Conversely, poor responders were children/adolescents who, despite receiving pharmacological treatment for at least 9 months, had an ADHD-RS-IV total score > 18. The comparison between good responders and poor responders was calculated using the chi-square or Fisher's exact test for categorical variables. For continuous variables, the Student's t test was used for normally distributed variables, and the Mann-Whitney test for non-normally distributed variables. *P*-values were unadjusted for multiplicity.

Results

Sample description and demographic characteristics

A total of 321 children/adolescents were enrolled in the study; 262 were recruited by child/adolescent psychiatrists, 59 by neuropediatricians. Table 1 summarizes the clinical and demographic baseline characteristics of the study sample. The age of the sample ranged between 6.3 and 18.0 years (mean [SD] 12.7 [2.9] years); most children/adolescents were male (78.5%) and 16 were younger than 8 years of age. The most frequent clinical presentation was combined ADHD type (61.4%), and the most common comorbidities were oppositional defiant disorder and anxiety disorders (19.9% and 17.8% of cases, respectively). At baseline, treating physicians rated children/adolescents as being mild to moderately ill in 73.9% of cases, and most had a good level of functioning with minor impairments (CGAS mean [SD] score = 74 [15.3]).

Table 1 Clinical and demographic baseline characteristics of the study sample (N = 321)

Characteristic	Cases
Age, years, mean (SD)	12.7 (2.9)
Age, years, range (P25, P75)	6.3–18.0 (10.6, 15.1)
Sex, n (%)	
Male	252 (78.5)
Female	69 (21.5)
ADHD presentation, n (%)	
Combined	197 (61.4)
Predominantly inattentive	112 (34.9)
Predominantly hyperactive-impulsive	12 (3.7)
ADHD-RS-IV score, mean (SD)	22.04 (10.3)
Duration of the disorder, years, mean (SD)	3.83 (2.5)
Current level of functioning (CGAS), mean (SD)	74 (15.3)
Lowest CGAS during the previous year, mean (SD)	56.1 (15.6)
Comorbidities, n (%)	
Oppositional defiant disorder	64 (19.9)
Other conduct disorders	19 (5.9)
Anxiety disorders	57 (17.8)
Addictions	6 (1.9)

ADHD attention-deficit/hyperactivity disorder; *ADHD-RS-IV* ADHD rating scale IV; *CGAS* Children's Global Assessment Scale; *P25* 25th percentile; *P75* 75th percentile; *SD* standard deviation

Most children/adolescents were currently living with their parents and siblings (63.6%); their relationship with their family was good in 53.0% of cases. However, because of the ADHD symptoms, 17.8% of parents had to give up their job to care for their child/adolescent, and 11.5% of children/adolescents had a caregiver other than their parents, of whom 54% were relatives.

Relationship with peers was good overall (59.5% of cases), but, in 43.0% of cases, parents reported that the child/adolescent had some type of social difficulty such as being led by others, provoking and annoying others, or being sore losers (e.g. becoming very upset or angry when he or she loses a game, contest, etc).

All children/adolescents were attending school except one who was unemployed; 51% were enrolled in partially State-funded institutions, 35% in public schools, and 14% in private institutions. At the academic level, 19.1% of children/adolescents required an adapted school curriculum, and 51.9% received reinforcement/tutoring lessons about 4 times/week (mean [SD] = 4.2 [3.8]). A total of 13.7% of children/adolescents had been expelled from school at least once, with a mean (SD) age at first expulsion of 12 (2.5) years, and a mean (SD) of 3.3 (4) expulsions. Finally, 33.6% repeated a grade (mean [SD] repetitions = 1.1 [0.3]), at a mean (SD) age of 10.6 (2.8) years for the first time.

Cost analysis

The average estimated total cost of ADHD per year per child/adolescent was €5732.64, with direct costs accounting for 60.2% of total costs (€3450.04) (Table 2).

The most frequently accessed health service was a visit to a psychiatrist, with a median of 4 visits per year (25th percentile [P25] = 2; 75th percentile [P75] = 6), followed by visits to a primary care center (median of 2 visits; P25 = 0; P75 = 4). Support from an educational psychologist or a psychologist (non-pharmacological treatment) was needed by 37.4% and 32.7% of children/adolescents, respectively, in the majority of cases held at private centers (75.8% and 62.8%, respectively), and represented 45.2% of direct costs and 27.2% of total costs. Pharmacotherapy accounted for 25.8% of direct costs and 15.5% of total costs. Stimulants, specifically MPH OROS (65.4%) and MPH IR (25.5%) were the most commonly prescribed drugs. The mean duration of treatments during the previous year was 288 and 252 days for MPH OROS and MPH IR, respectively (data not shown). Costs due to hospital admissions, diagnostic tests, and transportation to treatment centers represented 2% of total costs each.

Table 2 Estimates of annual resource use and costs in 321 children and adolescents with ADHD

Costs		Use of resource	Mean cost in € (SD)	Percentage of total cost
Direct medical costs	Visits to health services, mean (SD); median (P25, P75)		703.40 (785.64)	12.3%
	Primary care center	3.3 (5.8); 2 (0, 4)		
	Psychiatrist	5.02 (6.0); 4 (2, 6)		
	Another specialist[a]	1.59 (3.5); 0 (0, 2)		
	Hospital admissions, mean (SD)		95.42 (958.49)	1.7%
	Visits to emergency departments	0.3 (0.8)		
	Number of admissions	0.01 (0.1)		
	Days admitted	0.02 (0.2)		
	Stays in day hospital	0.54 (6.0)		
	Diagnostic tests, mean (SD)		98.43 (205.46)	1.7%
	Hemogram	0.46 (0.8)		
	Clinical chemistry	0.47 (0.9)		
	Urinalysis	0.16 (0.7)		
	NMR	0.08 (0.4)		
	EEG	0.09 (0.3)		
	ECG	0.2 (0.4)		
	CT scan	0.01 (0.1)		
	Evoked potentials	0.01 (0.1)		
	Pharmacotherapy,[b] n (%)		889.77 (674.72)	15.5%
	MPH OROS	210 (65.4)		
	MPH pellets	72 (22.4)		
	MPH IR	82 (25.5)		
	Atomoxetine	59 (18.4)		
	Clonidine	3 (0.9)		
	Other	37 (11.5)		
	Non-pharmacological treatment, n (%)		1561.14 (2768.53)	27.2%
	Educational psychologist	120 (37.4)		
	Psychologist	105 (32.7)		
Direct non-medical costs	Transportation to treatment center,[c] n (%)		101.88 (182.89)	1.8%
	Walking	27 (8.4)		
	Private car	223 (69.5)		
	Taxi	2 (0.6)		
	Public transport	68 (21.2)		
Total direct costs			3450.04 (3370.92)	60.2%
Indirect costs	Caregiving, hours/day, mean (SD)	4.6 (2.5)	1488.16 (5141.73)	26.0%
	Caregiving, days/week, mean (SD)	4.9 (1.7)		
	Sick leave, days, mean (SD)[d]		2.55 (45.7)	<1.0%
	Total sick leave	8.5 (2.12)		
	Leave due to ADHD	5 (7.1)		
	Time spent at medical visits[d]		791.89 (625)	13.8%
Total indirect costs			2282.60 (5391.28)	39.8%
Total costs			5732.64 (7211.39)	100%

[a]This includes neuropediatricians, but not psychologists/educational psychologists; [b]Children/adolescents were allowed to have more than one pharmacological treatment; [c]$n = 320$; [d]Applied to parents or caregivers of children/adolescents with ADHD
ADHD attention-deficit/hyperactivity disorder; *CT* computerized tomography; *ECG* electrocardiogram; *EEG* electroencephalogram; *IR* immediate release; *P25* 25th percentile; *P75* 75th percentile; *MPH* methylphenidate; *NMR* nuclear magnetic resonance; *SD* standard deviation

Among the indirect costs estimated, 65.2% was due to caregiver expenses, which were paid by a relative in 35.1% of cases (data not shown), and represented 26% of the total costs. Moreover, a parent or caregiver had to leave their job to care for the child/adolescent in 17.8% of cases, and the average number of lost working days in the previous year was 8.5, of which 5 (SD 7.1) days were due to ADHD itself (Fig. 1 and Table 2).

Impact of response to ADHD treatment

In the overall sample, 73.5% (n = 236) of children/adolescents received pharmacological treatment, and treating physicians considered that 58.8% (n = 139) were good responders.

There were no differences between good and poor responders with respect to type of treatment or treatment duration, but good responders (n = 139) had less severe ADHD measured at baseline, greater improvement from baseline, and were less frequently diagnosed with oppositional defiant disorder (Table 3 and Additional file 1: Table S1). Moreover, in poor responders (n = 97), the disorder had a more negative impact on several aspects of their lives, including poorer global functioning, with worse relationships with friends and family.

The difference in total annual costs of ADHD between groups was statistically significant, and higher for poor responders compared with good responders (mean [SD]: €7654 [€8966] versus €5517 [€6618]; P = 0.024). This was mainly due to significantly higher direct costs for poor responders versus good responders (mean [SD]: €4508 [€3922] versus €3258 [€2635]; P = 0.005), attributable to higher expenses in non-pharmacological treatment and transport (P = 0.012 and <0.0001, respectively) (Fig. 2). Finally, there was a trend towards a greater economic impact on indirect costs for poor responders (P = 0.058) driven by significantly longer time spent at visits (P = 0.011).

Discussion

In this study, we evaluated the economic impact of ADHD on the utilization of health care resources and societal costs in Europe as well as the costs of this neurodevelopmental disorder in children/adolescents from the societal perspective. In addition, we assessed how these costs differed between children/adolescents who adequately responded to pharmacological treatment compared with those for whom treatment response was poor.

Although few studies have assessed the economic impact of ADHD on the utilization of health care resources and societal costs in Europe, estimates of costs vary between studies depending on types of services included and methodology. The annual health care costs per child/adolescent with ADHD in Europe (adjusted to 2012 Euros) have been estimated to be between €716 and €3888 [11, 32]. The results of this study are in line with these estimates, with direct medical costs in Spain of €3450.04, accounting for 60.2% of all expenditures. However, it is largely recognized that, unlike many medical diseases, a significant proportion of the financial

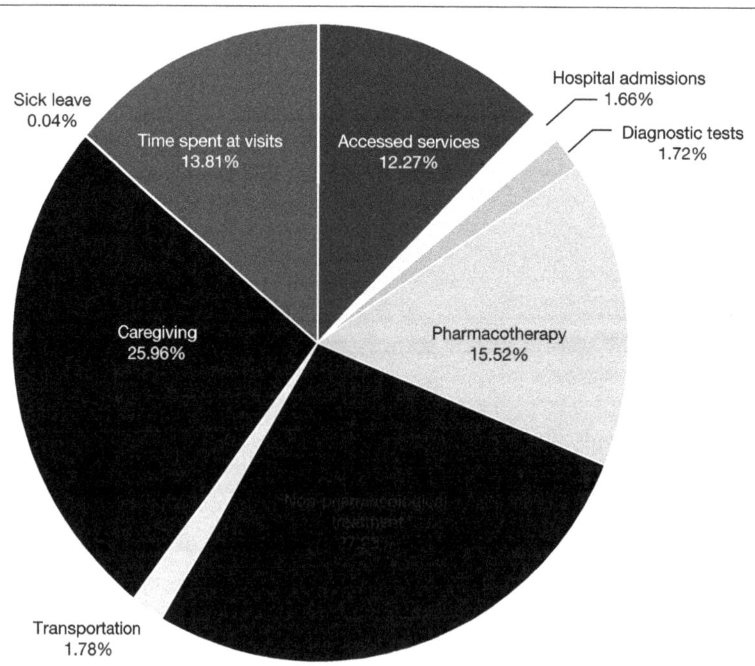

Fig. 1 National ADHD-related costs by cost categories

Table 3 Significant differences between children/adolescents with good response versus those with poor response to pharmacological treatment

	Good responders (n = 139)	Poor responders (n = 97)	P-value
Characteristics of the disease, mean (SD)			
Current level of functioning (CGAS)	78.6 (12.9)	67.9 (16.3)	<0.0001
Lowest CGAS score during the previous year	58.5 (14.2)	67.9 (16.3)	0.001
Current severity, n (%)			
Moderately-severely ill	36 (25.9)	63 (64.9)	<0.0001
Comorbidities, n (%)			
Oppositional defiant disorder	20 (14.4)	27 (27.8)	0.01
Other conduct disorders	7 (5.0)	8 (8.2)	0.40
Anxiety	21 (15.1)	24 (24.7)	0.07
Addictions	1 (0.7)	4 (4.1)	0.16
Impact on social functioning, n (%)			
Bad relationship with friends	1 (0.7)	15 (16.7)[a]	<0.0001
Bad relationship with family	7 (5.0)	22 (22.7)	<0.0001

[a]n = 90
CGAS Children's Global Assessment Scale, *SD* standard deviation

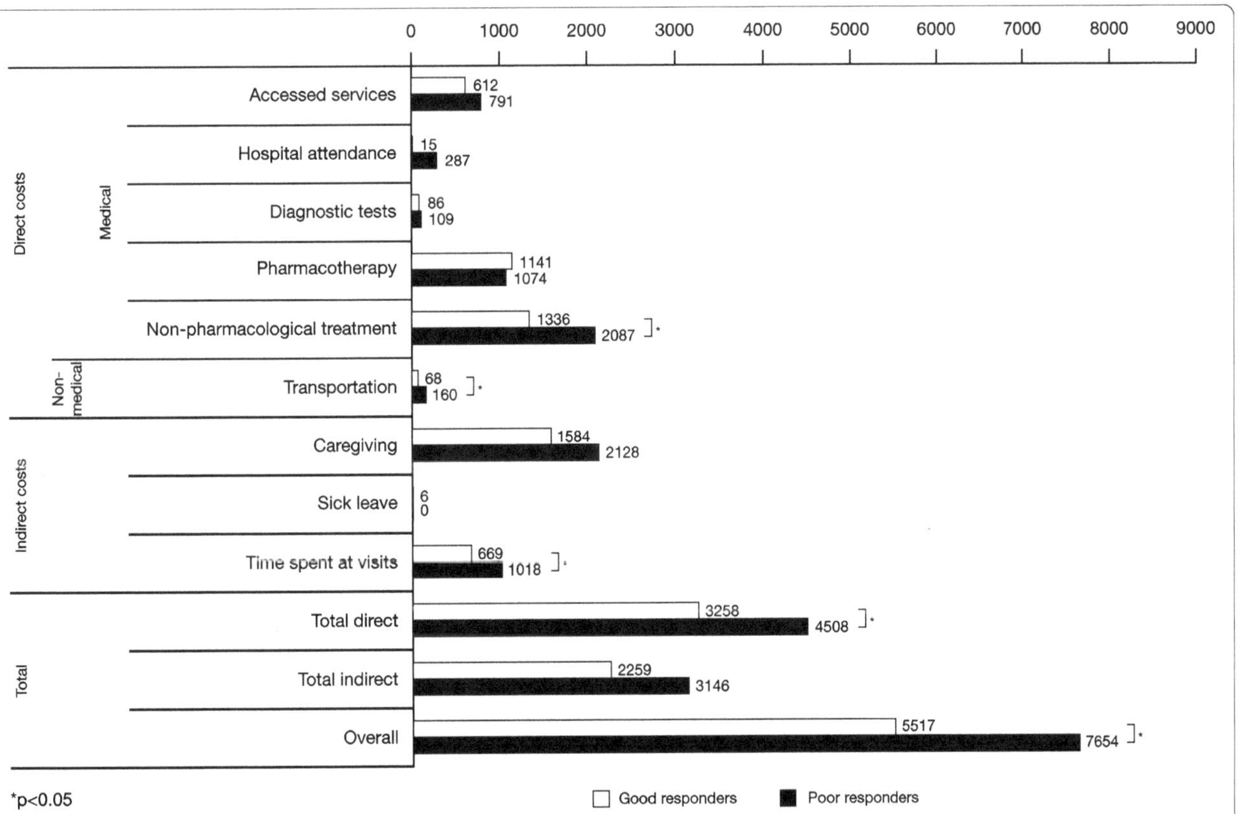

Fig. 2 ADHD costs (€) in children/adolescents with adequate pharmacological treatment response versus those for whom treatment failed

burden of psychiatric illnesses also arises from indirect costs [33]. The few available studies conducted in the European Union that estimated indirect costs of ADHD found values varying between €50 and €5596 per year, a difference that may be largely explained by the type of services considered [11, 34–36]. In the current study, indirect costs amounted to €2282.60, and were driven mainly by payment to a caregiver.

The main contributor to direct costs corresponded to non-pharmacological interventions (e.g. intervention by an educational psychologist or clinical psychologist), and accounted for 45.2% of total direct costs and 27.2% of total costs. Most cost-of-illness studies in ADHD include these services together with costs of other health care professionals, and therefore the specific weight of costs due to psychological interventions is difficult to compare. Nonetheless, these results are similar to a German study that considered the costs of behavioral therapy separately from other types of interventions, and reported that this expenditure represented 46.6% of costs for children/adolescents aged 6–17 years, and up to 74.4% in children ≤5 years of age [32]. Moreover, we did not consider special education needs, which might have contributed to an underestimation of the total costs in our study. Available European studies (conducted in the UK) that considered the costs of educational needs, such as special school, support teacher, or adapted school curriculum, reported them to be about 3-fold the sum of all other costs [36], or 44% of the total costs [18], and they were estimated to account for 30–40% of all expenditures in the US [16]. Although not directly comparable, our results seem to be in line with these estimates of the high burden due to special educational needs in children/adolescents with ADHD. The average proportion of costs of medication in the present study was 15.5%, which is in line with previous European studies that estimated that they range between 12% and 28.2% [32, 37–39].

One striking finding of our study was the high cost associated with the employment of a caregiver, which represented 65.2% of indirect costs, and 26% of all costs. Mental health-related problems in caregivers and families of children/adolescents with ADHD include stress, anxiety, and depression [40], but the financial burden on caregivers has not been routinely explored [1]. In our study, a parent had to leave their job to care for the child/adolescent in 17.8% of cases, thus hiding a significant unquantified productivity loss. Moreover, this shows that the costs we estimated to caregiving, although high, are largely an underestimation of the actual economic impact on families and society as a whole.

In this study, poor responders were observed to have worse global functioning, and poorer relationships with friends and family. This is in line with the results of several systematic reviews, which reported that treatment has a beneficial effect on multiple short- and long-term outcomes, including self-esteem, social functioning, academic performance, and antisocial behavior, among others, when compared with children/adolescents without ADHD or those with untreated ADHD [10, 22, 23]. Our results, however, also show that beyond symptom control, a poor response to treatment is an important component in the global negative impact of ADHD. This stresses the need for individualized treatment plans to optimize child/adolescent's outcomes, such as the incorporation of patient-oriented factors (e.g. age, ADHD subtype, comorbidities, and treatment/treatment response history) as well as the preferences and attitudes of children/adolescents and parents/caregivers to pharmacotherapy [41].

Poor responders were found to incur higher total financial expenses than good responders, a difference mainly due to direct medical costs, and particularly because of significantly higher costs of non-pharmacological treatment. Although not directly comparable, these results are in line with previous systematic reviews showing that treatment is associated with less use of ancillary services, including school-, health-, and work-related services; financial assistance services; use of the justice system; and fewer emergency room visits [22, 23].

The main advantage of the current study is that the studied population is representative of different regions in Spain and data were complete for almost all variables studied. However, the results must be interpreted in the light of considerable limitations. First, the cross-sectional nature of the study, with information obtained retrospectively through interview for some variables, means that results may be more sensitive to potential recall bias. Second, children/adolescents recruited in this study were treated by psychiatrists and neuropediatricians, and may therefore be representative of a subset of children/adolescents with more severe ADHD, thus incurring higher costs, as for adults [42]. Third, there are several factors that were not quantified in the study that might have contributed to an underestimation of the total ADHD-related costs. For example, we did not include additional indirect costs such as health-related problems among family members, although these may be considerable too, as suggested by a Dutch study that estimated annual average health care costs per family member as 14.3% of all health care costs [11, 37]. Moreover, we did not estimate costs associated with psychiatric/non-psychiatric comorbidities, which have been shown to cause a 6-fold increase in medical costs compared with 'pure' ADHD cases [37]. Although excluding comorbidities can lead to a significant underestimation of the total cost of illness, when it is difficult to separately assess the expenditures of closely related disorders, it can also potentially lead to an inflation of cost estimates [43]. In addition, we did not estimate ADHD-related costs due to the justice system, treatment of comorbid substance abuse, or traffic accidents. None of the available European studies have quantified these totals, but the costs of justice system service needs for children/adolescents with ADHD in the US were estimated to be about 1% of the total costs of ADHD [16].

Conclusions

ADHD is a highly prevalent disorder associated with a significant high personal, familial, and financial impact on the family, health system, and society. An adequate response to pharmacological treatment was associated with lower overall expenses in the management of the disorder.

Abbreviations

ADHD: Attention-deficit/hyperactivity disorder; ADHD-RS-IV: Attention-deficit/hyperactivity disorder rating scale, version IV; CGAS: Children's Global Assessment Scale; CRF: Case report form; DSM-5: Diagnostic and Statistical Manual of Mental Disorders, Fifth edition; DSM-IV-TR: Diagnostic and Statistical Manual of Mental Disorders, Fourth edition, Text Revision; IR: Immediate release; MPH: Methylphenidate; P25: 25th percentile; P75: 75th percentile; SD: Standard deviation

Acknowledgments

Under the direction of the authors, Mònica Gratacòs, for Caudex, provided writing assistance for this publication. Editorial assistance in formatting, proofreading, and copy editing of the manuscript, and coordination and collation of comments, was also provided by Caudex, funded by Shire International GmbH. Data from this manuscript have been presented at: 4th World Congress on ADHD (2013); 15th International Congress of ESCAP (2013); IX and X Congreso Nacional SENEP (2013 and 2014); XII Congreso AEPNYA (2014); and XVI World Congress of Psychiatry (2014).

Funding

Clinical research was funded by Shire Pharmaceuticals Ibérica Ltd (Spain). Editorial assistance was funded by Shire International GmbH. Although employees of Shire were involved in the design, collection, analysis, interpretation, and fact checking of information, the content of this manuscript, the ultimate interpretation, and the decision to submit it for publication in *BMC Psychiatry* was made by the authors independently. Alain Joseph from Shire reviewed and edited the manuscript for scientific accuracy.

Authors' contributions

JQ, JAR-Q, JSS, FM, AF-J, JM-R, MGG, MG, MJM, CS, JE, MT, MP, JC, JS, LG-O, JAA made substantial contributions to conception and design, or acquisition of data, or analysis and interpretation of data; JQ, JAR-Q, JSS, FM, AF-J, JM-R, MGG, MG, MJM, CS, JE, MT, MP, JC, JS, LG-O, JAA were involved in drafting the manuscript or revising it critically for important intellectual content. All authors read and approved the final version of the manuscript.

Consent for publication

Not applicable.

Competing interests

JQ: participated as speaker and/or acted as consultant for Grunenthal, Lilly, Shire, MSD, Janssen & Ferrer; received unrestricted educational and research support from Mutua Madrileña and Otsuka. JAR-Q: on the speakers bureau and/or acted as consultant for Eli Lilly, Novartis, Shire, Lundbeck, Ferrer, Medice, and Rubió; received travel awards from Rubió, Ferrer, Shire, and Eli Lilly; received unrestricted educational and research support from Eli Lilly, Shire, Rovi, Ferrer, Lundbeck, and Rubió. FM: received funding for collaborations for congress organization from Shire, Rubió, and Rovi. AF-J: received economic support to attend courses/congresses from Janssen, Eli Lilly, Rubio, Juste, Shire, and Otsuka; received fees for participation in medical congresses from Janssen, Eli Lilly, Rubio, Juste, and Shire; participated in advisory boards for Janssen, Eli Lilly, and Shire; received grants from Janssen, Eli Lilly, Rubio, and Shire. JM-R: received honoraria for being a speaker and acting on advisory boards from Shire and Janssen Pharmaceuticals. CS: received non-personal research funds for his department from Caja Navarra Foundation, Lundbeck, Shire, and Teva; served as consultant for Alicia Koplowitz Foundation, Editorial Médica Panamericana, Eli Lilly, EUNETHYDIS, Instituto de Salud Carlos III, Medice/Juste, NeuroTech Solutions Ltd., Rubió, and Shire; served on speakers bureaux on continuous medical education for Eli Lilly, Shire, Universidad Internacional Menéndez Pelayo, and Universidad Internacional de La Rioja (UNIR); received royalties from DOYMA, Editorial Médica Panamericana, and Mayo Ediciones. MT: received grant/research support from Shire Pharmaceuticals S.L., Rubio, Rovi, and Janssen. MP: participated as speaker for Lilly, Shire, and Rovi. JC: received consulting income and research support from Janssen, Shire, Ferrer, Lilly, and Lundbeck. JS and LG-O are employees of Shire. JSS, MGG, MG, MJM, and JE received support from Shire for this research. JAA: acted as consultant to or received honoraria or grants from Eli Lilly, Shire, Janssen Cilag, Rovi, Spanish Ministry of Health, Instituto de Salud Carlos III, Agència d'Informació, Avaluació i Qualitat en Salut (AIAQS), and the Alicia Koplowitz Foundation.

Author details

[1]Psychiatry Department, Hospital Universitario Infanta Leonor and Psychiatry and Medical Psychology Department, Complutense University, Madrid, Spain. [2]Department of Psychiatry, Hospital Universitari Vall d'Hebron, Barcelona, Spain; Biomedical Network Research Centre on Mental Health (CIBERSAM), Barcelona, Spain; and Department of Psychiatry and Legal Medicine, Universitat Autònoma de Barcelona, Bellaterra, Spain. [3]Child and Adolescent Psychiatry Department, Hospital Universitario Ramón y Cajal, Madrid, Spain and Psychiatry Department, Universidad de Alcalá, Madrid, Spain. [4]Hospital Universitario Fundación de Alcorcón, Madrid, Spain and Rey Juan Carlos I University, Madrid, Spain. [5]Department of Neuropediatrics, Hospital Universitario Quirón, Madrid, Spain. [6]UDPyPC, Hospital Universitario Dr. Peset and University of Valencia and University CEU-UCH, Valencia, Spain. [7]Child and Adolescent Psychiatry and Psychology Department, Institute of Neuroscience, Hospital Clinic, Barcelona, Spain. [8]Child and Adolescent Psychiatry and Psychology Department, Hospital Infantil Universitario Niño Jesús and Biomedical Network Research Centre on Mental Health (CIBERSAM), Madrid, Spain. [9]Child and Adolescent Psychiatry Department, Hospital Gregorio Marañón, Universidad Complutense, Madrid, Spain. [10]Child and Adolescent Psychiatry Unit, Department of Psychiatry and Medical Psychology, University of Navarra Clinic, Pamplona, Spain. [11]Neuropediatric Division, Pediatric Department, Complejo Hospitalario Universitario Santiago De Compostela, Santiago de Compostela, Spain. [12]Department of Neuropediatrics, Hospital La Fe, Valencia, Spain. [13]Hospital Parc Taulí, Sabadell, Spain and Autonomous University of Barcelona, Bellaterra, Spain. [14]Psychiatry and Mental Health Department, Hospital Universitario del Henares, Francisco de Victoria University, Madrid, Spain. [15]Shire, Madrid, Spain. [16]Child and Adolescent Psychiatry and Psychology Department, Hospital Sant Joan de Déu, Esplugues de Llobregat, 08950 Barcelona, Spain.

References

1. Flood E, Gajria K, Sikirica V, Dietrich CN, Romero B, Harpin V, et al. The Caregiver Perspective of Paediatric ADHD (CAPPA) survey: understanding sociodemographic and clinical characteristics, treatment use, and impact of ADHD in Europe. J Affect Disord. 2016;200:222–34.

2. Polanczyk G, Willcutt EG, Salum GA, Kieling C, Rohde LA. ADHD prevalence estimates across three decades: an updated systematic review and meta-regression analysis. Int J Epidemiol. 2014;43:434–42.
3. Willcutt EG. The prevalence of DSM-IV attention-deficit/hyperactivity disorder: a meta-analytic review. Neurotherapeutics. 2012;9:490–9.
4. American Psychiatric Association. Diagnostic and statistical manual of mental disorders, fifth edition (DSM-5). Arlington, VA: American Psychiatric Publishing; 2013.
5. Hodgkins P, Setyawan J, Mitra D, Davis K, Quintero J, Fridman M, et al. Management of ADHD in children across Europe: patient demographics, physician characteristics, and treatment patterns. Eur J Pediatr. 2013;172:895–906.
6. Coghill D, Soutullo C, d'Aubuisson C, Preuss U, Lindback T, Silverberg M, et al. Impact of attention-deficit/hyperactivity disorder on the patient and family: results from a European survey. Child Adolesc Psychiatry Ment Health. 2008;2:31.
7. Mrug S, Molina BS, Hoza B, Gerdes AC, Hinshaw SP, Hechtman L, et al. Peer rejection and friendships in children with attention-deficit/hyperactivity disorder: contributions to long-term outcomes. J Abnorm Child Psychol. 2012;40:1013–26.
8. Arnold LE, Hodgkins P, Kahle J, Madhoo M, Kewley G. Long-term outcomes of ADHD: academic achievement and performance. J Atten Disord. 2015;Jan 12; [Epub ahead of print]
9. Coghill D, Hodgkins P. Health-related quality of life of children with attention-deficit/hyperactivity disorder versus children with diabetes and healthy controls. Eur Child Adolesc Psychiatry. 2016;25:261–71.
10. Harpin V, Mazzone L, Raynaud JP, Kahle J, Hodgkins P. Long-term outcomes of ADHD: a systematic review of self-esteem and social function. J Atten Disord. 2016;20:295–305.
11. Young S, Fitzgerald M, Postma MJ. ADHD: Making the Invisible Visible. 2013. http://www.russellbarkley.org/factsheets/ADHD_MakingTheInvisibleVisible.pdf. Accessed 3 Feb 2017.
12. Dalsgaard S, Leckman JF, Mortensen PB, Nielsen HS, Simonsen M. Effect of drugs on the risk of injuries in children with attention deficit hyperactivity disorder: a prospective cohort study. Lancet Psychiatry. 2015;2:702–9.
13. Dalsgaard S, Ostergaard SD, Leckman JF, Mortensen PB, Pedersen MG. Mortality in children, adolescents, and adults with attention deficit hyperactivity disorder: a nationwide cohort study. Lancet. 2015;385:2190–6.
14. Knecht C, de Alvaro R, Martinez-Raga J, Balanza-Martinez V. Attention-deficit hyperactivity disorder (ADHD), substance use disorders, and criminality: a difficult problem with complex solutions. Int J Adolesc Med Health. 2015;27:163–75.
15. Shilon Y, Pollak Y, Aran A, Shaked S, Gross-Tsur V. Accidental injuries are more common in children with attention deficit hyperactivity disorder compared with their non-affected siblings. Child Care Health Dev. 2012;38:366–70.
16. Doshi JA, Hodgkins P, Kahle J, Sikirica V, Cangelosi MJ, Setyawan J, et al. Economic impact of childhood and adult attention-deficit/hyperactivity disorder in the United States. J Am Acad Child Adolesc Psychiatry. 2012;51: 990–1002.
17. Le HH, Hodgkins P, Postma MJ, Kahle J, Sikirica V, Setyawan J, et al. Economic impact of childhood/adolescent ADHD in a European setting: the Netherlands as a reference case. Eur Child Adolesc Psychiatry. 2013;23:587–98.
18. Khong B. The lifetime costs of attention deficit hyperactivity disorder (ADHD). 2017. https://www.centreformentalhealth.org.uk/costs-of-adhd. Accessed 4 Jul 2017.
19. Olesen J, Gustavsson A, Svensson M, Wittchen HU, Jonsson B. The economic cost of brain disorders in Europe. Eur J Neurol. 2012;19:155–62.
20. Catala-Lopez F, Ridao M, Sanfelix-Gimeno G, Peiro S. Cost-effectiveness of pharmacological treatment of attention deficit hyperactivity disorder in children and adolescents: qualitative synthesis of scientific evidence. Rev Psiquiatr Salud Ment. 2013;6:168–77.
21. Wu EQ, Hodgkins P, Ben-Hamadi R, Setyawan J, Xie J, Sikirica V, et al. Cost effectiveness of pharmacotherapies for attention-deficit hyperactivity disorder: a systematic literature review. CNS Drugs. 2012;26:581–600.
22. Arnold LE, Hodgkins P, Caci H, Kahle J, Young S. Effect of treatment modality on long-term outcomes in attention-deficit/hyperactivity disorder: a systematic review. PLoS One. 2015;10:e0116407.
23. Shaw M, Hodgkins P, Caci H, Young S, Kahle J, Woods AG, et al. A systematic review and analysis of long-term outcomes in attention deficit hyperactivity disorder: effects of treatment and non-treatment. BMC Med. 2012;10:99.
24. American Psychiatric Association. Diagnostic and statistical manual of mental disorders, fourth edition, text revision. Washington, DC: American Psychiatric Association; 2000.
25. DuPaul GJ, Power TJ, Anastopoulos AD, et al. ADHD rating scale-IV (for children and adolescents): checklists, norms, and clinical interpretation. New York, NY: Guilford Publications, Inc; 1998.
26. Guy W. ECDEU Assessment manual for psychopharmacology. Rockville, MD: Department of Health, Education and Welfare, National Institute of Mental Health; 1976.
27. Shaffer D, Gould MS, Brasic J, Ambrosini P, Fisher P, Bird H, et al. A children's global assessment scale (CGAS). Arch Gen Psychiatry. 1983;40:1228–31.
28. Reilly MC, Zbrozek AS, Dukes EM. The validity and reproducibility of a work productivity and activity impairment instrument. PharmacoEconomics. 1993; 4:353–65.
29. INE. Spanish National Institute of Statistics 2012. http://www.ine.es. Accessed 3 Feb 2017.
30. Ramos-Quiroga JA, Casas M. Achieving remission as a routine goal of pharmacotherapy in attention-deficit hyperactivity disorder. CNS Drugs. 2011;25:17–36.
31. Stein MA, Sarampote CS, Waldman ID, Robb AS, Conlon C, Pearl PL, et al. A dose-response study of OROS methylphenidate in children with attention-deficit/hyperactivity disorder. Pediatrics. 2003;112:e404.
32. Braun S, Zeidler J, Linder R, Engel S, Verheyen F, Greiner W. Treatment costs of attention deficit hyperactivity disorder in Germany. Eur J Health Econ. 2013;14:939–45.
33. Insel TR. Assessing the economic costs of serious mental illness. Am J Psychiatry. 2008;165:663–5.
34. De Ridder A, De Graeve D. Healthcare use, social burden and costs of children with and without ADHD in Flanders, Belgium. Clin Drug Investig. 2006;26:75–90.
35. Myren KJ, Thernlund G, Nylen A, Schacht A, Svanborg P. Atomoxetine's effect on societal costs in Sweden. J Atten Disord. 2010;13:618–28.
36. Telford C, Green C, Logan S, Langley K, Thapar A, Ford T. Estimating the costs of ongoing care for adolescents with attention-deficit hyperactivity disorder. Soc Psychiatry Psychiatr Epidemiol. 2013;48:337–44.
37. Hakkaart-van Roijen L, Zwirs BW, Bouwmans C, Tan SS, Schulpen TW, Vlasveld L, et al. Societal costs and quality of life of children suffering from attention deficient hyperactivity disorder (ADHD). Eur Child Adolesc Psychiatry. 2007;16:316–26.
38. Holden SE, Jenkins-Jones S, Poole CD, Morgan CL, Coghill D, Currie CJ. The prevalence and incidence, resource use and financial costs of treating people with attention deficit/hyperactivity disorder (ADHD) in the United Kingdom (1998 to 2010). Child Adolesc Psychiatry Ment Health. 2013;7:34.
39. Wehmeier PM, Schacht A, Rothenberger A. Change in the direct cost of treatment for children and adolescents with hyperkinetic disorder in Germany over a period of four years. Child Adolesc Psychiatry Ment Health. 2009;3:3.
40. Cadman T, Eklund H, Howley D, Hayward H, Clarke H, Findon J, et al. Caregiver burden as people with autism spectrum disorder and attention-deficit/hyperactivity disorder transition into adolescence and adulthood in the United Kingdom. J Am Acad Child Adolesc Psychiatry. 2012;51:879–88.
41. Hodgkins P, Dittmann RW, Sorooshian S, Banaschewski T. Individual treatment response in attention-deficit/hyperactivity disorder: broadening perspectives and improving assessments. Exp Rev Neurother. 2013;13:425–33.
42. Daley D, Jacobsen RH, Lange A-M, et al. Costing adult attention deficit disorder: impact on the individual and society. Oxford, UK: Oxford University Press; 2015.
43. Ward MM, Javitz HS, Smith WM, Bakst AA. Comparison of three approaches for attributing hospitalizations to specific diseases in cost analyses. Int J Technol Assess Health Care. 2000;16:125–36.

17

Evaluation of the diagnostic implications of Das-Naglieri cognitive assessment system in children with attention deficit hyperactivity disorder

Ling Qin, Hairun Liu*, Hong Zhang, Yanhong Fu and Dandan Li

Abstract

Background: Attention deficit hyperactivity disorder (ADHD) is a neurodevelopmental characterized by attention deficit, hyperactivity, emotional impulses and difficulty with cognitive functions. The Das-Naglieri Cognitive Assessment System (DN: CAS), as a theory-driven assessment kit, was explored based on Planning, Attention, Simultaneous, and Successive Theory (PASS). Recent researches have tried to explore the sensitivity and specificity of DN: CAS in diagnosing ADHD; nevertheless, these studies were performed in a small study population. The following study explores the cognitive functions in ADHD by the DN: CAS and to evaluate the DN: CAS's diagnostic value in ADHD.

Methods: A total of 135 children with ADHD and 140 healthy controls were enrolled to evaluate cognitive function by the DN: CAS. ROC curve and the area under the curve (AUC) were applied to evaluate the diagnostic value of DN: CAS on ADHD.

Results: Compared with healthy controls, children with ADHD had significantly lower scores in Planning, Simultaneous (Verbal-Spatial Relations), Attention in the four Subtests of DN: CAS, as well as the total scores. ROC analysis indicated that Planning and Attention of DN: CAS had good classification accuracy in diagnosing ADHD with AUCs of 0.808 and 0.730, respectively.

Conclusions: The planning and attention assessment of DN: CAS revealed high sensitivity and specificity in diagnosing ADHD, thus suggesting that DN: CAS might be an effective tool in diagnosing ADHD.

Keywords: Attention deficit hyperactivity disorder (ADHD), Das-Naglieri cognitive assessment system (DN:CAS), PASS, Cognitive assessment

Background

In China, approximately 4.31–5.83% of children are affected by ADHD, which is a neurodevelopmental disorder characterized by attention deficit, hyperactivity, emotional impulses and difficulty with cognitive functions [1, 2]. The American Academy of Child & Adolescent Psychiatry noted that the assessments for ADHD may include structured diagnostic interviews, parent and teacher report behavior rating scales, direct observations by doctor and cognitive tests. As cognitive neuroscience advances, most studies seem to demonstrate that the impairment of cognitive function is an important manifestation in ADHD [3–5]. Barkley constructed a theoretical model indicating that ADHD may be linked to four executive neuropsychological function impairments in 1997 [6]. These theories provided the basis for clinical diagnosis of ADHD and many cognitive assessment tools were used to evaluate the clinical symptoms of ADHD such as CPT test, Stroop test and Go/No Go task [7–10].

The Das-Naglieri cognitive assessment system (DN: CAS), as a theory-driven assessment kit, was explored based on PASS theory by JP. Das, which was applied to assess the cognitive function. PASS theory has

* Correspondence: liuhairun@sina.com
From the center of Cognitive and Sleeping, The people's hospital of Guangxi Zhuang autonomous region, Nanning 530021, Guangxi, China

reconceptualized intelligence as a process-driven understanding of cognitive abilities based on the following four cognitive processes: Planning, Attention, Simultaneous and Successive processing [11]. This theory has been linked to Luria's three functional units of the brain. Attention has been linked to the first structural unit, i.e. brain stem, midbrain and the brain; Simultaneous and Successive processing have been linked to the second structural unit, i.e. occipital, temporal, and parietal lobes; Planning has been linked with the third structural unit, i.e. the frontal lobe, and especially the prefrontal lobe in the same direction [12]. In his study, McCrea has reported on three patients with unilateral focalized stroke lesions that were examined longitudinally on the DN: CAS, suggesting that the DN: CAS subtests are not only unique but also sensitive and specific to focalized cortical lesions [13].

PASS theory, which is similar to Barkley's execution function defect theory, proposes that children with ADHD may be more impulsive in cognitive processing, which in turn can influence planning processing. Attention difficulties are expected to negatively affect attention processing. Some studies have demonstrated that children with ADHD assessed by DN: CAS have the lowest performance on Planning and Attention scores, whereas their Simultaneous and Successive processing scores appear normal [14, 15]. DN: CAS has been standardized in different languages including Chinese [16].

ADHD is a multifactorial disorder, and genetic factors might be associated with the risk of ADHD [17, 18]. Given the different genetic background, the aim of the present study was to explore the association of cognitive functions and ADHD, and to evaluate the DN: CAS's diagnostic value in Chinese children with ADHD.

Methods

Study population

A total of 135 children with ADHD and 140 controls were recruited in this study. The ADHD children were enrolled from People's hospital of Guangxi Zhuang Autonomous Region between Jan 2015 and Dec 2016. In addition, 140 healthy controls were enrolled from the same communities and schools. All study subjects were interviewed by two well-trained investigators at the Department of Psychiatry, who used K-SADS to conduct interview. ADHD was diagnosed according to American Psychiatric Association (APA) criteria (Diagnostic and statistical manual of mental disorders, 5th edition (DSM-5)). Medical history, clinical examination and APA diagnosis criteria evaluated by two independent psychiatrists were used to identify healthy controls as free of ADHD. Children with Intellectual Disability (The Full Scale IQ (FSIQ) < 85 by WISC-CR-II), Learning Disorder, Tic Disorders and Autism spectrum disorder were excluded from the study. The FSIQ was included in the present study.

The Ethics Committee of People's hospital of Guangxi Zhuang autonomous Region approved this study, and all study subjects agreed to participate in our research after they were debriefed about the study and after they signed the informed consent; for the children under 16-years of age, the consent was obtained from their guardians.

Instrument

DN:CAS Chinese version

The DN: CAS [16] was administered by a well-trained psychotherapist. This assessment tool includes four subscales, including Planning, Attention, Simultaneous Processing, and Successive Processing. The whole test is made up of 12 subtests, with each subscale containing three items. Two different sets of tests were carried out according to various age groups (5–7 year-olds and 8–17 year-olds).

Planning assessment was used to evaluate the efficiency in task solving, including Matching Numbers, Planned Codes and Planned Connections. Matching Numbers requires the test taker to find two identical numbers in the same row (e.g. find 2 identical numbers in a row such as 3–5–2-6-5-7-4). Arrangement in each row is well-designed in order to detect the benefit of the matching strategy during differentiation. Planned Codes require the test taker to code characters arranged in specific order with certain strategy, based on the way they've been previously thought (e.g. Codes for A, B and C are OX, XX, and XO, separately. The subject needs to convert a series of characters into corresponding codes). Planned Connections require the subject to connect randomly scattered numbers/numbers and letters in numerical or/and alphabetical order (e.g. 1–2–3-4/1-A-2-B-3-C).

Attention mainly assesses the ability to selectively focus on one part of the two-dimensional stimulus while ignoring the other part, including Expressive Attention, Number Detection and Receptive Attention. Expressive Attention refers to the ability to inhibit interfering stimuli in the procedure of expression (e.g. test taker is presented with cards containing the color names printed in colors that are different from the meaning of the printed word, and then the test taker is asked to say the color of the word instead of the word itself). Number Detection evaluates selective attention, switching attention and cognitive inhibition to distraction (e.g. test taker is presented with 3–6 targeted numbers together with several rows of numbers from 0 to 9 in the item, and then he/she is asked to find and underline figures that look exactly the same as targeted ones, from left to right in a row). Receptive Attention requires the subject to circle every pair of characters that look the same or that have the same pronunciation (e.g. circle AA but not AB, and circle Tt but not Tb).

Simultaneous processing requires the test taker to interconnect components of special items to get the correct answer. It includes Nonverbal Matrices, Verbal-Spatial Relations and Figure Memory. The test taker needs to figure out relation among the segments in the item, then to integrate them with abstract thinking and logical perception ability. There are three types of items in Nonverbal Matrices, i.e. graph filling, analogical reasoning and spatial vision. Each item contains graphs and geometrical elements with relations to either spatial organization or logical organization, and the subject reveals abstract reasoning by observing these relations (e.g. he/ she is asked to make a deduction and find out the absent figure based on the relationship among the five figures presented). In Verbal-Spatial Relations, the subject needs to choose a corresponding picture after he/she is given the description with underlying logical relationship (e.g. subject is presented with six pictures showing various spatial relationships between a ball and a desk, and asked to point out the correct picture). Figure Memory is a representative subtest of simultaneous processing. It includes two-dimensional or three-dimensional figures that are shown to subject, who is then asked to discriminate the simple figure from a complex one (e.g. subject is presented with a simple geometric figure for 5 s, which is then removed and the subject is asked to draw it).

Successive Processing requires individuals to replicate a particular event or sequence of events. It contains Word Series, Sentence Repetition and Sentence Questions. In this subscale, the subject needs to understand or repeat auditory information that is presented in specific order. The Word Series is made up of monosyllabic words (e.g. dog, pen, and book) whose length ranges from 2 to 9 alphabets. The administrator reads them in a speed of 1 s/alphabet and asks the subject to repeat in the same order. The Sentence Repetition requires for a duplication of the auditory sentence that is made up of color items and with no actual meaning (e.g. red is black). The Sentence Questions are used to evaluate the subject's understanding of the grammatical relations in the sentence by letting the subject to answer a question based on the stated sentence (e.g. 'White is blue. What is blue?' answer 'white').

Calculate raw scores in the 12 subtests separately, then convert them to scale scores. After that, add up the scale scores in each subscale and convert them to standardized scores.

Statistical analysis

Continuous variables were shown as the mean value ± SD. Normal distribution of data was analyzed using the Kolmogorov–Smirnov normality test. Data with normal distribution were compared by Student's t test and bonferroni correction. Those with unequal variance or without a normal distribution were analyzed by a Mann–Whitney rank sum test. Items of DN: CAS and FSIQ were compared by Student's t test, and statistical analyses were carried out using statistical analysis software package SPSS19.0 with the level of significance at $p < 0.05$.

ROC curve was used to measure classification performance (sensitivity and specificity) for the DN: CAS and statistical analyses were carried out using statistical analysis software MedCalc15.8 with the level of significance at $p < 0.05$.

Results

Characteristics of study population

The general characteristics of the ADHD and control group are presented in Table 1; there were not significant differences of age, gender and grade between ADHD group and control group. Comparing to control group children with ADHD had significantly lower scores in FSIQ.

The DN:CAS assessment of the ADHD and control group

In this study, children with ADHD had significantly lower scores in these subtests compared to control group: Planning ($T = -10.260$, $p < 0.01$), Simultaneous ($T = -2.406$, $p < 0.05$), Attention ($T = -7.075$, $p < 0.01$) of DN:CAS, while the total scores were also statically lower in ADHD group compared to controls ($T = -7.284$, $p < 0.01$). Compared with control group, ADHD children had worse performance in Matching Numbers ($T = -8.22$, $p < 0.01$), Planned Codes ($T = -5.779$, $p < 0.01$), Planned Connections ($T = -9.124$, $p < 0.01$) of Planning; Verbal-Spatial Relations ($T = -2.278$, $p < 0.01$) of Simultaneous and Expressive Attention ($T = -5.146$, $p < 0.01$); and Number Detection ($T = -6.608, p < 0.01$), Receptive Attention ($T = -4.059, p < 0.01$) (Table 2). The results showed that there were more cognitive deficits in ADHD group than in healthy subjects, especially in relation to planning and attention of DN: CAS.

Table 1 The general characteristics of Study Population

Variables	ADHD	Control	*P* valve
Age(years)	9.1 ± 2.1	9.3 ± 1.5	0.299
Gender(n)			0.755
Boys	112	114	
Girls	23	26	
Grade(n)			0.217
First grade	17	12	
Second grade	31	20	
Junior class	24	31	
Fourth grade	20	31	
Fifth grade	20	25	
Six grade	23	25	
FSIQ	98.33 ± 9.5	105.58 ± 14.9	0.000

Table 2 DN: CAS full scale and subscale means and standard deviations for ADHD groups and Control groups

CAS Subscales	ADHD		Control		t	*P* valve
	M	SD	M	SD		
Planning	23.19	5.15	29.59	5.19	−10.260	0.000
Matching Numbers	8.42	2.34	10.90	2.65	−8.218	0.000
Planned Codes	7.36	2.02	8.93	2.46	−5.779	0.000
Planned Connections	7.41	2.18	9.76	2.09	−9.124	0.000
Simultaneous	34.92	6.05	36.59	5.49	−2.406	0.017
Nonverbal Matrices	12.06	2.91	12.18	2.53	−0.363	0.717
Verbal-Spatial Relations	10.56	2.55	11.42	2.61	−2.785	0.006
Figure Memory	12.30	3.04	12.99	3.56	−1.725	0.086
Attention	25.73	5.52	30.38	5.37	−7.075	0.000
Expressive Attention	8.52	2.37	10.12	2.77	−5.146	0.000
Number Detection	8.50	1.98	10.08	1.99	−6.608	0.000
Receptive Attention	8.72	3.13	10.18	2.84	−4.059	0.001
Successive	32.47	6.25	33.44	5.32	−1.387	0.167
Word Series	16.27	2.73	16.81	2.63	−1.650	0.100
Sentence Repetition	7.08	2.19	7.48	1.85	−1.632	0.104
Sentence Questions	9.11	3.09	9.15	2.84	−0.109	0.913
Full Scale	116.30	16.17	129.99	14.99	−7.284	0.000

ROC analyses

Since our results revealed an association between planning and attention deficit and ADHD assessment by DN:CAS, we aimed to investigate the sensitivity and specificity of planning and attention assessment in diagnosing ADHD. The ROC analysis indicated that Planning and Attention assessment had good classification accuracy in ADHD diagnose with AUCs of 0.808 (95%CI: 0.756–0.853, $p < 0.01$) and 0.730 (95%CI: 0.673–0.782, $p < 0.01$) respectively. The cutoff point was drawn from the curve for Planning 25-point and for Attention 29-point for diagnostic measures (Table 3 and Fig. 1). Positive predictive value and negative predictive values for Planning were 72.6 and 79.3%; for Attention were 78.5 and 57.9%, respectively.

Discussion

The diagnosis of ADHD is mainly based on three categories of clinical symptoms, i.e. attention deficit, hyperactivity and impulsivity. Many scholars have tried to find

Table 3 ROC curves and other parameters of Planning and Attention

Test Variables	Area	*P* Value	95%CI	
			Lower	Upper
Planning	0.808	0.0301	0.756	0.853
Attention	0.730	0.0260	0.673	0.782

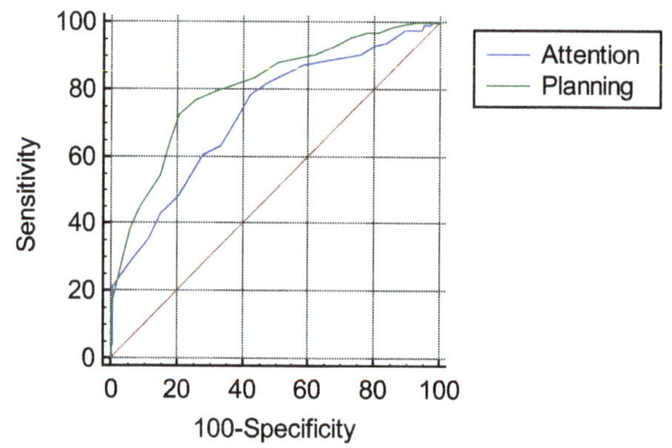

Fig. 1 The ROC Curve of the Planning and the Attention to diagnostic the ADHD ROC analysis indicated that Planning and Attention had good classification accuracy with AUCs of 0.808 (95% CI: 0.756–0.853, $p < 0.01$) and 0.730 (95% CI: 0.673–0.782, $p < 0.01$) respectively

an effective tool for diagnosis of ADHD, and from 1998, continuous performance tests (CPT) have been widely used in the diagnosis of ADHD. The CPT is used to assess attention and control ability [7, 8, 19]. Meanwhile, Go/No Go task is another test tool commonly used for ADHD diagnosis, which focuses on executive function but without assessing other cognitive functions [10]. Thus, the use of these tools has certain limitations in diagnosing ADHD and in evaluating the cognitive deficit in ADHD. The DN: CAS, a well-admissive theory-driven assessment kit consisting of four independent factors, which include Planning, Attention, Simultaneous and Successive processing in the PASS model, have been used to assess neurodevelopmental disorder in 5–17 year old children [15, 20]. To the best of our knowledge, the DN: CAS is the most comprehensive tool for assessment of cognitive processes, which is why we aimed to explore the association between ADHD diagnosis and the DN: CAS assessment.

Our results demonstrated that the ADHD gender incidence was 4.9 (112 boys): 1(23 girls), which was consistent with previous studies [1]. We found that ADHD children performed significantly worse in FSIQ and Planning including Matching Numbers, Planned Codes, Planned Connections; and Attention including Expressive Attention, Number Detection and Receptive Attention, which was consistent with the majority of recent researches [16, 20, 21]. According to PASS theory, Planning represents the ability to perform decision-making, selection and implementation, thanks to the corresponding brain regions that are located in frontal cortex [13, 22]. We found that ADHD subjects exhibited Planning defects in DN: CAS assessment, which was stated as EF impairment in Barkley's theoretical model [6]. While Attention subtests require a sustained focus for identification of a target stimulus, our study revealed the ADHD children had a weaker performance in the Attention compared to healthy children. In addition, compared with control subjects, ADHD children scored worse in Verbal-Spatial Relations of Simultaneous, which was inconsistent with previous studies [14, 16]. According to PASS theory, Simultaneous is a cognitive process by which the individual integrates separate stimuli into a single group, and Simultaneous requires the children to understand logical-grammatical relationships [20]. Our results indicated that ADHD subjects might have deficit in Simultaneous processing of Verbal-Spatial reasoning.

Since the ADHD children appeared to have obvious defects in DN: CAS assessment, especially in planning and attention, ROC analysis was applied to evaluate the sensitivity and specificity of planning and attention assessment in diagnosing ADHD. The AUC of Planning was 0.808 when the cut-off point was set at 25-points, where the sensitivity was 72.6% and specificity was 79.3%; the AUC of Attention was 0.730, when the cut-off point was set at 29-points, where the sensitivity was 78.5% and specificity was 57.9%. The obtained results indicated that the planning and attention assessment of DN: CAS had high sensitivity and specificity in diagnosing ADHD, which suggested that DN: CAS might be an effective tool for diagnosing ADHD, especially in a clinical setting. This study also provided a useful indication for the treatment of ADHD by using remedial programmers; their specific focus will be the amelioration of EF deficit.

Limitation

This study had some limitations. First, selection bias might exist in enrollment; Secondly, we recruited the ADHD cases without any comorbidities in order to reduce the possible bias from study subject's stratification, we need to enlarge the study population of ADHD in the future; thirdly, larger sample needed to be carried out to verify the diagnostic value of DN:CAS in ADHD diagnosis.

Conclusion

The planning and attention assessment of DN: CAS had highly sensitivity and specificity in diagnosing ADHD, which was encouraged that DN: CAS might be an effective tool in diagnosing ADHD.

Abbreviations

ADHD: attention deficit hyperactivity disorder; APA: American Psychiatric Association criteria; CPT: continuous performance tests; DN: CAS: Das-Naglieri cognitive assessment system; DSM-5: Diagnostic and statistical manual of mental disorders 5th edition; FSIQ: Full Scale IQ; PASS: Planning, Attention, Simultaneous, and Successive Theory

Acknowledgments

None.

Funding

This work was supported by the Scientific Research and Technology Development Program of Guangxi (1355005-5-5).

Declarations

This work was supported by the Scientific Research and Technology Development Program of Guangxi (1355005-5-5), and no other relationships/conditions/circumstances that present potential conflict of interest.

Authors' contributions

Conception and design of the study: LQ and HRL. Data acquisition: HZ, YHF, DDL Data management and analysis: HRL. Manuscript drafting/editing: HRL. All authors read and approved the final manuscript.

Consent for publication

Not applicable.

Competing interests

The authors declare that they have no competing interests.

References

1. Faraone SV, Sergeant J, Gillberg C, Biederman J. The worldwide prevalence of ADHD: is it an American condition? World Psychiatry. 2003;2(2):104–13.
2. Polanczyk GV, Willcutt EG, Salum GA, Kieling C, Rohde LA. ADHD prevalence estimates across three decades: an updated systematic review and meta-regression analysis. Int J Epidemiol. 2014;43(2):434–42.
3. Tillman CM, Bohlin G, Sorensen L, Lundervold AJ. Intellectual deficits in children with ADHD beyond central executive and non-executive functions. Arch. Clin. Neuropsychol. 2009;24(8):769–82.
4. Velez-van-Meerbeke A, Zamora IP, Guzman G, Figueroa B, Lopez Cabra CA, Talero-Gutierrez C. Evaluating executive function in schoolchildren with symptoms of attention deficit hyperactivity disorder. Neurologia (Barcelona, Spain). 2013;28(6):348–55.
5. Berenguer Forner C, Rosello Miranda B, Baixauli Fortea I, Garcia Castellar R, Colomer Diago C, Miranda Casas A. ADHD symptoms and peer problems: mediation of executive function and theory of mind. Psicothema. 2017; 29(4):514–9.
6. Barkley RA. Behavioral inhibition, sustained attention, and executive functions: constructing a unifying theory of ADHD. Psychol Bull. 1997;121(1): 65–94.
7. Krieger V, Amador-Campos JA. Assessment of executive function in ADHD adolescents: contribution of performance tests and rating scales. Child Neuropsychol. 2017:1–25.
8. Lundervold AJ, Stickert M, Hysing M, Sorensen L, Gillberg C, Posserud MB. Attention deficits in children with combined autism and ADHD: a CPT study. J Atten Disord. 2016;20(7):599–609.
9. Sorensen L, Plessen KJ, Adolfsdottir S, Lundervold AJ. The specificity of the Stroop interference score of errors to ADHD in boys. Child Neuropsychol. 2014;20(6):677–91.
10. Newman E, Jernigan TL, Lisdahl KM, Tamm L, Tapert SF, Potkin SG, Mathalon D, Molina B, Bjork J, Castellanos FX, et al. Go/no go task performance predicts cortical thickness in the caudal inferior frontal gyrus in young adults with and without ADHD. Brain Imaging Behav. 2016;10(3):880–92.
11. Perez-Alvarez F, Timoneda-Gallart C. PASS neurocognitive dysfunction in attention deficit. Rev Neurol. 2001;32(1):30–7.
12. Deilami M, Jahandideh A, Kazemnejad Y, Fakour Y, Alipoor S, Rabiee F, Pournesaie GS, Heidari RN, Mosavi SA. The effect of neurofeedback therapy on reducing symptoms associated with attention deficit hyperactivity disorder: a case series study. Basic Clin Neurosci. 2016;7(2):167–71.
13. McCrea SM. A cognitive neuropsychological examination of the Das-Naglieri cognitive assessment system subtests: a report of three stroke cases studied longitudinally during recovery. Int J Neurosci. 2009;119(4):553–99.

14. Van Luit JE, Kroesbergen EH, Naglieri JA. Utility of the PASS theory and cognitive assessment system for Dutch children with and without ADHD. J Learn Disabil. 2005;38(5):434–9.
15. Nakashima N, Yamashita Y, Hirata R, Nagamitsu S, Matsuishi T. Kana reading disability and Das-Naglieri cognitive assessment system findings in children with attention deficit hyperactivity disorder. Pediatri Int. 2012;54(6):849–53.
16. Deng CP, Liu M, Wei W, Chan RC, Das JP. Latent factor structure of the Das-Naglieri cognitive assessment system: a confirmatory factor analysis in a Chinese setting. Res Dev Disabil. 2011;32(5):1988–97.
17. Kuntsi J, Pinto R, Price TS, van der Meere JJ, Frazier-Wood AC, Asherson P. The separation of ADHD inattention and hyperactivity-impulsivity symptoms: pathways from genetic effects to cognitive impairments and symptoms. J Abnorm Child Psychol. 2014;42(1):127–36.
18. Tannock R. Attention deficit hyperactivity disorder: advances in cognitive, neurobiological, and genetic research. J Child Psychol Psychiatry. 1998;39(1): 65–99.
19. Mesquita C, Nazar BP, Pinna CM, Rabelo B, Serra-Pinheiro MA, Sergeant J, Mattos P. How can continuous performance test help to assess inattention when mood and ADHD symptoms coexist? Psychiatry Res. 2016;243:326–30.
20. Naglieri JAGS, Iseman JS. Schwebach.: performance of children with attention deficit hyperactive disorder and anxiety/depresión on the WISC-III and cognitive assessment system (CAS). J Psychoeduc Assess. 2003;21:32–43.
21. Canivez GL, Gaboury AR. Construct validity and diagnostic utility of the cognitive assessment system for ADHD. J Atten Disord. 2016;20(6):519–29.
22. Posner J, Siciliano F, Wang Z, Liu J, Sonuga-Barke E, Greenhill L. A multimodal MRI study of the hippocampus in medication-naive children with ADHD: what connects ADHD and depression? Psychiatry Res. 2014; 224(2):112–8.

Sequential treatment of ADHD in mother and child (AIMAC study): importance of the treatment phases for intervention success in a randomized trial

Christopher Hautmann[1,2*†], Manfred Döpfner[1,2†], Josepha Katzmann[2], Stephanie Schürmann[1,2], Tanja Wolff Metternich-Kaizman[1,2], Charlotte Jaite[3], Viola Kappel[3], Julia Geissler[4], Andreas Warnke[4], Christian Jacob[5,6], Klaus Hennighausen[7^], Barbara Haack-Dees[7], Katja Schneider-Momm[7], Alexandra Philipsen[8,9], Swantje Matthies[8], Michael Rösler[10], Wolfgang Retz[10,11], Alexander von Gontard[12], Esther Sobanski[13,14], Barbara Alm[13], Sarah Hohmann[15], Alexander Häge[15], Luise Poustka[15,16,17], Michael Colla[18,19], Laura Gentschow[18], Christine M. Freitag[12,20], Katja Becker[15,21] and Thomas Jans[4]

Abstract

Background: The efficacy of parent-child training (PCT) regarding child symptoms may be reduced if the mother has attention-deficit/hyperactivity disorder (ADHD). The AIMAC study (ADHD in Mothers and Children) aimed to compensate for the deteriorating effect of parental psychopathology by treating the mother (Step 1) before the beginning of PCT (Step 2). This secondary analysis was particularly concerned with the *additional* effect of the Step 2 PCT on child symptoms after the Step 1 treatment.

Methods: The analysis included 143 mothers and children (aged 6–12 years) both diagnosed with ADHD. The study design was a two-stage, two-arm parallel group trial (Step 1 treatment group [TG]: intensive treatment of the mother including psychotherapy and pharmacotherapy; Step 1 control group [CG]: supportive counseling only for mother; Step 2 TG and CG: PCT). Single- and multi-group analyses with piecewise linear latent growth curve models were applied to test for the effects of group and phase. Child symptoms (e.g., ADHD symptoms, disruptive behavior) were rated by three informants (blinded clinician, mother, teacher).

Results: Children in the TG showed a stronger improvement of their disruptive behavior as rated by mothers than those in the CG during Step 1 (Step 1: TG vs. CG). In the CG, according to reports of the blinded clinician and the mother, the reduction of children's disruptive behavior was stronger during Step 2 than during Step 1 (CG: Step 1 vs. Step 2). In the TG, improvement of child outcome did not differ across treatment steps (TG: Step 1 vs. Step 2).

(Continued on next page)

* Correspondence: christopher.hautmann@uk-koeln.de
†Christopher Hautmann and Manfred Döpfner contributed equally to this work.
^Deceased
[1]Department of Child and Adolescent Psychiatry, Psychosomatics and Psychotherapy, Medical Faculty of the University of Cologne, Cologne, Germany
[2]School of Child and Adolescent Cognitive Behavioral Therapy (AKiP), University Hospital Cologne, Pohligstraße 9, 50969 Cologne, Germany

(Continued from previous page)
Conclusions: Intensive treatment of the mother including pharmacotherapy and psychotherapy may have small positive effects on the child's disruptive behavior. PCT may be a valid treatment option for children with ADHD regarding disruptive behavior, even if mothers are not intensively treated beforehand.

Keywords: Mothers, Children, Adult treatment, Parent training, Efficacy

Background

The general efficacy of behavioral interventions for children with attention-deficit/hyperactivity disorder (ADHD), including parent training, has been comprehensively investigated [1–3]. However, as treatment success varies across families [4], several studies investigated the moderating role of parental ADHD in the efficacy of behavioral parent training. This introduction builds in part on two comprehensive reviews summarizing the findings from this research area [5, 6].

The heritability of ADHD is high [7] and many children with ADHD have parents who show ADHD symptoms themselves [8, 9]. Furthermore, parents with ADHD are more likely to have deficits in parenting than parents without ADHD [10–12].

Most importantly, parental ADHD has been linked to reduced efficacy of behavioral parent training. Diminished effects have been reported for child ADHD symptoms and behavioral problems [13, 14] as well as for parenting [13, 15]. However, there are also studies reporting no deteriorating effect of parental ADHD on child benefit from treatment [13, 15, 16], which may at least partly be explained by less affected parents and more personalized treatment approaches in the respective studies [5].

For adults with ADHD, the current first-line treatment option is pharmacotherapy [17, 18]. Effect sizes of stimulants on ADHD symptoms are in the medium to large range [19, 20] and are comparable to those reported for children and adolescents [21]. Cognitive behavioral therapy has been less intensively investigated [18, 22], but the available evidence shows some positive findings [23–26].

Treatment of ADHD in adults (pharmacotherapy, cognitive behavioral therapy) may also affect parenting and child outcome. Only a small number of trials have investigated this issue with regard to pharmacotherapy. The current evidence is mixed [27–29] and it has been suggested that the effects of pharmacotherapy on parenting might be limited and insufficient [5]. To our knowledge, the effects of cognitive-behavioral interventions in adults have not yet been evaluated with respect to child outcomes.

Some studies tested the combined effect of parent ADHD treatment and behavioral parent training in terms of improving child outcome [30–32]. In such cases, the adult treatment might serve two different purposes: First, it may have a (limited) more or less direct effect on parenting and on child outcome (via parenting); and second, improvements in neurocognitive functioning might help parents to participate in and benefit from the training (e.g., sustaining attention during the sessions) and to fulfill accompanying requirements (e.g., homework).

In a study by Babinski et al. [30], the combination of pharmacotherapy for adults and behavioral parent training revealed no treatment advantage over behavioral parent training alone with regard to observed parenting and child behavior. However, parents only received stimulants before and after the parent training intervention period. Therefore, the study was able to provide information about the short-term effects of stimulants on parenting, but not about the potential treatment advantage of medication for training participation.

The AIMAC (ADHD in Mothers and Children) study tested the efficacy of combined mother and child ADHD treatment in a randomized controlled trial with an active control group [32–34]. In the first phase (Step 1), mothers of the treatment group (TG) received group psychotherapy plus stimulant medication, while mothers of the control group (CG) received supportive counseling only. In the second phase (Step 2), treatment of the mother was maintained and mothers of both groups were additionally provided with the same individual parent-child training. The results revealed that after Step 2, mothers of the TG showed a stronger ADHD symptom reduction, but no group differences were detected regarding children's ADHD symptoms and disruptive behavior [32].

The current study constitutes a supplemental analysis of the AIMAC study by Jans et al. [32]. The previous main analysis focused on the comparison of the CG and TG (between-group analysis) concerning the combined effect of the mother and child treatment. As the main analysis revealed no group differences on important child domains, the present re-analysis aimed to establish the relative importance of the two treatment phases (Step 1, Step 2). For this purpose, the observed total change was split not only by group but also by treatment phase. Comparisons were conducted between groups (Step 1: CG vs. TG; Step 2: CG vs. TG) as well as within groups (CG: Step 1 vs. Step 2; TG: Step 1 vs. Step 2). The latter analyses served as a type of within-group control design (e.g., stronger child symptom reduction during Step 2 compared to Step 1 would have been considered as evidence for the efficacy of the parent-child training).

We were particularly interested in two research questions (primary testing approach in parentheses): (i) Is parent-child training useful for mothers with ADHD who have been minimally or intensively treated beforehand (CG: Step 1 vs. Step 2; TG: Step 1 vs. Step 2)? (ii) Do children benefit from intensive pharmacological and psychological treatment of the mother (Step 1: TG vs. CG)?

The first question concerned the efficacy and importance of the parent-child training in the treatment groups, a subject that is crucial for treatment planning and that is unresolved with regard to mothers with ADHD. On the one hand, for parents with ADHD, the efficacy of parent-child training has been called into question and is often considered to be reduced; on the other hand, non-significant findings have also been reported, and it has been suggested that for personalized parent training, the treatment effects might not be attenuated even in mothers with ADHD [5]. Furthermore, the main analysis of the AIMAC study did not reveal group differences on important child domains, despite the successful treatment of the mothers of the TG (e.g., ADHD symptoms, disruptive behavior) [32]. Contrary to our own previous hypotheses, we therefore assumed post hoc that the parent-child treatment actually did work in both treatment groups due to the individualized approach. Particularly for the CG, where the mother's treatment was of low intensity, we expected the within-group control comparison to be significant, meaning that we would find a stronger symptom reduction during the Step 2 parent-child training than during the Step 1 treatment of the mother (CG: Step 1 vs. Step 2). For the TG, we also considered the parent-child training to be effective. However, regarding the within-group comparison (TG: Step 1 vs. Step 2), clear hypotheses were more difficult to derive for the TG, as here, the Step 1 treatment of the mother was more intense and at least for pharmacotherapy in adults, (limited) effects on parenting and child symptoms have been reported [27, 29]. We thus considered it more likely that a more homogenous and less distinct pattern of change would be observed across the treatment phases for the TG (TG: Step 1 vs. Step 2) and therefore, if additional effects were to be observed, we expected them to be rather small.

The second research question concerned the effects of the pharmacotherapy and psychological treatment of the mothers in the TG on the child's symptoms when compared with supportive counseling for the mother (Step 1: TG vs. CG). ADHD pharmacotherapy for adults has shown some positive indirect effects on their children, but the sustainability of the impact has been questioned [5]. To our knowledge, the effect of adult psychotherapy on children has not been investigated so far, and nor has the combination of pharmacotherapy and psychotherapy been tested. We consider this to be the first trial to investigate this subject using a randomized design (Step 1: TG vs. CG). Due to the indirect effect of the treatment on the child, we expected to find rather small effects in favor of the TG.

Methods

Design

The design consisted of a blinded randomized multicenter parallel-group trial with two treatment arms (TG, CG). Families were allocated to the treatment arms by block randomization at a ratio of 1:1 and were stratified by center.

Sites

The trial was conducted at five specialized units of university hospitals in Germany (Berlin, Freiburg, Homburg, Mannheim, Würzburg) and was coordinated by the University Hospital of Würzburg. Families were primarily recruited from patients who were referred to the hospitals but were also recruited via local child psychiatrists and newspaper and website advertising.

Inclusion and exclusion criteria

Inclusion and exclusion criteria concerned mothers and their children and have been reported in detail elsewhere [32–34]. Mothers had to fulfill the following inclusion criteria: (a) age 18 to 60 years; (b) diagnosis of ADHD according to the *Diagnostic and Statistical Manual of Mental Disorders* (4th ed.; DSM-IV) [35]; (c) a score ≥ 30 on the Wender Utah Rating Scale, German short version (WURS-K) [36]. Exclusion criteria for mothers were: (a) IQ < 85; (b) psychotherapy for ADHD, methylphenidate treatment or parent-child training within the last 6 months before baseline assessment; (c) current psychotherapeutic or psychopharmacological treatment, (d) methylphenidate intolerance; (e) indication for inpatient treatment; (f) insufficient German language skills; (g) severe comorbid psychological disorder (e.g., schizophrenia, bipolar disorder); (h) medical contraindication (e.g., seizures, thyroid function, pregnancy).

Child inclusion criteria were: (a) age 6 to 12 years; (b) diagnosis of ADHD according to DSM-IV criteria; (c) no medication or stable medication for at least 4 weeks before baseline assessment. Exclusion criteria were: (a) IQ ≤ 80; (b) indication for inpatient treatment; (c) insufficient German language skills; (d) severe comorbid psychological disorder (e.g., pervasive developmental disorder, psychosis).

Sample

The AIMAC study sample has been described in detail elsewhere [32, 34]. Briefly, during the trial, 444 families were contacted and pre-screened, 206 were assessed for eligibility, and 144 families were randomized. The current analysis is based on the full analysis set (FAS), considering only families with the primary outcome (child's combined ADHD-ODD score) available at baseline ($n = 143$) [32].

Across the treatment groups, mothers were on average 38.30 ($SD = 5.70$) years old. Regarding DSM-IV ADHD diagnoses, 65.7% showed the combined type, 23.8% the predominantly inattentive type and 10.5% the predominantly hyperactive-impulsive type. At least one current or past comorbid disorder was detected in 71.3% of the mothers, with a single episode of major depressive disorder (26.6%) and recurrent major depressive disorder (21.7%) being the most prevalent conditions. Prior to the start of the study, 55.9% of the mothers had already received psychiatric or psychotherapeutic treatment and 14.0% had been previously treated with some stimulant medication (methylphenidate, amphetamine, other) and 0.7% had been prescribed atomoxetine.

In the FAS sample, children were predominantly male (73.4%) and were on average 9.44 ($SD = 1.71$) years old. With respect to the DSM-IV diagnosis of ADHD, 52.4% of the children showed the combined type, 39.2% the predominantly inattentive type and 8.4% the predominantly hyperactive-impulsive type. At least one current comorbid disorder was apparent in about half of the children (47.6%), with oppositional defiant disorder (ODD) being the most prevalent condition (30.1%). Prior to the start of the trial, 81.1% of the children had received psychiatric or psychological treatment. Furthermore, 53.8% had previously received stimulant medication (methylphenidate, amphetamine, other) and 2.8% had been treated with atomoxetine. During the trial, 74.8% of the children received ongoing psychopharmacological medication that had been prescribed before the start of the study and was to be kept stable.

Intervention

Intervention steps

The intervention comprised three steps in both intervention arms (Step 1, Step 2, Step 3; see Additional file 1: Figure S1). Step 1 served for the treatment of the mothers and lasted for 3 months. Mothers of the TG received multimodal treatment for adults with ADHD (group psychotherapy, psychopharmacotherapy) while mothers of the CG received supportive counseling. In Step 2, the treatment of the mothers was continued and the parent-child training began. The second period also lasted for 3 months, and the treatment protocol of the parent-child training was identical for both the TG and CG. Step 3 lasted for 6 months and served as a maintenance period for mother and child treatment.

Treatment for mothers was on a weekly basis (12 sessions) during Step 1 and every 4 weeks thereafter (10 sessions during Step 2 and Step 3). Parent-child training during Step 2 was scheduled every week (12 sessions) and two booster sessions were offered thereafter (Step 3). For reasons of simplicity, in the following, the Step 1 treatment phase is called mother treatment and the Step 2 treatment phase is called parent-child training.

ADHD treatment for mothers – TG

Group psychotherapy for mothers of the TG was based on a treatment manual founded in cognitive behavioral therapy and dialectical behavior therapy [25, 37]. Topics of the sessions are psychoeducation, mindfulness training, organizational skills, self-management, emotional regulation, impulse control, stress management and interpersonal problems. Each session was planned to last for 2 h, with groups comprising six to nine parents, and to include homework. Based on the needs of each patient, up to three individual sessions were offered.

Mothers of the TG additionally received pharmacological treatment with long-acting methylphenidate (Medikinet® retard) [38]. Therapy was started with 10 mg/d and was individually adjusted to daily dosages of up to 1.3 mg/kg. Multiple dosages per day were allowed.

ADHD treatment for mothers – CG

Mothers of the CG received individual supportive counseling. Sessions lasted for 15 to 20 min and topics were based on the individual needs of the mothers. Counseling was conducted in a non-directive manner and mothers were encouraged to find solutions to their problems on their own.

ADHD treatment for children

Parent-child training was based on the German treatment manual THOP (Therapieprogramm für Kinder mit hyperkinetischem und oppositionellem Problemverhalten [Therapy program for children with hyperkinetic and oppositional problem behavior]) [39] for children with hyperkinetic and oppositional problem behavior, which has been shown to be effective in the short term and have lasting effects in the long term [40–42]. The treatment included the following topics: developmental model of behavioral problems, identification of most concerning child problems, enhancing positive parent-child interaction, rules, effective commands, positive consequences and negative consequences, time-out and token economy [40]. The individual training was held in 1-h sessions and focused primarily on mothers and their children; however, fathers and teachers were included whenever needed and feasible.

Assessment and informants

Assessments were conducted at baseline (T1), immediately after Step 1 about 3 months from baseline (T2), after Step 2 about 6 months from baseline (T3), and after the Step 3 maintenance period about 12 months from baseline (T4). A follow-up assessment took place after a maintenance period of approximately 1 year (T5).

The current analysis concerned the assessments T1 to T3, which spanned Step 1 (T1–T2) and Step 2 (T2–T3). Other measurement occasions were disregarded as not all outcome measures of analysis were collected at all assessment points.

The analysis included the ratings of three informants (blinded clinician, mother, teacher). The blinded clinician was not involved in the treatment and conducted clinical interviews with the mother and the child. Her or his rating was blind to the treatment condition, but given the nature of interviews with families, blindness to the time of the assessment may not have been ensured in all cases.

Outcome measures

Assessment of child symptoms

The selection of instruments considered for this analysis concerned child externalizing behavior and its impact on the family, including reports of all three informants (blinded clinician, mother, teacher).

Kiddie-Sads-Present and Lifetime Version (K-SADS)

The K-SADS is a semi-structured interview developed to assess psychopathology in children aged 6 to 18 years [43, 44]. It was conducted by the blinded clinician, who interviewed mothers and children separately regarding the child's behavior during the past 2 weeks. Besides categorical diagnostics, the interview can also be used for dimensional assessment [45]. The three scales Inattention (Inattention; nine items), Hyperactivity/Impulsivity (Hyp/Imp; nine items) and Oppositional Defiant Disorder (ODD; eight items) are reported.

Strengths and Difficulties Questionnaire (SDQ)

The SDQ is a questionnaire to assess behaviors, emotions and relationships in children [46]. The version for parents and teachers of children aged 4 to 17 years was used and was rated by both informants. For this analysis, the scales Hyperactivity (Hyperactivity; five items), Conduct Problems (Conduct; five items) and Emotional Symptoms (Emotional; five items) are reported.

Home Situation Questionnaire (HSQ)

The HSQ is a questionnaire to assess externalizing behavior of children in specific situations [47, 48]. Items were rated by mothers, and the total scale (Total; 16 items) was used.

Family Impact Questionnaire (FIQ)

The FIQ is a questionnaire to measure the impact of child externalizing behavior on family functioning [49]. Results of three scales Impact on Social Life (Social; 11 items), Positive Feelings Toward Child (Positive; seven items) and Negative Feelings Toward Child (Negative; nine items) based on ratings of the mothers are reported.

Assessment of maternal symptoms

The instruments concerned the ADHD symptoms of the mothers. Reports of the blinded clinician and the mothers were considered.

Conners' Adult ADHD Rating Scales–Observer: Long Version (CAARS–O)

The CAARS–O are designed to assess ADHD symptom domains in adults rated by significant others (e.g., relatives, professionals) [50]. For the study, the questionnaire was completed by the blinded clinician. Results of the subscales Inattention and Memory Problems (Inattention; 12 items), Hyperactivity/Restlessness (Hyperactivity; 12 items) and Impulsivity/Emotional Lability (Impulsivity; 12 items) are reported.

Conners' Adult ADHD Rating Scales–Self-Report: Long Version (CAARS–S)

The CAARS–S were developed analogously to the CAARS–O [50] and were rated by the mothers.

Statistical analysis

All analyses were performed using the statistical software R (Version 3.4) [51], and for structural equation modeling in particular, the specific R package lavaan was used (Version 0.5) [52]. Change over time was investigated by piecewise latent growth models [53, 54]. The TG and CG were first analyzed separately (single-group analysis) and then jointly (multi-group analysis; for a graphical representation, see Additional file 1: Figure S2). To describe the growth process, three latent variables were considered for each treatment group, one random intercept and two fixed slope factors. The means of the first fixed slope factor (CG: $\alpha_2^{(CG)}$; TG: $\alpha_2^{(TG)}$) represented the change during the Step 1 treatment of the mother in each of the treatment groups (T1 to T2), and the means of the second fixed slope factor (CG: $\alpha_3^{(CG)}$; TG: $\alpha_3^{(TG)}$) indicated the change during the Step 2 parent-child training (T2 to T3).

The mean of the random intercept factor (CG: $\alpha_1^{(CG)}$; TG: $\alpha_1^{(TG)}$) represented the average outcome at baseline (T1).

During the modeling process, a series of nested models were analyzed to test for differences among factor means (null hypotheses [H_0] in parentheses). The first step of the analysis (single-group analysis) focused on the comparison of the Step 1 change with the Step 2 change in the respective treatment groups (within-group analysis; CG H_0: $\alpha_2^{(CG)} = \alpha_3^{(CG)}$; TG H_0: $\alpha_2^{(TG)} = \alpha_3^{(TG)}$). For each treatment group, two models were analyzed and compared by a Chi-square difference test, one with the means of the two slope factors freely estimated and one with the means constrained to be equal. Equal growth rates would indicate that the observed change during the Step 1 treatment of the mother and the Step 2 parent-child training did not significantly differ and consequently, that no additional effect of the parent-child training could be shown in a particular treatment group.

In the next step of the examination, the treatment groups were tested jointly (multi-group analysis) in order to conduct comparisons among them (between-group analysis). The analysis was based on the final models of the former single-group analyses. The purpose of the between-group analysis was to compare the change rates in the CG and TG during the Step 1 treatment of the mother (H_0: $\alpha_2^{(CG)} = \alpha_2^{(TG)}$) as well as to compare the change rates among the treatment groups during the Step 2 parent-child training (H_0: $\alpha_3^{(CG)} = \alpha_3^{(TG)}$). The Step 1 comparison was of particular interest, because it served as a test for the efficacy of the intensive treatment of the mother in the TG relative to the CG. The analytical procedure was analogous to the within-group comparison; models with freely estimated means and models with the means constrained to be equal were estimated and were compared by Chi-square difference test. In this case, equal growth rates would show that the change during a respective treatment period was comparable between the groups. The between-group analysis additionally included a comparison of the means of the intercept factors in the CG and TG (H_0: $\alpha_1^{(CG)} = \alpha_1^{(TG)}$), which served as a test for differences at the beginning of the treatment (T1).

Results for standardized variables as well as unstandardized variables (see Additional file 1) are reported. For standardization, a z-transformation was conducted with the grand mean and the grand standard deviation over time and group of all available data [55]. The transformation was conducted to increase the interpretability of the coefficients. Given this type of standardization and the fact that the means of the two slope factors represented the average change during Step 1 and Step 2, we interpreted them like a Cohen's *d* effect size measure.

Model fit was considered satisfactory when, for the Chi-square (χ^2) test, $p > .05$ and the comparative fit index (*CFI*) > .90. The root mean square error of approximation (*RMSEA*) was not used, because all models had small degrees of freedom and, moreover, had a small sample size [56]. Missing data were handled by full-information maximum likelihood [57]. For a person to be considered for analysis, at least one of the three assessment points (T1–T3) had to be available.

Results

Descriptive statistics of the CG and TG for outcome measures before and after Step 1 and Step 2 treatment are reported in Additional file 1: Table S1. Depending on the outcome measure, 57–66 families from the CG and 65–77 families from the TG were included.

Results of the final latent growth curve models for standardized variables are provided for child outcome (Table 1) and mother outcome (Table 2). Reported are the means of the latent slope factors for the CG ($\alpha_2^{(CG)}, \alpha_3^{(CG)}$) and TG ($\alpha_2^{(TG)}, \alpha_3^{(TG)}$), which represent change in groups during Step 1 and Step 2. The results concern the final models after constraints among the means of the latent factors had been tested in the within- and the between-group analysis. All coefficients with an asterisk (*) indicate that the means are significantly different from zero. Further, coefficients of equal size indicate equality constraints among the parameters and show that the parameters did not significantly differ across time or group. For example, for K-SADS ODD (Table 1), change rates across groups and periods were all considered to be equal except for the CG during the Step 2 treatment ($\alpha_2^{(CG)} = \alpha_2^{(TG)} = \alpha_3^{(TG)} = -0.16$; $\alpha_3^{(CG)} = -0.53$). Although the within- and between-group analyses were integrated, for reasons of convenience, the results are described separately in the following.

Results for unstandardized variables of child and mother outcome are provided in Additional file 1: Table S2. This table also contains additional information about model fit (χ^2 test, *CFI*) and the means of the latent intercept factor α_1.

Within-group analysis

In the within-group analysis, the equality of the Step 1 and Step 2 slope factor means was tested within the groups. This primarily served as a test for the additional effects of the Step 2 parent-child training in the TG and the CG after the Step 1 treatment of the mother. In the CG and for child outcome (Table 1), $\alpha_2^{(CG)}$ and $\alpha_3^{(CG)}$ did not significantly differ, except for child disruptive behavior rated by the blinded clinician (K-SADS ODD) and the mother (SDQ Conduct). For these two measures, a stronger symptom decrease was observed during the Step 2 parent-child training compared to the previous

Table 1 Change in Child Outcome Variables During Step 1 Treatment of the Mother and Step 2 Parent-Child Training for Standardized Variables

Outcome & informant	Control group		Treatment group	
	$\alpha_2^{(CG)}$	$\alpha_3^{(CG)}$	$\alpha_2^{(TG)}$	$\alpha_3^{(TG)}$
K-SADS blinded clinician				
Inattention	−0.42*	− 0.42*	− 0.42*	− 0.42*
Hyp/Imp	− 0.25*	− 0.25*	− 0.25*	− 0.25*
ODD	− 0.16*	− 0.53*	− 0.16*	− 0.16*
SDQ mother				
Hyperactivity	−0.30*	− 0.30*	− 0.30*	− 0.30*
Conduct	− 0.05	−0.24*	− 0.24*	− 0.24*
Emotional	− 0.19*	− 0.19*	− 0.19*	− 0.19*
HSQ mother				
Total	−0.27*	− 0.27*	− 0.27*	− 0.27*
FIQ mother				
Social	−0.14*	− 0.14*	− 0.14*	− 0.14*
Negative	− 0.20*	− 0.20*	− 0.20*	− 0.20*
Positive	0.04	0.04	0.04	0.04
SDQ teacher				
Hyperactivity	−0.11*	− 0.11*	− 0.11*	− 0.11*
Conduct	− 0.17*	− 0.17*	− 0.17*	− 0.17*
Emotional	− 0.13*	− 0.13*	− 0.13*	− 0.13*

Note. Results concern the final model of a series of nested piecewise linear latent growth models (within- and between-group analysis). In the case of equal coefficients (i.e., α_2 and α_3 in TG and CG), change rates did not significantly differ across treatment groups and/or steps and were constrained to be equal. $\alpha_2^{(CG)}$ = mean of latent slope factor representing average change in CG during Step 1 (T1 to T2); $\alpha_3^{(CG)}$ = mean of latent slope factor indicating average change in CG during Step 2 (T2 to T3); $\alpha_2^{(TG)}$ = mean of latent slope factor representing average change in TG during Step 1 (T1 to T2); $\alpha_3^{(TG)}$ = mean of latent slope factor indicating average change in TG during Step 2 (T2 to T3); *K-SADS* Kiddie-Sads-Present and Lifetime Version with the scales Inattention, Hyperactivity/Impulsivity and Oppositional defiant disorder, *SDQ* Strengths and Difficulties Questionnaire with the scales Hyperactivity, Conduct Problems and Emotional Symptoms, *HSQ* Home Situation Questionnaire, *FIQ* Family Impact Questionnaire with the scales Impact on Social Life, Positive Feelings Toward Child and Negative Feelings Toward Child
*$p < .05$

Step 1 treatment of the mother, indicating additional treatment effects of the parent-child training in the CG. For mother outcome in the CG (Table 2), no differences between $\alpha_2^{(CG)}$ and $\alpha_3^{(CG)}$ were detected.

Regarding the TG and child outcome (Table 1), no differences between $\alpha_2^{(TG)}$ and $\alpha_3^{(TG)}$ were found, and therefore no evidence for any additional effect of the parent-child training after the Step 1 intensive treatment of the mother. In contrast, varying change rates in the TG during Step 1 and Step 2 were obtained for ADHD symptoms of the mothers (Table 2) rated by the blinded clinician (CAARS–O Inattention, CAARS–O Impulsivity) and the mothers themselves (CAARS–S Inattention, CAARS–S Hyperactivity, CAARS–S Impulsivity). Both informants reported a stronger symptom reduction during the Step 1 treatment of the mother compared to the Step 2 parent-child training.

Table 2 Change in Mother Outcome Variables During Step 1 Treatment of the Mother and Step 2 Parent-Child Training for Standardized Variables

Outcome & informant	Control group		Treatment group	
	$\alpha_2^{(CG)}$	$\alpha_3^{(CG)}$	$\alpha_2^{(TG)}$	$\alpha_3^{(TG)}$
CAARS–O blinded clinician				
Inattention	−0.19*	− 0.19*	− 0.60*	− 0.19*
Hyperactivity	− 0.20*	− 0.20*	− 0.35*	− 0.35*
Impulsivity	− 0.25*	− 0.25*	− 0.62*	− 0.25*
CAARS–S mother				
Inattention	−0.18*	− 0.18*	− 0.58*	− 0.18*
Hyperactivity	− 0.24*	− 0.24*	− 0.55*	− 0.24*
Impulsivity	− 0.23*	− 0.23*	− 0.62*	− 0.23*

Note. Results concern the final model of a series of nested piecewise linear latent growth models (within- and between-group analysis). In the case of equal coefficients, change rates did not significantly differ across treatment groups and/or steps and were constrained to be equal. $\alpha_2^{(CG)}$ = mean of latent slope factor representing average change in CG during Step 1 (T1 to T2); $\alpha_3^{(CG)}$ = mean of latent slope factor indicating average change in CG during Step 2 (T2 to T3); $\alpha_2^{(TG)}$ = mean of latent slope factor representing average change in TG during Step 1 (T1 to T2); $\alpha_3^{(TG)}$ = mean of latent slope factor indicating average change in TG during Step 2 (T2 to T3); *CAARS–O* Conners' Adult ADHD Rating Scales–Observer: Long Version with the scales Inattention and Memory Problems, Hyperactivity/Restlessness and Impulsivity/Emotional Lability, *CAARS–S* Conners' Adult ADHD Rating Scales–Self-Report: Long Version with scales analogous to CAARS–O
*$p < .05$

Between-group analysis

This analysis considered two comparisons: First, the contrast of the Step 1 slope factor means of the CG and TG (H_0: $\alpha_2^{(CG)} = \alpha_2^{(TG)}$) and second, the comparison of the Step 2 factor means of both groups (H_0: $\alpha_3^{(CG)} = \alpha_3^{(TG)}$). The Step 1 comparison was of particular interest for this analysis, as it served as a test for the efficacy of the intensive treatment of the mother in the TG relative to the CG. For child outcome (Table 1), differences between groups were detected only for disruptive behavior during Step 1 in ratings of the mothers (SDQ Conduct) and during Step 2 in ratings of the blinded clinicians (K-SADS ODD). More specifically, throughout Step 1, mothers of the CG reported no symptom change, while mothers of the TG rated a reduction (SDQ Conduct). This indicated the efficacy of the intensive treatment of the mother in the TG relative to the CG regarding the child's disruptive behavior. In ratings of the blinded clinicians, group differences emerged at Step 2 during parent-child training and were in favor of the CG in terms of a stronger reduction of disruptive behavior (K-SADS ODD).

With respect to ADHD symptoms of mothers (Table 2) during Step 1, there was a consistent treatment advantage for the TG in ratings of the blinded clinicians (CAARS–O Inattention, CAARS-O Hyperactivity, CAARS–O Impulsivity) as well as in reports of the mothers (CAARS–S Inattention, CAARS-S Hyperactivity, CAARS–S Impulsivity). Subsequently, during Step 2, the TG benefit was only assessed for hyperactivity reported by the blinded clinicians (CAARS-O Hyperactivity).

Effect size and informants

Factor means ($\alpha_2^{(CG)}$, $\alpha_3^{(CG)}$, $\alpha_2^{(TG)}$, $\alpha_3^{(TG)}$) of the standardized observed variables (Tables 1 and 2) were considered as effect size measures and were interpreted like Cohen's *d* (see Statistical analysis section). The effect sizes varied depending on different factors including the outcome measure, the informant, and the treatment period. For child symptoms (Table 1), on a descriptive level, the strongest change was observed for disruptive behavior in the CG during Step 2 as rated by the blinded clinician, with an effect size in the medium range (K-SADS ODD). In contrast, as expected, teachers reported comparatively low effect sizes for child symptoms in general (SDQ). For ADHD symptoms of the mother (Table 2), the most pronounced change was detected in the TG during Step 1 treatment of the mother rated by the blinded clinicians (CAARS–O) as well as the mothers (CAARS–S), with effect sizes in the medium range.

Model fit and intercept factor

Model fit criteria were not fulfilled for all outcome variables in multi-group analysis (Additional file 1: Table S2). Therefore, for each variable, we inspected which group (CG, TG) was the source for insufficient model fit and did not achieve model fit criteria when analyzed in single-group analysis. However, we refrained from any post-hoc model specifications because the consideration of correlated residuals often resulted in model errors.

The between-group analysis also included a comparison of the intercept factor means α_1 that indicated the average outcome at baseline (Additional file 1: Table S2). Except for one scale in mother rating (FIQ Social), no group differences were detected between the CG and TG.

Discussion

The AIMAC study aimed to test, in a randomized trial, whether an intensive treatment for mothers with ADHD including pharmacotherapy and group psychotherapy, improves outcomes for ADHD parent-child training. Previous analyses showed that ADHD symptoms could be successfully reduced in mothers with intensive Step 1 treatment compared to minimal treatment. However, the combination of intensive treatment of the mother and subsequent parent-child training revealed no treatment advantage regarding ADHD symptoms and disruptive behavior of the child [32].

This secondary analysis was particularly concerned with the efficacy of the parent-child training in the AIMAC study. The results of our analysis suggest that the parent-child training may be a valid treatment option and may help to reduce the disruptive behavior (but not ADHD symptoms) of the child even for mothers who are not intensively treated beforehand. This can be concluded from the within-group analysis of the CG in reports of the blinded clinician and the mothers (CG: Step 1 vs. Step 2). The results are of practical importance as they suggest that children's disruptive behavior may improve from parent-child training even if the mothers still show ADHD symptoms and do not receive the best available treatment in advance. Previous research findings on this topic have been mixed [5, 6]. As suggested in previous reviews, the positive results in this trial may be explained by the personalized approach we used in order to accommodate the training to the needs of the parents [5]. The individualized treatment planning may have helped the mothers to compensate for ADHD-related deficits and to participate in the training.

The efficacy of the parent-child training in the CG may also contribute to the understanding of why, in previous studies, the two treatment groups may not have differed when the total change across both treatment steps was analyzed [32]. Our results suggest that what the CG may have missed out on in terms of improvement during the first phase of the study (due to the lower intensity of the treatment of the mother), was likely made up for during the second phase when the parent-child training was offered. For the TG, by contrast, there is a tendency, across informants, that the improvement of the disruptive behavior already began earlier, during the treatment of the mother, and was more equally distributed over the two treatment steps. TG families might therefore have had less room for improvement at the beginning of the parent-child training. Furthermore, although we found no evidence for an additional effect of the parent-child training in the TG, we would not conclude that this treatment approach was less relevant for these children. The parent-child training might have been important to maintain the initial Step 1 treatment gains, and the limitations of our analytical approach have to be considered (see limitations section).

The second research question concerned the efficacy of the intensive treatment of the mother (pharmacotherapy, psychotherapy) regarding child symptoms. Compared to supportive counseling in the CG, children of the TG showed a treatment advantage regarding disruptive behavior in the ratings of the mothers at the end of the first treatment phase (Step 1: TG vs. CG). To our knowledge, this is the first study to demonstrate a treatment advantage of the combined effect of adult pharmacotherapy and psychotherapy on the child outcome. We consider this finding to be robust, as we tested against an active control condition in which at least some common treatment factors were realized (e.g., hope, therapeutic alliance). One might speculate further that the effect of the adult treatment in the TG on the disruptive behavior of the child was mediated by improved parenting practices, which are considered to be the link between neuropsychological functioning of the parent and the psychopathology of the child [11]. However, the effect of the adult treatment on the child was rather small.

Positive effects for child disruptive behavior were observed in ratings of the blinded clinician and the mother but not in teacher ratings. The latter may be explained by a lack of generalization of the improvement to different settings. This is a common finding and has been reported in other studies as well [58]. Although we consider the blinded clinician perspective to be valuable, restrictions also need to be considered here. As clinical ratings were largely based on a parent interview, their assessment might have been biased towards the perspective of the mother [32].

Of further interest is our observation of a reduction of child ADHD symptoms in both treatment groups. For each treatment group and step, the improvement was in the small to medium range for ratings of the blinded clinician and the mothers. For ratings of the teachers, the effects were negligible. However, we could not highlight any group or phase to be superior to the other (within- and between-group comparison). As a consequence, the internal validity of the findings is low and the results remain somewhat inconclusive. It might be that all interventions are effective, but it is not possible to estimate their treatment advantage compared to merely waiting, and other explanations for the symptom reductions are possible as well (e.g., regression to the mean).

One potentially important factor in explaining these results for child ADHD symptoms is child pharmacotherapy which already existed before the trial. Three quarters of the children were maintained on medication throughout the study. As indicated by rather low baseline values, this probably reduced the room for improvement in child ADHD symptoms and consequently the likelihood of detecting treatment effects. For many children, the results therefore rather reflect the additional effect of study treatments beyond that of an existing medication. However, in recent moderator analyses, ongoing child medication was found to have no explanatory power [59].

This study has several limitations. First, the analysis relied in part on a within-group control design, which is less optimal for drawing firm conclusions than the randomized between-group comparison. To test the additional treatment effect of the parent-child training, the change rates of the two treatment phases were contrasted. This test is based implicitly on the assumption that the change during the first step is maintained in the second step, which in our case was a very conservative assumption particularly for the efficacy of the parent-child training in the TG. Second, model fit criteria were quite liberal and, moreover, were not reached in all outcome variables. Multiple factors may be responsible for misfit in growth curve models [60, 61], including misspecifications in the mean structures (e.g., functional form of the mean growth trajectory) and the covariance structures (e.g., covariance of residuals). As change during Step 1 and Step 2 was determined by two assessment points only, we could not investigate other growth forms besides the linear models. We also abstained from any post-hoc model modifications regarding the covariance structure (e.g., adding correlated residuals), because the consideration of correlated residuals often resulted in model errors. Furthermore, we were primarily interested in the mean growth trajectory, which is less affected by possible misspecifications in the covariance structure [60]. Third, our results do not always completely correspond to previous findings of the study (e.g., SDQ Conduct) [32]. Among other things, this is due to differences in the research question and varying statistical models. In Jans et al. [32] the focus was on the between-group differences (CG vs. TG). For this a linear regression approach was used and the outcome at certain time points was predicted by the treatment group along with other covariates including the baseline assessment. In contrast for the current analysis we also were interested in the within-group perspective (Step 1 vs. Step 2 in CG and TG). For this change scores (T1 to T2; T2 to T3) were estimated by piecewise latent growth curve models that could be contrasted not only between but also within the treatment groups. A detailed discussion about other and more general concerns regarding this study has been provided elsewhere [32, 62].

Conclusions

We conclude from our findings that parent-child training may be effective to reduce children's disruptive behavior even if parental ADHD is not intensively treated beforehand. This is in contrast to some previous findings. The discrepant results may be explained by different methodological approaches, although we hypothesize that the positive effects in this analysis were mainly attributable to the fact that the parent-child training was individualized, which may have helped the parents to compensate for ADHD-related deficits and to enhance their treatment participation. Future studies should investigate the importance of personalized treatment approaches for parents with ADHD in more detail and under experimental control. We also found that the combination of pharmacotherapy and psychotherapy for mothers improved children's disruptive behavior, at least from the perspective of the participating mothers. However, the effects were rather small and may not be sufficient to fully support the child. This finding is in line with previous studies investigating the effect of adult pharmacotherapy on children in isolation. The results of our analysis add to the existing knowledge that even a multimodal approach for ADHD in parents might not be sufficient for their children. Therefore, if both parent and child are diagnosed with ADHD, a child-centered approach is recommended in any case.

Abbreviations

ADHD: Attention-deficit/hyperactivity disorder; AIMAC: ADHD in Mothers and Children; study under investigation; CAARS-L: Conners' Adult ADHD Rating Scales–Self-Report: Long Version; questionnaire rated by mothers; CAARS-O: Conners' Adult ADHD Rating Scales–Observer: Long Version; questionnaire rated by blinded clinicians; CFI: Comparative fit index; CG: Control group; receives supportive counseling during Step 1 and parent-child training in Step 2; DSM-IV: Diagnostic and Statistical Manual of Mental Disorders (4th ed.); FAS: Full analysis set; sample that considers only families with the primary outcome available at baseline; FIQ: Family Impact Questionnaire; questionnaire rated by mothers; H_0: Null hypothesis; HSQ: Home Situation Questionnaire; questionnaire rated by mothers; K-SADS: Kiddie-Sads-Present and Lifetime Version; semi-structured interview rated by blinded clinician; ODD: Oppositional defiant disorder; RMSEA: Root mean square error of approximation; SDQ: Strengths and Difficulties Questionnaire; questionnaire rated by mothers and teachers; Step 1: First treatment phase of 3 months; encompasses treatment of the mother; Step 2: Second treatment phase of 3 months; encompasses parent-child training and continued treatment of the mother; Step 3: Third treatment phase of 3 months; encompasses maintenance period for the mother and the child treatment; T1: Assessment at baseline; T2: Assessment immediately after Step 1 about 3 months after T1; T3: Assessment immediately after Step 2 about 6 months after T1; T4: Assessment immediately after Step 3 about 12 months after T1; T5: Follow-up assessment approximately 1 year after Step 3; TG: Treatment group; receives group psychotherapy and stimulant medication during Step 1 and parent-child training in Step 2; THOP: Therapieprogramm für Kinder mit hyperkinetischem und oppositionellem Problemverhalten (Therapy program for children with hyperkinetic and oppositional problem behavior); a German treatment manual; WURS-K: Wender Utah Rating Scale, German short version, questionnaire rated by mothers

Acknowledgements

The authors would like to gratefully thank all the participating families and all of our partners for their cooperation as well as Erika Graf from the University of Freiburg for providing advice regarding the statistical analysis. Editorial assistance was provided by Sarah Mannion. In memoriam Klaus Hennighausen.

Funding

The AIMAC study is part of a multicenter research network on the psychotherapy of ADHD funded by the German Federal Ministry of Education and Research (BMBF) Grants 01GV0605 and 01GV0606. The BMBF had no role in the design of the study, in the data collection, analysis and interpretation of the results and in writing the manuscript.

Authors' contributions

CH analyzed the data, and together with MD, interpreted the findings and drafted a first version of the manuscript. JK and JG revised the manuscript critically and made important contributions to the text. SS and TWMK were responsible for supervision of the parent-child training. AW and TJ were principal investigators of the trial and designed the trial together with AP, who followed AW as head of the research network "ADHDnet" on the psychotherapy of ADHD in adults and children. Members of the clinical research teams at the study sites were AW, TJ, ChaJ, VK, KH, BHD, KSM, AvG, SH, AH, LP, CMF, and KB (primarily involved in the assessment of children and the implementation of parent-child training) as well as AP, ChrJ, SM, MR, WR, ES, BA, MC, and LG (primarily involved in the assessment and treatment of mothers). All authors were involved in finalizing the manuscript and approved the final version.

Consent for publication

Not applicable.

Competing interests

Barbara Alm gave lectures for Eli Lilly.

Katja Becker is trained in behavioral as well as family therapy and is member of the executive committee of a training institute for behavioral therapy for physicians as well as psychologists (Institut für Verhaltenstherapie und Verhaltensmedizin). She was on the Advisory Board of Eli Lilly/Germany (up to 2014) and was paid for public speaking by Shire (one scientific lecture in December 2015). No research/clinical trials sponsored by pharmaceutical industry within the last 5 years.

Manfred Döpfner received consulting income and research support from Lilly, Medice, Shire, Janssen Cilag, Novartis, and Vifor and research support from the German Research Foundation, German Ministry of Education and Research, and German Ministry of Health. He received income as Head, supervisor, and lecturer at the School of Child and Adolescent Behavior Therapy at the University Hospital Cologne and as a consultant for Child Behavior Therapy at the National Association of Statutory Health Insurance Physicians (Kassenärztliche Bundesvereinigung). He also received royalties from treatment manuals, books and psychological tests published by Beltz, Elsevier, Enke, Guilford, Hogrefe, Huber, Kohlhammer, Schattauer, Springer, and Wiley.

Christine M. Freitag has been a scientific adviser for Desitin and Roche regarding Autism Spectrum Disorder (ASD). She receives royalties for books and intervention manuals on ADHD and ASD. She has received research funding from the German Research Foundation (DFG), German Federal Ministry of Education and Research (BMBF), and the European Commission.

Alexander Häge received speaker's fees, was on advisory boards or has been involved in clinical trials by Shire, E. Lilly, Janssen-Cilag, Otsuka, Lundbeck and Servier.

Christopher Hautmann is trained in cognitive behavioral therapy.

Klaus Hennighausen did not report any conflicts of interest with respect to other articles on the AIMAC study.

Sarah Hohmann received a speaker's fee from Shire in 2015.

Josepha Katzmann is trained in cognitive behavioral therapy.

Swantje Matthies received speaker's fees from 2007 to 2009 and was involved as a study physician in clinical trials conducted by Janssen-Cilag and Lilly. She is currently involved in clinical trials conducted by Janssen and Lundbeck.

Alexandra Philipsen has served on advisory boards, given lectures, performed phase 3 studies, or received travel grants within the last 3 years from Eli Lilly and Co, Janssen-Cilag, MEDICE Arzneimittel Putter GmbH and Co KG, Novartis, and Shire; and has authored books and articles on psychotherapy published by Elsevier, Hogrefe, Schattauer, Kohlhammer, Karger, Springer, and Oxford University Press.

Luise Poustka has received conference attendance support and speaker's fees from Lilly, Shire and Medice.
Wolfgang Retz receives royalties for diagnostic instruments and treatment manuals for adult ADHD published by Hogrefe, Elsevier and Kohlhammer.
Michael Rösler is a member of the speaker's bureau of Medice, Shire and Lilly. He is a member of the advisory board of Medice and Shire.
Stephanie Schürmann is an author of the treatment manual THOP. Through the development of materials and supervision, she collaborated with Eli Lilly and Shire.
Esther Sobanski has been a member of the advisory board of Shire Deutschland and Medice.
Andreas Warnke has not had contact with relevant companies for the last 5 years. He is a former President of the World Federation of ADHD; no conflict of interest with regard to this project and article.
Tanja Wolff Metternich-Kaizman is an author of a behavioral prevention program and of an ADHD guide, both published by Hogrefe, Göttingen. Through the development of materials and supervision, she collaborated with Eli Lilly and Shire. The same companies provided a grant for the ADHD Competence Network Cologne, of which she is a member.
Michael Colla, Julia Geissler, Laura Gentschow, Barbara Haack-Dees, Christian Jacob, Charlotte Jaite, Thomas Jans, Viola Kappel, Katja Schneider-Momm and Alexander von Gontard are not aware of any conflicts that might be perceived as affecting the objectivity of this article.

Author details

[1]Department of Child and Adolescent Psychiatry, Psychosomatics and Psychotherapy, Medical Faculty of the University of Cologne, Cologne, Germany. [2]School of Child and Adolescent Cognitive Behavioral Therapy (AKiP), University Hospital Cologne, Pohligstraße 9, 50969 Cologne, Germany. [3]Department of Child and Adolescent Psychiatry and Psychotherapy, Charité – Universitätsmedizin Berlin, Freie Universität Berlin, Humboldt-Universität zu Berlin, and Berlin Institute of Health (BIH), Berlin, Germany. [4]Department of Child and Adolescent Psychiatry, Psychosomatics and Psychotherapy, Center for Mental Health, University Hospital of Würzburg, Würzburg, Germany. [5]Department of Psychiatry, Psychosomatics and Psychotherapy, Center for Mental Health, University Hospital of Würzburg, Würzburg, Germany. [6]Department of Psychiatry, Psychosomatics and Psychotherapy, Medius Clinic, Kirchheim, Germany. [7]Department of Child and Adolescent Psychiatry, Psychotherapy and Psychosomatics, Medical Faculty and Medical Center – University of Freiburg, Freiburg, Germany. [8]Department of Psychiatry and Psychotherapy, Medical Center – University of Freiburg, Faculty of Medicine, University of Freiburg, Freiburg, Germany. [9]Department of Psychiatry and Psychotherapy, University Hospital Bonn, Bonn, Germany. [10]Institute for Forensic Psychology and Psychiatry, Saarland University Faculty of Medicine, Homburg/Saar, Germany. [11]Department of Psychiatry and Psychotherapy, University Medical Center Mainz, Mainz, Germany. [12]Saarland University Hospital: Department of Child and Adolescent Psychiatry and Psychotherapy, Saarland University Faculty of Medicine, Homburg/Saar, Germany. [13]Clinic for Psychiatry and Psychotherapy, Central Institute of Mental Health Mannheim, Medical Faculty Mannheim, University of Heidelberg, Mannheim, Germany. [14]Department of Child and Adolescent Psychiatry and Psychotherapy, Johannes Gutenberg University Mainz, Mainz, Germany. [15]Department of Child and Adolescent Psychiatry and Psychotherapy, Central Institute of Mental Health, Medical Faculty Mannheim, University of Heidelberg, Mannheim, Germany. [16]Department of Child and Adolescent Psychiatry, University Medicine Göttingen, Göttingen, Germany. [17]Department of Child and Adolescent Psychiatry, Medical University of Vienna, Vienna, Austria. [18]Department of Psychiatry and Psychotherapy, Campus Benjamin Franklin, Charité – Universitätsmedizin Berlin, Berlin, Germany. [19]Department of Psychiatry, University Medical Center Rostock, Rostock, Germany. [20]Department of Child and Adolescent Psychiatry, Psychosomatics and Psychotherapy, Frankfurt University Hospital, Frankfurt, Germany. [21]Department of Child and Adolescent Psychiatry and Psychotherapy, Philipps University Marburg, Marburg, Germany.

References

1. Coates J, Taylor JA, Sayal K. Parenting interventions for ADHD: a systematic literature review and meta-analysis. J Atten Disord. 2015;19:831–43. https://doi.org/10.1177/1087054714535952.
2. Daley D, van der Oord S, Ferrin M, Danckaerts M, Doepfner M, Cortese S, et al. Behavioral interventions in attention-deficit/hyperactivity disorder: a meta-analysis of randomized controlled trials across multiple outcome domains. J Am Acad Child Adolesc Psychiatry. 2014;53:835–47. https://doi.org/10.1016/j.jaac.2014.05.013.
3. Hodgson K, Hutchinson AD, Denson L. Nonpharmacological treatments for ADHD: a meta-analytic review. J Atten Disord. 2014;18:275–82. https://doi.org/10.1177/1087054712444732.
4. van der Oord S, Daley D. Moderators and mediators of treatments for youth with ADHD. In: Maric M, Prins PJM, Ollendick TH, editors. Moderators and mediators of youth treatment outcomes. New York: Oxford University Press; 2015. p. 123–45.
5. Chronis-Tuscano A, Wang CH, Woods KE, Strickland J, Stein MA. Parent ADHD and evidence-based treatment for their children: review and directions for future research. J Abnorm Child Psychol. 2017;45:501–17. https://doi.org/10.1007/s10802-016-0238-5.
6. Wang CH, Mazursky-Horowitz H, Chronis-Tuscano A. Delivering evidence-based treatments for child attention-deficit/hyperactivity disorder (ADHD) in the context of parental ADHD. Curr Psychiatry Rep. 2014;16:1–8. https://doi.org/10.1007/s11920-014-0474-8.
7. Larsson H, Chang Z, D'Onofrio BM, Lichtenstein P. The heritability of clinically diagnosed attention deficit hyperactivity disorder across the lifespan. Psychol Med. 2014;44:2223–9. https://doi.org/10.1017/S0033291713002493.
8. Dentz A, Romo L, Konofal E, Parent V. Self-rated ADHD symptoms among biological mothers or fathers of children with confirmed ADHD in a French population. Psychol Rep. 2016;118:277–91. https://doi.org/10.1177/0033294115626640.
9. Starck M, Grünwald J, Schlarb AA. Occurrence of ADHD in parents of ADHD children in a clinical sample. Neuropsychiatr Dis Treat. 2016;12:581–8. https://doi.org/10.2147/NDT.S100238.
10. Babinski DE, Pelham WE Jr, Molina BSG, Gnagy EM, Waschbusch DA, Wymbs BT, et al. Maternal ADHD, parenting, and psychopathology among mothers of adolescents with ADHD. J Atten Disord. 2016;20:458–68. https://doi.org/10.1177/1087054712461688.
11. Johnston C, Mash EJ, Miller N, Ninowski JE. Parenting in adults with attention-deficit/hyperactivity disorder (ADHD). Clin Psychol Rev. 2012;32: 215–28. https://doi.org/10.1016/j.cpr.2012.01.007.
12. Park JL, Hudec KL, Johnston C. Parental ADHD symptoms and parenting behaviors: a meta-analytic review. Clin Psychol Rev. 2017;56:25–39. https://doi.org/10.1016/j.cpr.2017.05.003.
13. Chronis-Tuscano A, O'Brien KA, Johnston C, Jones HA, Clarke TL, Raggi VL, et al. The relation between maternal ADHD symptoms & improvement in child behavior following brief behavioral parent training is mediated by change in negative parenting. J Abnorm Child Psychol. 2011;39:1047–57. https://doi.org/10.1007/s10802-011-9518-2.
14. Sonuga-Barke EJS, Daley D, Thompson M. Does maternal ADHD reduce the effectiveness of parent training for preschool children's ADHD? J Am Acad Child Adolesc Psychiatry. 2002;41:696–702. https://doi.org/10.1097/00004583-200206000-00009.
15. Harvey E, Danforth JS, McKee TE, Ulaszek WR, Friedman JL. Parenting of children with attention-Defecit/hyperactivity disorder (ADHD): the role of parental ADHD symptomatology. J Atten Disord. 2003;7:31–42. https://doi.org/10.1177/108705470300700104.
16. van den Hoofdakker BJ, Nauta MH, van der Veen-Mulders L, Sytema S, Emmelkamp PMG, Minderaa RB, et al. Behavioral parent training as an adjunct to routine care in children with attention-deficit/hyperactivity disorder: moderators of treatment response. J Pediatr Psychol. 2010;35:317–29. https://doi.org/10.1093/jpepsy/jsp060.
17. Kooij SJJ, Bejerot S, Blackwell A, Caci H, Casas-Brugué M, Carpentier PJ, et al. European consensus statement on diagnosis and treatment of adult ADHD: the European network adult ADHD. BMC Psychiatry. 2010;10:1–24. https://doi.org/10.1186/1471-244X-10-67.
18. National Institute for Health and Care Excellence. Attention deficit hyperactivity disorder: diagnosis and management. 2016. Report No.: CG72.
19. Bitter I, Angyalosi A, Czobor P. Pharmacological treatment of adult ADHD. Curr Opin Psychiatry. 2012;25:529–34. https://doi.org/10.1097/YCO.0b013e328356f87f.
20. Moriyama TS, Polanczyk GV, Terzi FS, Faria KM, Rohde LA. Psychopharmacology and psychotherapy for the treatment of adults with

ADHD-a systematic review of available meta-analyses. CNS Spectr. 2013;18: 296–306. https://doi.org/10.1017/S109285291300031X.

21. Santosh PJ, Sattar S, Canagaratnam M. Efficacy and tolerability of pharmacotherapies for attention-deficit hyperactivity disorder in adults. CNS Drugs. 2011;25:737–63. https://doi.org/10.2165/11593070-000000000-00000.
22. De Crescenzo F, Cortese S, Adamo N, Janiri L. Pharmacological and non-pharmacological treatment of adults with ADHD: a meta-review. Evid Based Ment Health. 2017;20:4–11. https://doi.org/10.1136/eb-2016-102415.
23. He JA, Antshel KM. Cognitive behavioral therapy for attention-deficit/hyperactivity disorder in college students: a review of the literature. Cogn Behav Pract. 2016. https://doi.org/10.1016/j.cbpra.2016.03.010.
24. Young S, Amarasinghe JM. Non-pharmacological treatments for ADHD: a lifespan approach. J Child Psychol Psychiatry. 2010;51:116–33. https://doi.org/10.1111/j.1469-7610.2009.02191.x.
25. Philipsen A, Jans T, Graf E, Matthies S, Borel P, Colla M, et al. Effects of group psychotherapy, individual counseling, methylphenidate, and placebo in the treatment of adult attention-deficit/hyperactivity disorder: a randomized clinical trial. JAMA Psychiatry. 2015;72:1199–210. https://doi.org/10.1001/jamapsychiatry.2015.2146.
26. Groß V, Lücke C, Graf E, Lam AP, Matthies S, Borel P, et al. Effectiveness of psychotherapy in adult ADHD: what do patients think? Results of the COMPAS study. J Atten Disord. 2017. https://doi.org/10.1177/1087054717720718.
27. Chronis-Tuscano A, Seymour KE, Stein MA, Jones HA, Jiles CD, Rooney ME, et al. Efficacy of osmotic-release oral system (OROS) methylphenidate for mothers with attention-deficit/hyperactivity disorder (ADHD): preliminary report of effects on ADHD symptoms and parenting. J Clin Psychiatry. 2008; 69:1938–47. https://doi.org/10.4088/JCP.v69n1213.
28. Wietecha L, Young J, Ruff D, Dunn D, Findling RL, Saylor K. Atomoxetine once daily for 24 weeks in adults with attention-deficit/hyperactivity disorder (ADHD): impact of treatment on family functioning. Clin Neuropharmacol. 2012;35:125–33. https://doi.org/10.1097/WNF.0b013e3182560315.
29. Waxmonsky JG, Waschbusch DA, Babinski DE, Humphrey HH, Alfonso A, Crum KI, et al. Does pharmacological treatment of ADHD in adults enhance parenting performance? Results of a double-blind randomized trial. CNS Drugs. 2014;28:665–77. https://doi.org/10.1007/s40263-014-0165-3.
30. Babinski DE, Waxmonsky JG, Pelham WE. Treating parents with attention-deficit/hyperactivity disorder: the effects of behavioral parent training and acute stimulant medication treatment on parent–child interactions. J Abnorm Child Psychol. 2014;42:1129–40. https://doi.org/10.1007/s10802-014-9864-y.
31. Chronis-Tuscano A, Wang CH, Strickland J, Almirall D, Stein MA. Personalized treatment of mothers with ADHD and their young at-risk children: a SMART pilot. J Clin Child Adolesc Psychol. 2016;45:510–21. https://doi.org/10.1080/15374416.2015.1102069.
32. Jans T, Jacob C, Warnke A, Zwanzger U, Groß-Lesch S, Matthies S, et al. Does intensive multimodal treatment for maternal ADHD improve the efficacy of parent training for children with ADHD? A randomized controlled multicenter trial. J Child Psychol Psychiatry. 2015;56:1298–313. https://doi.org/10.1111/jcpp.12443.
33. Jans T, Philipsen A, Graf E, Ihorst G, Gerlach M, Warnke A. Does the treatment of maternal attention deficit and hyperactivity disorder (ADHD) enhance the efficacy of a behavioural parent training for the treatment of their children's ADHD? Study protocol of a randomized controlled multicentre trail. Atten Defic Hyperact Disord. 2009;1:33–45. https://doi.org/10.1007/s12402-009-0004-4.
34. Jans T, Graf E, Jacob C, Zwanzger U, Groß-Lesch S, Matthies S, et al. A randomized controlled multicentre trial on the treatment for ADHD in mothers and children: enrolment and basic characteristics of the study sample. Atten Defic Hyperact Disord. 2013;5:29–40. https://doi.org/10.1007/s12402-012-0092-4.
35. American Psychiatric Association. Diagnostic and statistical manual of mental disorders. 4th ed. Washington, DC: American Psychiatric Association; 1994.
36. Rösler M, Retz-Junginger P, Retz W, Stieglitz R-D. Homburger ADHS-Skalen für Erwachsene. Göttingen: Hogrefe; 2007.
37. Hesslinger B, Philipsen A, Richter H, Ebert D. Psychotherapie der ADHS im Erwachsenenalter: Ein Arbeitsbuch. Göttingen: Hogrefe; 2004.
38. MEDICE. Medikinet retard SPC. 2013.
39. Döpfner M, Schürmann S, Frölich J. Therapieprogramm für Kinder mit hyperkinetischem und oppositionellem Problemverhalten (THOP). Weinheim: Beltz Psychologie Verlags Union; 2007.
40. Döpfner M, Breuer D, Schürmann S, Wolff Metternich T, Rademacher C, Lehmkuhl G. Effectiveness of an adaptive multimodal treatment in children with attention-deficit hyperactivity disorder - global outcome. Eur Child Adolesc Psychiatry. 2004;13(Suppl. 1):i117–i29. https://doi.org/10.1007/s00787-004-1011-9.
41. Döpfner M, Ise E, Wolff Metternich-Kaizman T, Schürmann S, Rademacher C, Breuer D. Adaptive multimodal treatment for children with attention-deficit/hyperactivity disorder: an 18 month follow-up. Child Psychiatry Hum Dev. 2015;46:44–56. https://doi.org/10.1007/s10578-014-0452-8.
42. Döpfner M, Ise E, Breuer D, Rademacher C, Wolff Metternich-Kaizman T, Schürmann S. Long-term course after adaptive multimodal treatment for children with ADHD. J Atten Disord. 2016. https://doi.org/10.1177/1087054716659138.
43. Delmo C, Weiffenbach O, Gabriel M, Stadler C, Poustka F. Diagnostisches Interview Kiddie-Sads-Present and Lifetime Version (K-SADS-PL); 2001. http://www.adhs-essen.com/PDF/K-SADS_Fragebogen.pdf.
44. Kaufman J, Birmaher B, Brent D, Rao U, Ryan N. Diagnostic interview: Kiddie-Sads-Present and Lifetime Version (K-SADS-PL). Pittsburgh: University of Pittsburgh; 1996.
45. Jans T, Weyers P, Schneider M, Hohage A, Werner M, Pauli P, et al. The kiddie-SADS allows a dimensional assessment of externalizing symptoms in ADHD children and adolescents. Atten Defic Hyperact Disord. 2009;1:215–22. https://doi.org/10.1007/s12402-009-0013-3.
46. Goodman R. The strengths and difficulties questionnaire: a research note. J Child Psychol Psychiatry. 1997;38:581–6. https://doi.org/10.1111/j.1469-7610.1997.tb01545.x.
47. Barkley RA, Edelbrock C. Assessing situational variation in children's problem behaviors: the home and school situations questionnaires. In: Prinz R, editor. Advances in behavioral assessment of children and families. Greenwich: JAI Press; 1987. p. 157–76.
48. Breuer D, Döpfner M. Die Erfassung von problematischen Situationen in der Familie. Prax Kinderpsychol Kinderpsychiatr. 1997;46:583–96.
49. Donenberg G, Baker BL. The impact of young children with externalizing behaviors on their families. J Abnorm Child Psychol. 1993;21:179–98. https://doi.org/10.1007/BF00911315.
50. Conners CK, Erhardt D, Sparrow E. Conners' adult ADHD rating scales (CAARS): technical manual. North Tonawanda: Multi Health Systems; 1999.
51. R Core Team. R: A language and environment for statistical computing. Vienna: R Foundation for Statistical Computing; 2017.
52. Rosseel Y. lavaan: An R package for structural equation modeling. J Stat Softw. 2012;48:1–36. https://doi.org/10.18637/jss.v048.i02.
53. Bollen KA, Curran PJ. Latent curve models: a structural equation perspective. Hoboken: Wiley; 2006.
54. Preacher KJ, Wichman AL, MacCallum RC, Briggs NE. Latent growth curve modeling. Thousand Oaks: Sage; 2008.
55. Little TD. Longitudinal structural equation modeling. New York: Guilford Press; 2013.
56. Kenny DA, Kaniskan B, McCoach DB. The performance of RMSEA in models with small degrees of freedom. Sociol Methods Res. 2015;44:486–507. https://doi.org/10.1177/0049124114543236.
57. Raykov T. Analysis of longitudinal studies with missing data using covariance structure modeling with full-information maximum likelihood. Struct Equ Modeling. 2005;12:493–505. https://doi.org/10.1207/s15328007sem1203_8.
58. Hautmann C, Dose C, Duda-Kirchhof K, Greimel L, Hellmich M, Imort S, et al. Behavioral versus nonbehavioral guided self-help for parents of children with externalizing disorders in a randomized controlled trial. Behav Ther. 2018;49:951–65. https://doi.org/10.1016/j.beth.2018.02.002.
59. Jaite C, van Noort BM, Vloet TD, Graf E, Kappel V, Geissler J, et al. A multicentre randomized controlled trial on trans-generational attention deficit/hyperactivity disorder (ADHD) in mothers and children (AIMAC): an exploratory analysis of predictors and moderators of treatment outcome. Z Kinder Jugendpsychiatr Psychother. https://doi.org/10.1024/1422-4917/a000602.
60. Wu W, West SG, Taylor AB. Evaluating model fit for growth curve models: integration of fit indices from SEM and MLM frameworks. Psychol Methods. 2009;14:183–201. https://doi.org/10.1037/a0015858.

Nicotine dependence in Croatian male inpatients with schizophrenia

Marina Šagud[1,2*], Bjanka Vuksan-Ćusa[2,3,4], Nenad Jakšić[2], Alma Mihaljević-Peleš[1,2], Maja Živković[5], Suzana Vlatković[5], Tea Prgić[6], Darko Marčinko[1,2] and Wei Wang[7]

Abstract

Background: Patients with schizophrenia have the highest known rates of cigarette smoking, but less is known about their smoking behavior and the differences across geographical regions, including Croatia.
The aim of this study was to compare patterns of nicotine dependence between patients with schizophrenia and healthy individuals, and to determine the relationship between clinical presentation and the severity of smoking.

Methods: This cross-sectional study included 182 recently hospitalized male inpatients and 280 healthy males, who were daily smokers. All participants have fulfilled the Fagerstrom Test for Nicotine Dependence (FTND). Patients were also evaluated by the Positive and Negative Syndrome Scale (PANSS).

Results: Patients had higher FTND total score ($p = 0.010$), smoked their first cigarette earlier in the morning ($p = 0.000$), consumed higher number of cigarettes ($p = 0.000$), while healthy subjects had more difficulties to refrain from smoking in places where it is forbidden ($p = 0.000$) and smoked more even when they were sick ($p = 0.000$). While severe dependence was more prevalent in the patient group, light dependence was more frequent in control subjects ($p = 0.04$). Smoking behavior was not associated with either PANSS total score or any of its subscales and items.

Conclusions: Smokers with schizophrenia differ from healthy smokers in both smoking behavior and level of dependence. Longitudinal studies are needed to shed more light on the complex relationship between smoking and psychopathology in schizophrenia.

Keywords: Nicotine dependence, Smoking behavior, Schizophrenia, FTND

Background

Smoking is one of the largest risk-factors for premature mortality from non-communicable diseases in general population [1]. Patients with schizophrenia have the highest known rates of cigarette smoking and it was consistently reported in different parts of the world [2–6]. Such high prevalence of smoking contributes to premature mortality in those patients, which does not lessen over time [7]. Men appear to be even at higher risk for those unfortunate findings compared to women [1, 7].

However, less is known whether the level of nicotine dependence differs in smokers with schizophrenia compared to healthy individuals, and how smoking interacts with symptoms of the disease. For example, among smokers who smoked at least 20 cigarettes per day, and had similar levels of nicotine dependence, those with schizophrenia or schizoaffective disorder had higher number of puffs smoked per cigarette, larger cigarette total puff volume, shorter inter-puff interval duration as well as higher carbon monoxide boosts, compared to participants who had no major mental illness [8]. Similarly, smokers with schizophrenia had higher four-minute nicotine boost and a higher dose of nicotine per cigarette than persons without mental illness in the previous year [9]. Moreover, male patients with schizophrenia had higher proportion of smoking more than 10 cigarettes daily, and lower proportion of individuals who

* Correspondence: marinasagud@mail.com
[1]School of Medicine, University of Zagreb, Zagreb, Croatia
[2]Department of Psychiatry, University Hospital Center Zagreb, Kišpatićeva 12, 10 000 Zagreb, Croatia

stopped smoking [10] compared to males with negative history for psychiatric disorders. The relationship between illness severity and smoking indices is incompletely understood. Previous studies have reported mixed results on the association between smoking and the intensity of symptoms. While majority of studies suggested that smokers with schizophrenia had more severe symptoms [10–15], one study reported similar overall symptomatology [15], while a series of studies reported milder symptoms in smokers than in nonsmokers [16–18]. In patients with first-episode schizophrenia, smokers had higher positive and negative syndrome scale (PANSS) total score and PANSS positive subscale scores and similar PANSS negative and PANSS general scores, in comparison to patients who were nonsmokers [10]. Among patients with several psychiatric disorders, including schizophrenia, smokers were more likely than nonsmokers to report hallucinations, delusions and subjective thought disorder and had worse negative symptoms [11]. In patients with schizophrenia, smokers with severe nicotine dependence had greater PANSS positive, while smokers with mild nicotine dependence had higher PANSS negative scores, respectively, compared to patients who did not smoke [12]. In another study on patients with schizophrenia, smokers had higher PANSS positive score than nonsmokers, while tobacco smoking was associated with more positive symptomatology, and less negative symptoms. [13]. Moreover, PANSS total scores and the PANSS general psychopathology scores were higher in non-smokers compared to smokers while PANSS positive and negative scores were similar between smokers and non-smokers with schizophrenia [14]. In patients with treatment-resistant schizophrenia (TRS), smokers had higher PANSS total score and PANSS negative score than nonsmokers, while there were no differences in two groups in PANSS positive and general scores [15]. Smoking status was not associated with PANSS total score in a sample consisted of patients with schizophrenia and bipolar disorder, although no data on PANSS subscales were presented [5]. On the opposite, in male inpatients with schizophrenia, smokers had lower PANSS positive scores, with no differences in the PANSS total score or the negative and general psychopathology subscales compared with non-smokers [16]. Notably, in this study, smokers who smoked more cigarettes had lower intensity of negative symptoms [16]. In the two studies on male patients with schizophrenia, current smokers had lower PANSS negative scores than never smokers [17] and never smokers and former smokers [18]. The discrepancies across those studies might arise from many methodological issues, such as different measures of psychopathology, sample sizes, age and sex differences, study settings (outpatients versus inpatients) and the presence of comorbid substance abuse. For example, psychopathology was estimated by The Diagnostic Interview for Psychosis [11] and PANSS total score and its subscales [10] as well as only PANSS total score [5]. Of note, smokers with schizophrenia have also received higher daily doses of antipsychotics [12, 14] than nonsmokers. While larger doses are logically related to higher severity of symptoms, they could also result from smoking-induced hepatic metabolism of some antipsychotics, such as clozapine and olanzapine [19]. Interestingly, in the sample of patients with TRS, smokers and nonsmokers did not differ in terms of mean daily antipsychotic dose [15]. Majority of those studies analyzed the association of smoking versus non-smoking status with psychopathology [5, 10, 11, 14, 15, 13], while few have investigated the influence of severity of nicotine dependence on psychopathology [16].

The relationship between schizophrenia and nicotine dependence is complex [20] and includes some shared genetic vulnerability [21]. Reasons for such high prevalence of cigarette smoking in patients with schizophrenia are still unclear [20]. So far, dopamine appears to play a major role in this relationship. It is well-known that schizophrenia is linked to elevated dopamine levels in dorsal striatum and reduced cortical dopamine release [reviewed in [22]. Nicotine increases dopamine levels in striatum by stimulating its release via nicotinic receptors, and decreasing its degradation by inhibiting monoamine oxidase type A and B. [reviewed in [20]. Clinical consequences include behavioral stimulation, antidepressant effects and decrease of drug-induced extrapyramidal adverse events [reviewed in [20]. More recently, it has been reported that smoking also induced cortical dopamine release, at least in subjects who smoked ≥10 cigarettes daily and had no current psychiatric disorder [23].

There are differences across countries in both smoking prevalence and smoking behavior in general population [24], schizophrenic patients [25] and control samples [2]. For example, smoking prevalence in general population varied significantly across 18 European countries, ranging from 40.9% in Bulgaria to 16.3% in Sweden [26]. In Croatian general population the rate of current smoking was 26.6%, which was similar to European average of 27% [26] and to frequency of smoking in other European transitional countries [27].

Interestingly, smokers in countries with lower smoking prevalence such as Sweden, had higher nicotine dependence levels compared to those from countries with higher prevalence of smoking, such as Germany [24]. Healthy persons from United States had higher rates of heavy nicotine dependence compared to Spanish control sample [2].

Men had higher smoking prevalence than women, in European countries including Croatia [26], and unlike women, Croatian men did not show decreasing trend in smoking prevalence [27]. Croatian men also had higher prevalence of heavy smoking compared to women [28], which is in line with data from other regions. For example, in healthy persons, males had higher FTND total scores [24, 29], and higher nicotine and cotinine levels [29] than females. In patients with schizophrenia severe nicotine dependence was associated with male gender [30]. Patients with schizophrenia from Spain had higher smoking prevalence compared to those from Germany, Greece and Italy [25].

To the best of our knowledge, no study has compared smoking behavior in Croatian patients with schizophrenia and healthy individuals. Given the above gender and regional differences in smoking indices, and complex relationship between smoking and schizophrenia, more investigation is needed to verify factors associated with nicotine dependence in schizophrenia, in different countries. The aim of the present study was to contribute to the current knowledge of smoking behavior in schizophrenia, and to investigate smoking behavior in Croatian patients. Specific objectives were to:

1) compare patterns of nicotine dependence between patients with schizophrenia and healthy controls
2) determine the pattern between nicotine dependence and psychopathology in patients with schizophrenia

Methods

Study setting and subjects

This cross-sectional study was carried out in University Hospital Centre Zagreb, Department of Psychiatry, and Psychiatric Hospital Popovača. Inclusion criteria were: male inpatients aged 18 to 65 years, diagnosed with schizophrenia, who were current smokers. Since daily smoking is considered to be a sign of nicotine addiction [25], smokers were defined as individuals who declared to smoke at least one cigarette daily. Given the observed differences in smoking patterns observed in both healthy subjects [24, 29] and individuals with schizophrenia [25, 30] only males were enrolled. Exclusion criteria were: intellectual disability and other conditions affecting the current capacity to participate in the evaluation, such as moderate to severe agitation and/or aggression, catatonic features, patients with first-episode psychosis, substance abuse and dependence in the previous year other than nicotine and caffeine dependence, and any severe and/or unstable comorbid somatic or neurological disorder. Although subjects with the most severe clinical presentations were not included because of insufficient cooperation and understanding of questions and purpose of the study, there were no cut-off values in overall disease severity for the exclusion of patients.

Incusion criteria for healthy group were: males who were daily smokers, and exclusion criteria were: current or previous psychiatric disorders, comorbid substance use (other than nicotine and caffeine), as well as somatic (inclusive neurological) disorders.

Assessment

Diagnosis of schizophrenia was confirmed by the Structured Clinical Interview (SCID) [31] based on the DSM-IV criteria (American Psychiatric Association, 1994). The level of nicotine dependence was measured by the Fagerstrom Test for Nicotine Dependence (FTND) [32], which is composed of six questions about daily cigarette consumption. It assesses the extent of cigarette smoking and smoking behavior. This questionnaire is the most widely used measure of nicotine dependence [33] and is also a reliable tool for the assessment of smoking behavior in schizophrenia [34]. Both patients and control group have fulfilled the FTND. The Cronbach alpha coefficients in the healthy and patient group were 0.76 and 0.68, respectively, indicating adequate internal reliability (having in mind the low number of items comprising this scale).

Symptom severity in patients was evaluated by structured interview for PANSS, including the PANSS positive, PANSS negative, PANSS general psychopathology subscale [35] and PANSS Cognitive subscale [36]. The average total score was 114.35 (SD = 21.609).

For this study, participants were divided in three groups according to the levels of tobaccodependence: (1) smokers with low dependence (FTND 0–4) (2) smokers with moderatedependence (FTND = 5) and (3) smokers with severe dependence (FTND≥6).

The investigation was approved by local Ethics Committee and was carried out in accordance with the Helsinki declaration (1975). All patients have signed informed consent approved by Ethics Committee prior to inclusion. The investigation was a part of a project "Predictors of treatment response in schizophrenia", BM1.45, sponsored by the University of Zagreb.

Statistical analysis

We ran all the statistical analyses in the SPSS version 19 (SPSS, Chicago, IL). Descriptive statistics contained means (M) and standard deviations (SD). Internal reliability of the FTND was described by Cronbach alpha coefficients. Mann-Whitney U test, Chi-square test and independent samples t-test were used to examine the potential differences in age and tobacco dependence parameters between schizophrenia patients and healthy control subjects. Pearson correlations were computed to examine the zero-order relationship among the investigated variables. The level of statistical significance was set at $P < 0.05$.

Results

Overall, 182 patients and 280 healthy individuals took part in this investigation. The average length of treatment was 17.49 years (SD = 8.395), while the average number of previous psychiatric hospitalizations was 5.91 (SD = 4.730).

The average age was 42.20 years (SD = 11.974) for patients and 40.26 years (SD = 10.250) for healthy participants. The difference in their average age was not statistically significant ($t = 1.784$, df = 436, $p = 0.075$).

The differences between the groups (patients and healthy controls) in the total score on the FTND scale, individual items as well as the three tobacco dependence categories, are shown in Tables 1 and 2.

As presented in Table 1, patients had significantly higher total score on the tobacco dependence measure, compared to healthy subjects. On the individual items, patients scored higher on items 1 (they tended to smoke their first cigarette earlier after waking up) and 4 (they smoked more cigarettes a day). Higher percentage of healthy controls compared to patients found it harder to refrain from smoking in places where it is forbidden (item 2) and they smoked more even when they were sick (item 6). No differences were observed in items 3 and 5.

In addition, based on the chi-square test ($\chi^2 = 6.416$, $p < .04$) (Table 2) patients were more often categorized as severely dependent on tobacco, whereas healthy controls were more often in the low dependence category. There was no difference in the frequencies of moderate dependence category among groups. The exact distribution of patients and healthy controls in the three nicotine dependence categories is shown in Table 2.

Finally, there was no significant correlation between age and FTND total score in both groups, and there was also no correlation between the PANSS total score and positive and negative scores with FTND total score in the patient group ($p > 0.05$). However, negative correlations between item 2 on FTND scale and PANSS total score, as well as PANSS positive and general subscores, were observed, as presented in Table 3.

Discussion

Main findings of the present study are:

1) Smokers with schizophrenia had higher FTND score compared to healthy smokers,
2) Smokers with schizophrenia had higher rates of severe dependence while healthy smokers had higher rates of light dependence,
3) On the individual FTND items, patients with schizophrenia scored higher on items 1 and 4, healthy individuals scored higher on items 2 and 6, while there were no significant differences on items 3 and 5.

Severity of nicotine dependence in patients and healthy controls

We confirmed previous reports of increased FTND scores in patients with schizophrenia compared to healthy individuals [34, 37] and increased frequency of heavy smoking compared with general population [3]. However, our findings disagree with similar prevalence of heavy smoking and FTND score in healthy persons and first-episode patients [10], and with even higher FTND scores in healthy controls [38]. The differences might be related to age, since the prevalence of smoking in patients with schizophrenia increases with age [5, 39]. Smokers with schizophrenia were older than non-smokers [17]. Given the self-medication hypothesis of smoking in schizophrenia [20], it might be speculated that older patients smoked more often in order to alleviate extrapyramidal and depressive symptoms, which are related to longer disease duration [40, 41]. However, other studies on individuals with schizophrenia have reported that smokers were actually younger than non-smokers [14, 16]. Because schizophrenia is highly heterogonous disorder, longitudinal studies are needed to investigate whether and how the pattern of smoking changes throughout its course.

The average age in both of our groups corresponds to age-range which had the highest prevalence of smoking in European general population [26]. The discrepancy

Table 1 Comparisons between the schizophrenia patients and healthy controls in the investigated tobacco dependence parameters

	Schizophrenia patients ($n = 182$)	Healthy controls ($n = 280$)	U / X^2(df)	P
FTND total (mean (SD))	5.60 (2.312)	4.98 (2.690)	21,911	**.010**
FTND item 1 (mean (SD))	2.07 (1.044)	1.59 (1.027)	17,951	**.000**
FTND item 2 (proportions of *yes* answers)	40.7%	60%	16.542 (1)	**.000**
FTND item 3 (proportions of *yes* answers)	70.3%	72.1%	0.178 (1)	.673
FTND item 4 (mean (SD))	1.55 (.857)	1.17 (.825)	19,227	**.000**
FTND item 5 (proportions of *yes* answers)	47.8%	38.9%	3.556 (1)	.060
FTND item 6 (proportions of *yes* answers)	40.1%	60.7%	18.782 (1)	**.000**

FTND Fagerstrom Test for Nicotine Dependence, *U* Mann Whitney test, *X^2(df)* Chi-square test and degrees of freedom; Significant *P* values are highlighted in bold

Table 2 Frequencies of schizophrenia patients and healthy controls in the three tobacco dependence categories

	Mild tobacco dependence	Moderate tobacco dependence	Severe tobacco dependence
Patients with schizophrenia	58 (31.9%)	25 (13.7%)	99 (54.4%)
Healthy controls	119 (42.5%)	41 (14.6%)	120 (42.9%)

Chi-square test (X^2) = 6.416; df = 2; p = 0.041

with reference [38], might arise from differences in smoking limitation. While in the latter study there was a restriction of smoking, in our hospitals there is facility where patients are allowed to smoke. More smoking restrictions might discourage light smokers to consume cigarettes, but not individuals who are more heavily dependent [24].

In the present study, compared to healthy individuals, smokers with schizophrenia had also higher prevalence of severe, and lower prevalence of mild nicotine dependence. There is some evidence that severe nicotine dependence may have distinct biological changes [42, 43]. However, the present study did not measure biological markers.

Differences in smoking behavior between patients and healthy individuals

Several differences in smoking behavior were observed between group of patients and healthy subjects.

Item 1-How soon after you wake up do you smoke your first cigarette?

Our patients had higher scores on item 1, which has correlated with a difficulty in maintaining abstinence due to emerging withdrawal symptoms [44], and was repeatedly found related to nicotine dependence in general population [29], while data on patients with schizophrenia are missing. For example, FTND items 1, 4 and 5 were the best predictors of cotinine concentrations in general population [45]. This item was even proposed to be a good single-item measure of nicotine dependence

Table 3 Pearson correlations between FTND scores and values on the PANSS diagnostic scale

Variables	PANSS – total	PANSS – P	PANS S –N	PANSS – G
FTND 1	.04	.02	.04	.04
FTND 2	–.18*	–.17*	–.13	–.16*
FTND 3	–.03	–.09	.04	–.02
FTND 4	–.02	.05	–.04	–.06
FTND 5	–.08	–.09	–.09	–.03
FTND 6	–.02	.02	–.04	–.02
FTND total	–.06	–.05	–.04	–.05

FTND Fagerstrom Test for Nicotine Dependence, *PANSS* Positive and Negative Syndrome Scale *P* positive symptoms subscale, *N* negative symptoms subscale, *G* general psychopathology subscale
*statistically significant correlations ($P <= .036$)

[46]. Therefore, our findings smoking in European genre severe nicotine dependence in schizophrenia [3], particularly in males.

Item 2-Do you find it difficult to refrain from smoking in places where it is forbidden?

While higher inhibition of smoking in patients compared to control group might appear counterintuitive, this finding could result from different settings. Our hospital facilities had smoking areas, and unlike healthy persons, patients had no smoking restrictions. On the contrary, smoking ban at workplace was found to decrease both average number of daily cigarette consumption and proportion of heavy smokers in Croatian healthcare stuff [47]. While majority of patients were unemployed and all healthy participants had regular jobs, those two groups might have been differently affected by smoke-free laws. Alternatively, higher levels of nicotine dependence were related to lower inhibitory capacity in healthy persons [48, 49] and individuals with different psychiatric conditions [49].

Item 3-Which cigarette do you hate most to give up?

This item, which differentiates first morning cigarette from any other during the day, had similar scores in patients and controls. It is another FTND item focusing on morning smoking as an indicator of greater nicotine dependence, which is related to the preference of first cigarette in the morning. Some authors have raised concern that FTND may deflate nicotine dependence scores among smokers with schizophrenia [33]. Differences in restrictions to smoking between patients and controls also need to be taken into account in the interpretation of this finding.

Item 4. The number of cigarettes, smoked per day

This item, together with item 1, is supposed to reflect the best nicotine dependence. The sum of those 2 items is referred to as the heaviness of smoking index [3, 50], and had the greatest impact on exposure to nicotine and carbon monoxide [51]. Patients in the present study had higher scores in both items 1 and 4, which is consistent with meta-analysis that patients with schizophrenia smoke "heavier" than smokers in general population [3] and with other reports of higher number of cigarettes smoked daily in patients in first-episode psychosis [52] and schizophrenia [53].

Item 5. Do you smoke more frequently during the first hours after awakening than during the rest of the day?

No differences were found between groups on the item 5 score. Since both items 3 and 5 refer to higher priority of morning smoking compared to the rest of the day, both groups appear to have had similar levels of morning cigarette craving. Smokers with schizophrenia, however, use tobacco during the night, and therefore may maintain sufficient nicotine levels to suppress morning withdrawal symptoms [33]. Although the current study did not measure nighttime smoking, similar scores in items 3 and 5 might simply reflect less nocturnal smoking in healthy individuals.

Item 6. Do you smoke even if you are so ill that you are in bed most of the day?

This item addresses persistence in maintaining nicotine concentrations during waking hours. In the present study, healthy persons scored higher on FTND items related to difficulties in restraining from smoking at certain places (item 2) and situations (item 6). It might be that, unlike healthy smokers, smokers with schizophrenia do not even attempt to refrain from smoking. In fact, patients with schizophrenia had impaired impulse control compared to healthy persons [54], and among patients, smokers exhibited even higher rates of impulsivity [55] and had different motives to smoke, such as "increased need of stimulation" and lower scores of "sociability" [56]. Therefore, variations in impulse control and motivation for smoking might help explain the higher score on items 2 and 6 in healthy controls.

Nicotine dependence and severity of symptoms

We observed no associations between smoking severity and PANSS total score and any of its subscales or individual items. Those findings contrast previous reports of lower negative symptom severity in patients with higher levels of nicotine dependence [57–60] and positive correlations between FTND and PANSS negative scale, and several PANSS general items [61]. Our results are in line with other authors who observed no correlations between FTND total score [38], presence of severe nicotine dependence [30] and number of cigarettes per day [10], with any of PANSS items.

Those discrepancies might arise from disease severity, patient age, definitions of severity of nicotine dependence and comorbidity. Patients in majority of studies had the average PANSS total score lower than 60 [57–59], 80 [10, 30, 38], and 82 [60]. Our patients had more severe clinical presentation, as reflected by their PANSS total score of 114. The only study that also included acutely psychotic patients, with an average PANSS score of 105 [61], reported a positive correlation between FTND and PANSS negative scale, and items of unusual thought content, disorientation, poor attention, and poor impulse control [61]. While all those studies, including the current one, were cross-sectional, longitudinal studies are needed to determine whether the association between heaviness of smoking and severity of symptoms changes during phases of illness.

Another explanation might include gender, given that men had higher nicotine dependence in healthy individuals [24, 29] and in patients with schizophrenia [30], and other addictions. While cannabis and alcohol consumption were related to more positive symptoms [62, 63], and less prominent negative symptoms [62], those comorbidities might also influence severity of symptoms and contribute to discrepant findings. The definition of heavy smoking has also varied across studies. For example, [58] defined heavy smokers as those who smoked at least one pack of cigarettes per day, while we used FTND definition.

Limitations

Due to cross-sectional design, causal relationship cannot be established. Groups were not controlled for other variables, such as education, financial status, and doses of antipsychotics. Smoking data were based on self-report and, given that patients were acutely psychotic, results might not be completely accurate. Given that PANSS rating was performed by 5 psychiatrists, who were in most cases also treating psychiatrists for those patients, potential bias cannot be excluded. In addition, given than only men without recent substance abuse were included, those findings might not be generalizable to women and / or patients with current substance abuse. Another limitation is that sociodemographic data for healthy control group were not collected.

Conclusions

Our results extend previous findings of higher levels of nicotine dependence in patients with schizophrenia compared to healthy persons, to patients from Croatia, according to the hypothesis [25] that "schizophrenia is associated with increased smoking among smokers". Our findings also highlight the differences in their smoking behavior compared to healthy smokers. In spite of those variations, degree of nicotine dependence was not associated with the severity of the disease or any particular symptoms. Given the high prevalence of both smoking and severe nicotine dependence in patients with schizophrenia, future investigations comparing smoking behavior in remitted patients versus those in acute relapse are needed.

Abbreviations

FTND: Fagerstrom Test for Nicotine Dependence; PANSS: Positive and Negative Syndrome Scale

Acknowledgements

We express our gratitude to the staff of the Department of Psychiatry, University Hospital Centre Zagreb, for their assistance and support.

Funding

The investigation was a part of a project "Predictors of treatment response in schizophrenia", BM1.45, sponsored by the University of Zagreb.

Authors' contributions

MŠ, BVĆ, AMP, SV and MŽ have recruited the patients, collected their demographic data, dispensed FTND questionnaires and performed PANSS ratings, NJ performed statistical analysis, TP recruited healthy individuals and distributed FTND questionnaires, MŠ and NJ prepared the first draft of the article, while MŠ, BVĆ, NJ, AMP, MŽ, SV, TP, DM and WW actively participated in the interpretation of data and have read and approved the final version of the manuscript.

Consent for publication

Not applicable

Competing interests

Not applicable

Author details

[1]School of Medicine, University of Zagreb, Zagreb, Croatia. [2]Department of Psychiatry, University Hospital Center Zagreb, Kišpatićeva 12, 10 000 Zagreb, Croatia. [3]School of Medicine, University of Osijek, Osijek, Croatia. [4]School of Medicine, University of Mostar, Mostar, Bosnia and Herzegovina. [5]Psychiatric Clinic Vrapče, Zagreb, Croatia. [6]Department of Psychiatry, General Hospital Vinkovci, Vinkovci, Croatia. [7]Department of Clinical Psychology and Psychiatry, Zhejiang University College of Medicine, Hangzhou, China.

References

1. Stringhini S, Carmeli C, Jokela M, Avendaño M, Muennig P, Guida F, Ricceri F, d'Errico A, Barros H, Bochud M, Chadeau-Hyam M, Clavel-Chapelon F, Costa G, Delpierre C, Fraga S, Goldberg M, Giles GG, Krogh V, Kelly-Irving M, Layte R, Lasserre AM, Marmot MG, Preisig M, Shipley MJ, Vollenweider P, Zins M, Kawachi I, Steptoe A, Mackenbach JP, Vineis P, Kivimäki M, LIFEPATH consortium. Socioeconomic status and the 25 × 25 risk factors as determinants of premature mortality: a multicohort study and meta-analysis of 1.7 million men and women. Lancet. 2017;389(10075):1229–37.
2. de Leon J, Becoña E, Gurpegui M, Gonzalez-Pinto A, Diaz FJ. The association between high nicotine dependence and severe mental illness may be consistent across countries. J Clin Psychiatry. 2002;63(9):812–6.
3. de Leon J, Diaz FJ. A meta-analysis of worldwide studies demonstrates an association between schizophrenia and tobacco smoking behaviors. Schizophr Res. 2005;76(2–3):135–57.
4. Myles N, Newall H, Nielssen O, Large M. The association between cannabis use and earlier age at onset of schizophrenia and other psychoses: meta-analysis of possible confounding factors. Curr Pharm Des. 2012;18(32):5055–69.
5. Dickerson F, Stallings CR, Origoni AE, Vaughan C, Khushalani S, Schroeder J, Yolken RH. Cigarette smoking among persons with schizophrenia or bipolar disorder in routine clinical settings, 1999–2011. Psychiatr Serv. 2013;64(1):44–50.
6. Bressington D, Mui J, Tse ML, Gray R, Cheung EF, Chien WT. Cardiometabolic health, prescribed antipsychotics and health-related quality of life in people with schizophrenia-spectrum disorders: a cross-sectional study. BMC Psychiatry. 2016;16(1):411.
7. Hjorthøj C, Stürup AE, JJ MG, Nordentoft M. Years of potential life lost and life expectancy in schizophrenia: a systematic review and meta-analysis. Lancet Psychiatry. 2017;4(4):295–301.
8. Tidey JW, Rohsenow DJ, Kaplan GB, Swift RM. Cigarette smoking topography in smokers with schizophrenia and matched non-psychiatric controls. Drug Alcohol Depend. 2005;80(2):259–65.
9. Williams JM, Gandhi KK, Lu SE, Kumar S, Shen J, Foulds J, Kipen H, Benowitz NL. Higher nicotine levels in schizophrenia compared with controls after smoking a single cigarette. Nicotine Tobacco Res. 2010; 12(8):855 9.
10. Zhang XY, Chen DC, Xiu MH, Haile CN, He SC, Luo X, Zuo L, Rosenheck R, Kosten TA, Kosten TR. Cigarette smoking, psychopathology and cognitive function in first-episode drug-naive patients with schizophrenia: a case-control study. Psychol Med. 2012:1–10.
11. Cooper J, Mancuso SG, Borland R, Slade T, Galletly C, Castle D. Tobacco smoking among people living with a psychotic illness: the second Australian survey of psychosis. Aust N Z J Psychiatry. 2012; 46(9):851–63.
12. Krishnadas R, Jauhar S, Telfer S, Shivashankar S, McCreadie RG. Nicotine dependence and illness severity in schizophrenia. Br J Psychiatry. 2012;201(4):306–12.
13. Mallet J, Le Strat Y, Schürhoff F, Mazer N, Portalier C, Andrianarisoa M, Aouizerate B, Berna F, Brunel L, Capdevielle D, Chereau I, D'Amato T, Denizot H, Dubreucq J, Faget C, Gabayet F, Lançon C, Llorca PM, Misdrahi D, Rey R, Roux P, Schandrin A, Urbach M, Vidailhet P, Fond G, Dubertret C, FACE-SZ (FondaMental Academic Centers of Expertise for Schizophrenia) group. Cigarette smoking and schizophrenia: a specific clinical and therapeutic profile? Results from the FACE-Schizophrenia cohort. Prog Neuropsychopharmacol Biol Psychiatry. 2017;79(Pt B):332–9.
14. Nedic Erjavec G, Uzun S, Nikolac Perkovic M, Kozumplik O, Svob Strac D, Mimica N, Hirasawa-Fujita M, Domino EF, Pivac N. Cortisol in schizophrenia: no association with tobacc smoking, clinical symptoms or antipsychotic medication. Prog Neuro-Psychopharmacol Biol Psychiatry. 2017;77:228–35.
15. Iasevoli F, Balletta R, Gilardi V, Giordano S, de Bartolomeis A. Tobacco Smoking in treatment-resistant schizophrenia patients is associated with impaired cognitive functioning, more severe negative symptoms, and poorer social adjustment. Neuropsychiatr Dis Treat. 2013; 9:1113–20.
16. An HM, Tan YL, Tan SP, Shi J, Wang ZR, Yang FD, Huang XF, Soars JC, Kosten TR, Zhang XY. Smoking and serum lipid profiles in schizophrenia. Neurosci Bull. 2016;32(4):383–8.
17. Zhang XY, Liang J, Chen DC, Xiu MH, He J, Cheng W, Wu Z, Yang FD, Haile CN, Sun H, Lu L, Kosten TA, Kosten TR. Cigarette smoking in male patients with chronic schizophrenia in a Chinese population: prevalence and relationship to clinical phenotypes. PLoS One. 2012; 7(2):e30937.
18. Zhang XY, Chen DC, Tan YL, Tan SP, Luo X, Zuo L, Rao W, Yu Q, Kou C, Allen M, Correll CU, Wu J, Soares JC. A functional polymorphism in the interleukin-1beta and severity of nicotine dependence in male schizophrenia: a case-control study. J Psychiatr Res. 2015;64:51–8.
19. Tsuda Y, Saruwatari J, Yasui-Furukori N. Meta-analysis: the effects of smoking on the disposition of two commonly used antipsychotic agents, olanzapine and clozapine. BMJ Open. 2014;4(3):e004216.
20. Sagud M, Mihaljević-Peles A, Mück-Seler D, Pivac N, Vuksan-Cusa B, Brataljenović T, Jakovljević M. Smoking and schizophrenia. Psychiatr Danub. 2009;21(3):371–5.
21. Chen J, Bacanu SA, Yu H, Zhao Z, Jia P, Kendler KS, Kranzler HR, Gelernter J, Farrer L, Minica C, Pool R, Milaneschi Y, Boomsma DI, Penninx BW, Tyndale RF, Ware JJ, Vink JM, Kaprio J, Munafò M, Chen X, Cotinine meta-analysis group, FTND meta-analysis group. Genetic Relationship between Schizophrenia and Nicotine Dependence. Sci Rep. 2016;6:25671.
22. Howes OD, McCutcheon R, Owen MJ, Murray RM. The role of genes, stress, and dopamine in the development of schizophrenia. Biol Psychiatry. 2017; 81(1):9–20.
23. Wing VC, Payer DE, Houle S, George TP, Boileau I. Measuring cigarette smoking-induced cortical dopamine release: a [^{11}C]FLB-457 PET study. Neuropsychopharmacology. 2015;40(6):1417–27.
24. Fagerström K, Furberg H. A comparison of the Fagerström test for nicotine dependence and smoking prevalence across countries. Addiction. 2008;103(5):841–5.
25. De Leon J, Diaz FJ. Genetics of schizophrenia and smoking: an approach to studying their comorbidity based on epidemiological findings. Hum Genet. 2012;131(6):877–901.
26. Gallus S, Lugo A, La Vecchia C, Boffetta P, Chaloupka FJ, Colombo P, Currie L, Fernandez E, Fischbacher C, Gilmore A, Godfrey F, Joossens L, Leon ME, Levy DT, Nguyen L, Rosenqvist G, Ross H, Townsend J, Clancy

L. Pricing policies and control of tobacco in Europe (PPACTE) project: cross-national comparison of smoking prevalence in 18 European countries. Eur J Cancer Prev. 2014;23(3):177–85.

27. Padjen I, Dabić M, Glivetić T, Biloglav Z, Biočina-Lukenda D, Lukenda J. The analysis of tobacco consumption in Croatia–are we successfully facing the epidemic? Cent Eur J Public Health. 2012;20(1):5–10.
28. Samardzić S, Pristas I, Mravinac GV. Charactersitics of heavy smsokers in Croatia. Coll Antropol. 2009;33(Suppl 1):61–6.
29. Van Overmeire IP, De Smedt T, Dendale P, Nackaerts K, Vanacker H, Vanoeteren JF, Van Laethem DM, Van Loco J, De Cremer KA. Nicotine Dependence and Urinary Nicotine, Cotinine and Hydroxycotinine Levels in Daily Smokers. Nicotine Tob Res. 2016;18(9):1813–9.
30. Rey R, D'Amato T, Boyer L, Brunel L, Aouizerate B, Berna F, Capdevielle D, Chereau I, Chesnoy-Servanin G, Denizot H, Dorey JM, Dubertret C, Dubreucq J, Faget C, Gabayet F, Lancon C, Mallet J, Misdrahi D, Passerieux C, Schandrin A, Schürhoff F, Urbach M, Vidailhet P, Llorca PM, Fond G, FACE-SZ (FondaMental Academic Centers of Expertise for Schizophrenia) group. Nicotine dependence is associated with depression and childhood trauma in smokers with schizophrenia: results from the FACE-SZ dataset. Eur Arch Psychiatry Clin Neurosci. 2017; [Epub ahead of print]
31. First MB, Spitzer RL, Gibbon M, Williams JBW, Davies M, Borus J, Howes MJ, Kane J, Pope HG, Rounsaville B. The structured clinical interview for DSM-III-R personality disorders (SCID-II). Part II: multi-site test-retest reliability study. J Personal Disord. 1995;9(2):92–104.
32. Heatherton TF, Kozlowski LT, Frecker RC, Fagerström KO. The Fagerström Test for Nicotine Dependence: a revision of the Fagerström Tolerance Questionnaire. Br J Addict. 1991;86(9):1119–2.
33. Prochaska JJ, Leek DN, Hall SE, Hall SM. Cognitive interviews for measurement evaluation of the Fagerström Test for Nicotine Dependence (FTND) in smokers with schizophrenia spectrum disorders. Addict Behav. 2007;32(4):793–802.
34. Weinberger AH, Reutenauer EL, Allen TM, Termine A, Vessicchio JC, Sacco KA, Easton CJ, McKee SA, George TP. Reliability of the Fagerström Test for Nicotine Dependence, Minnesota Nicotine Withdrawal Scale, and Tiffany Questionnaire for Smoking Urges in smokers with and without schizophrenia. Drug Alcohol Depend. 2007;86(2–3):278–82.
35. Kay SR, Fiszbein A, Opler LA. The positive and negative syndrome scale (PANSS) for schizophrenia. Schizophr Bull. 1987;13(2):261–76.
36. Tuinier S, Eschauzier JC, JIM E, WMA V. Response and remission in schizophrenia: the limited value of new remissioin criteria. Clinical Neuropsychiatry. 2008;5(2):83–9.
37. Freeman TP, Stone JM, Orgaz B, Noronha LA, Minchin SL, Curran HV. Tobacco smoking in schizophrenia: investigating the role of incentive salience. Psychol Med. 2014;44(10):2189–97.
38. Kishi T, Fukuo Y, Okochi T, Kawashima K, Moriwaki M, Furukawa O, Musso GM, Fujita K, Correll CU, Iwata N. Relationship between nicotine dependence and the endophenotype-related trait of cognitive function but not acoustic startle reponses in Japanese patients with schizophrenia. Hum Psychopharmacol. 2013;28(3):220–9.
39. Salokangas RK, Honkonen T, Stengård E, Koivisto AM, Hietala J. Cigarette smoking in long-term schizophrenia. Eur Psychiatry. 2006;21(4):219–23.
40. Morgante F, Barbui C, Tinazzi M, Italian DIP, Study Group. Parkinsonian axial signs in schizophrenia. Parkinsonism Relat Disord. 2017;36:89–92.
41. Schennach R, Obermeier M, Seemüller F, Jäger M, Schmauss M, Laux G, Pfeiffer H, Naber D, Schmidt LG, Gaebel W, Klosterkötter J, Heuser I, Maier W, Lemke MR, Rüther E, Klingberg S, Gastpar M, Spellmann I, Musil R, Möller HJ, Riedel M. Add-on antidepressants in the naturalistic treatment of schizophrenia Spectrum disorder - when, who, and how? Pharmacopsychiatry. 2017;50(4):136–14.
42. Fond G, Berna F, Andrianarisoa M, Godin O, Leboyer M, Brunel L, Aouizerate B, Capdevielle D, Chereau I, D'Amato T, Denizot H, Dubertret C, Dubreucq J, Faget C, Gabayet F, Llorca PM, Mallet J, Misdrahi D, Passerieux C, Richieri R, Rey R, Schandrin A, Urbach M, Vidailhet P, Boyer L, Schürhoff F, FACE-SZ (FondaMental academic centers of expertise for schizophrenia) group. Chronic low-grade peripheral inflammation is associated with severe nicotine dependence in schizophrenia: results from the national multicentric FACE-SZ cohort. Eur Arch Psychiatry Clin Neurosci. 2017; [Epub ahead of print]
43. Li Y, Yuan K, Cai C, Feng D, Yin J, Bi Y, Shi S, Yu D, Jin C, von Deneen KM, Qin W, Tian J. Reduced frontal cortical thickness and increased caudate volume within fronto-striatal circuits in young adult smokers. Drug Alcohol Depend. 2015;151:211–9.
44. DiFranza JR, Wellman RJ, Savageau JA, Beccia A, Ursprung WW, McMillen R. What aspect of dependence does the fagerström test for nicotine dependence measure? ISRN Addict 2012;2013:906276.
45. Fu M, Martínez-Sánchez JM, Agudo A, Pascual JA, Ariza C, Moncada A, Fernández E, Study Investigators DCOT. Nicotine depedence and salivary cotinine concentration in daily smokers. Eur J Cancer Prev. 2012;21(1):96–102.
46. Transdisciplinary Tobacco Use Research Center (TTURC) Tobacco Dependence, Baker TB, Piper ME, DE MC, Bolt DM, Smith SS, Kim SY, Colby S, Conti D, Giovino GA, Hatsukami D, Hyland A, Krishnan-Sarin S, Niaura R, Perkins KA, Toll BA. Time to first cigarette in the morning as an index of ability to quit smoking: implications for nicotine dependence. Nicotine Tob Res. 2007;9(Suppl 4):S555–70.
47. Gazdek D, Samardzic S. Croatian smoke-free law and smoking habits among employees of health care facilities in Koprivnica-Križevci County. Croat Med J. 2013;54(4):407–10.
48. Billieux J, Gay P, Rochat L, Khazaal Y, Zullino D, Van der Linden M. Lack of inhibitory control predicts cigarette smoking dependence: evidence from a non-deprived sample of light to moderate smokers. Drug Alcohol Depend. 2010;112(1–2):164–7.
49. Flaudias V, Picot MC, Lopez-Castroman J, Llorca PM, Schmitt A, Perriot J, Georgescu V, Courtet P, Quantin X, Guillaume S. Executive Functions in Tobacco Dependence: Importance of Inhibitory Capacities. PLoS One. 2016;11(3):e0150940.
50. Heatherton TF, Kozlowski LT, Frecker RC, Rickert W, Robinson J. Measuring the heaviness of smoking: using self-reported time to the first cigarette of the day and number of cigarettes smoked per day. Br J Addict. 1989;84(7):791–9.
51. Muhammad-Kah RS, Hayden AD, Liang Q, Frost-Pineda K, Sarkar M. The relationship between nicotine dependence scores and biomarkers of exposure in adult cigarette smokers. Regul Toxicol Pharmacol. 2011; 60(1):79–83.
52. Hickling LM, Perez-Iglesias R, Ortiz-García de la Foz V, Balanzá-Martínez V, McGuire P, Crespo-Facorro B, Ayesa-Arriola R. Tobacco smoking and its association with cognition in first episode psychosis patients. Schizophr Res. 2017; [Epub ahead of print]
53. Van Haren NE, Koolschijn PC, Cahn W, Schnack HG, Hulshoff Pol HE, Kahn RS. Cigarette smoking and progressive brain volume loss in schizophrenia. Eur Neuropsychopharmacol. 2010;20(7):454–8.
54. Nolan KA, D'angelo D, Hoptman MJ. Self-report and laboratory measures of impulsivity in patients with schizophrenia or schizoaffective disorder and healthy controls. Psychiatry Res. 2011;187(1–2):301–3.
55. Kao YC, Liu YP, Cheng TH, Chou MK. Cigarette smoking in outpatients with chronic schizophrenia in Taiwan: relationships to socio-demographic and clinical characteristics. Psychiatry Res. 2011;190(2–3):193–9.
56. Barr AM, Procyshyn RM, Hui P, Johnson JL, Honer WG. Self-reported motivation to smoke in schizophrenia is related to antipsychotic drug treatment. Schizophr Res. 2008;100(1–3):252–60.
57. Zhang XY, Chen DC, Tan YL, Luo X, Zuo L, Lv MH, Shah NN, Zunta-Soares GB, Soares JC. Smoking and BDNF Val66Met polymorphism in male schizophrenia: a case-control study. J Psychiatr Res. 2015;60:49–55.
58. Zhang XY, Chen DC, Tan YL, Xiu MH, Cui J, Hui L, Yang FD, Kosten TR. Socio-demographic and clinical characteristics of heavy and non-heavy smokers among schizophrenia inpatients in a Chinese Han population. Psychopharmacology. 2014;231(1):305–14.
59. Yee A, Bt Nek Mohamed NN, Binti Hashim AH, Loh HS, Harbajan Singh MK, Ng CG, Jambunathan ST. The effect of nicotine dependence on psychopathology in patients with schizophrenia. Biomed Res Int. 2015;2015:730291.
60. Misiak B, Kiejna A, Frydecka D. Assessment of cigarette smoking status with respect to symptomatic manifestation in first-episode schizophrenia patients. Compr Psychiatry. 2015;58:146–51.
61. Patkar AA, Gopalakrishnan R, Lundy A, Leone FT, Certa KM, Weinstein SP. Relationship between tobacco smoking and positive and negative symptoms in schizophrenia. J Nerv Ment Dis. 2002;190(9):604–1.
62. Compton MT, Whicker NE, Hochman KM. Alcohol and cannabis use in urban, African American, first-episode schizophrenia-spectrum patients: associations with positive and negative symptoms. J Clin Psychiatry. 2007; 68(12):1939–45.

Experiences of an internet-based support and coaching model for adolescents and young adults with ADHD and autism spectrum disorder

Helena Sehlin[1,2*], Britt Hedman Ahlström[3], Gerhard Andersson[4,5] and Elisabet Wentz[1]

Abstract

Background: There is a great demand for non-medical treatment and support targeting the needs of adolescents and young adults with autism spectrum disorder (ASD) and attention-deficit/hyperactivity disorder (ADHD). There is also a lack of qualitative studies providing in-depth insight into these individuals' own experiences within this area. The current study aimed to explore how adolescents and young adults with ADHD, ASD or both experienced taking part in an internet-based support and coaching intervention.

Methods: Sixteen participants with ASD, ADHD or both who had participated in an 8-week internet-based support and coaching model, were interviewed using semi-structured interviews. Data was analyzed using qualitative content analysis.

Results: Analysis yielded three themes; *Deciding to participate*, *Taking part in the coaching process* and *The significance of format*. Various motives for joining were expressed by participants, such as viewing the technology as familiar and appealing and expecting it to be better suited to their situation. There was also a previously unfulfilled need for support among participants. In deciding to take part in the intervention the coaches' competence and knowledge were considered essential, often in the light of previously negative experiences. Taking part in the coaching process meant feeling reassured by having someone to turn to in view of shared obstacles to seeking and receiving help. The support was used for talking through and receiving advice on matters related to their diagnosis. Findings further revealed appreciation for aspects relating to the format such as communicating through the written word, being in one's own home and an experience of immediacy. Some disadvantages were voiced including incomplete personal interaction and failing technology. There were also suggestions for greater flexibility.

Conclusions: The in-depth qualitative data obtained from this study suggest that the current model of support and the internet-based format have specific qualities that could play an important role in the support of adolescents and young adults with ADHD and ASD. Although not a replacement for face-to-face interaction, it could be a promising complement or alternative to other support and treatment options.

Keywords: ADHD, Autism, Coaching, Support, Internet-based, Adolescent, Adult, Qualitative, Experiences

* Correspondence: helena.sehlin@regionhalland.se
[1]Gillberg Neuropsychiatry Centre, Institute of Neuroscience and Physiology, University of Gothenburg, Gothenburg, Sweden
[2]Kungsbacka Clinic of Adult Psychiatry, Department of Psychiatry, Kungsbacka, Region Halland, Sweden
Full list of author information is available at the end of the article

Background

Attention-deficit/hyperactivity disorder (ADHD) and autism spectrum disorder (ASD) are both neurodevelopmental disorders with an early childhood debut [1]. Contrary to previous beliefs, recent research has shown that the majority of individuals with ADHD still meet diagnostic criteria in adulthood, affecting 2–4% of the adult population [2–5]. For ASD the prevalence rate for adults is 1% [6]. Although separate disorders ADHD and ASD often share certain cognitive impairments, such as problems with executive function [7]. There is also a considerable overlap between them which has led to a joint conception known as ESSENCE (Early Symptomatic Syndromes Eliciting Neurodevelopmental Clinical Examinations) [1] and to ASD and ADHD no longer being mutually exclusive in the *Diagnostic and Statistical Manual of Mental Disorders* [8].

Awareness about the persistence of symptoms in ADHD and ASD over the life span has increased the demand for treatment and support options specifically targeting the needs of adolescents and adults [9–12]. Medication such as psychostimulants are regarded effective for adult ADHD but are not always sufficient and the number of controlled studies concerning stimulant medication for emerging adults is scarce [13, 14]. Mounting evidence supports the use of multimodal treatment including psychoeducation and cognitive behavioural therapy [15]. Several qualitative studies have shown that despite medication being helpful, adolescents and adults with ADHD in European countries and in the U.S. still report difficulties within several areas, and experience a strong need for psychological treatment or psychoeducation that is often unmet by healthcare [16–18]. Importantly, there are no pharmacological treatments available for core symptoms in ASD, and research into support for the adult population is considerably lacking [9]. Current recommendations include interventions such as cognitive behavioural therapy and social skills training [19]. A qualitative study [10] examining experiences reported by adults with ASD in the U.S. identified factors on several levels (patient/provider/system level) that negatively impacted the accessibility and experiences of received health care for this group.

More recently, interest has increased in coaching to aid individuals with ADHD [20–22]. Coaching is a diverse field and a single operationalized definition is hard to find [22, 23]. Target areas can include individualized support, encouragement and structure, psychoeducation; providing information about ADHD and the outcomes of living with it, as well as developing strategies to handle problems in everyday living [22–25]. A limited number of studies, including a few qualitative ones, have specifically focused on coaching for adolescents and adults with ADHD [24–27]. These previous studies are all important but also acknowledge methodological limitations such as narrow sample sizes and possible confounding variables. However, they show some initial support for the concept of coaching as helpful for individuals with ADHD. A qualitative study concerning the experiences of college students with ADHD also showed a preference for the term "coaching" and strategy-based interventions over ones including the term "therapy" [18]. A few studies have suggested that coaching could be helpful for individuals with ASD within social skills training or as support within an academic setting [28, 29].

Telehealth and internet-based mental health interventions have received increased interest over the past decade as a complement to current treatment options [30–32]. For people with ASD and ADHD core aspects of the condition can sometimes pose a barrier in traditional health care. Problems with eye contact, reading body language and in processing simultaneous perceptual modalities often make face-to-face contact challenging for individuals with ASD [33, 34]. Furthermore, difficulties with structure, motivation, procrastination and time management can lead to high dropout rates and problems with treatment adherence for individuals with ADHD [35, 36]. In remote geographical areas there is often a shortage of practitioners specialized in ASD and/or ADHD. There is almost no published research on internet interventions within mental health for individuals with these disorders. One recent study, however, showed encouraging results for an internet-based cognitive behavioral therapy program designed for adults with ADHD [37].

The critical period of transition from adolescence into adulthood can be difficult for those with ASD and ADHD. Less external structure from home and/or school and increased demands to independently manage the tasks of daily living pose significant executive function challenges for these individuals [18, 24, 38–41]. Therefore, adolescents and young adults with these conditions often require alternatives to medical help to deal with different aspects of their daily life. There is however a great shortage of both qualitative and quantitative studies within this area. Most notably there is a need for qualitative studies examining these individuals' own perspectives on treatment and support [9, 10, 16, 19].

Finding forms of support that are acceptable and accessible for these individuals is imperative. Towards this objective, the aim of this study was to use a qualitative methodology to examine the experiences of adolescents and young adults with ADHD, ASD or both who had participated in an 8-week internet-based support and coaching intervention.

Methods

Design

This qualitative interview study was part of a multicentre study evaluating the intervention "NP Young Coaching", an internet-based support and coaching model (IBSC) for adolescents and young adults with ASD and ADHD [12]. The intervention (IBSC) took place at two study centres in the southwest of Sweden between the autumn of 2010 and winter 2014. Interviews were carried out up until the spring of 2015.

Internet-based support and coaching

The internet-based support and coaching model used was developed by E.W. and tested in a pilot study [12]. The model builds on coaching and psychoeducative techniques in order to facilitate the individual's understanding and handling of his/her everyday life problems [23, 42]. The model entails using professionals with extensive knowledge about ADHD and ASD. It includes an initial face-to-face meeting with an appointed coach followed by eight weeks of internet-based coaching. Coaching consists of two weekly scheduled chat-sessions á 30–60 min which typically take place from the participants´ homes by using a specially designed chat program. Two sessions (week 3 and week 6 of the intervention) are live meetings with the coach at their home clinic. Coaches and participants can also communicate via an e-mail function. Before the intervention starts, participants choose two preliminary topics that they want to focus on during chat-sessions [12].

Settings and procedure

The IBSC multicentre study

After the pilot study, the model was tested in a multicentre study including participants from a psychiatric outpatient clinic specialized in adults with ASD and ADHD, and a Habilitation service centre serving children, adolescents and adults. Participants were adolescents or young adults, aged 15 to 32 years, with a confirmed DSM–IV diagnosis of ADHD, ASD or both. Participants included both individuals who recently received a neuropsychiatric evaluation as well as individuals who had previously been assigned the diagnosis. All neuropsychiatric evaluations had been performed at well-established clinics with multi-professional teams. Hence, the participants´ symptoms were regarded as leading to clinically significant impairment as described in the diagnostic criteria of the DSM-IV for these disorders. Exclusion criteria were other current serious or dominant disorders (e. g. psychosis, alcohol or substance abuse and/or conduct disorder/antisocial personality disorder). This was established by using the Structured Clinical Interview for DSM-IV Axis I Disorders (SCID-I) [43] and the antisocial personality disorder part of the Structured Clinical Interview for DSM-IV Axis II Disorders (SCID-II) [44]. Major depression was an exclusion criterion if the participant was judged in need of another treatment or not suitable/able to comply with the format of the intervention. Finally, individuals with severe dyslexia and mental retardation/intellectual disability were excluded. A total of 30 individuals were included in the IBSC multicentre study; $n = 13$ at the psychiatric outpatient clinic and $n = 17$ at the Habilitations service centre. Of these, two from the psychiatric clinic and four from the Habilitation service centre did not complete their participation in the IBSC.

Coaches were all experienced in working with ASD and ADHD but came from different occupational backgrounds. At the psychiatric outpatient clinic coaches comprised two educational therapists, one clinical psychologist and one trained social worker. At the Habilitation service centre two special education teachers and one trained social worker were coaches. All of them were employed at the study centres.

Participants and recruitment process for the interviews

A consecutive sampling method was applied. All individuals who took part in the IBSC multicentre study, including individuals who had dropped out, were asked to participate in the interview-study during visits at their home clinic. They received verbal and written information about the study and study personnel, and if they agreed to participate an interview date was set up at their home clinic. Depending on when the participants were enrolled in the original study, the interview could take place from three months and up to 21 months (median 8.5 months) after receiving the intervention. Seventeen participants agreed to be interviewed. One of these did not show up even though several interview dates were set up, resulting in a total of 16 individuals participating (See Table 1). Participants ranged in age from 15 to 32 years (mean = 23 [SD = 5]) and consisted of 56% males and 44% females. Reasons for declining participation were not shared. A monetary compensation for participation was offered, partly to cover any associated travel expenses.

Data collection

Data was collected between the autumn of 2012 and spring of 2015 through single individual qualitative narrative interviews carried out at the clinic closest to their home. One interview took place in the home of the participant at their request. During one interview, the participant's mother was present. A semi-structured interview guide was used. It included questions about thoughts; experiences and expectations participants may have had before, during and after receiving IBSC, benefits and disadvantages compared to other forms of support as well as likes and dislikes. The perceived significance of the coaches' training and knowledge about ASD and ADHD was inquired about. The interviewer encouraged participants to speak freely and to regard the interview as a conversation with the purpose of capturing their subjective experience. Six interviews were conducted by the first author (HS), a female clinical psychologist employed at one of the study centres. As she had previously been involved as a

Table 1 Clinical and sociodemographic characteristics of participants ($n = 16$)

Participant	Study Centre (1/2)	Diagnosis	Level of education (completed or ongoing)	Occupation	Civil state & living situation	Geographical Area	Completed participation in IBSC
1	1	ALC + ADHD	Compulsory School	Student	Single, living with parents	Rural	Yes
2	1	AS	Upper Secondary School	Sick leave	In a relationship, one person household	Urban	Yes
3	1	AA	Upper Secondary School	Student	Single, living with parents	Urban	Yes
4	1	ADHD	Upper Secondary School	Sick leave	In a relationship, co-habitation	Rural	Yes
5	1	AD + ADHD	Upper Secondary School	Student	Single, living with parents	Rural	Yes
6	1	ADHD + DCD	University	Student	Single, living with parents	Rural	Yes
7	2	AS	University	Student	In a relationship, one person household	Urban	Yes
8	2	AS + ADHD	Upper Secondary School	Student	Single, one person household	Urban	Yes
9	2	ALC + ADHD	Has not completed Compulsory School	Student	Single, living with parents	Urban	Yes
10	2	AS	Compulsory School	Student	Single, living with parents	Urban	Yes
11	2	AS + ADHD	Compulsory School	Work Experience Placement	In a relationship, one person household	Urban	Yes
12	2	ADHD	Upper Secondary School	Unemployed	Single, one person household	Rural	Yes
13	2	ADHD	Compulsory School	Working	Married, living with partner and/or children	Rural	No
14	2	AD	Upper Secondary School	Student	Single, living with parents	Urban	Yes
15	2	AS + ADHD	University	Work Experience Placement	Single, one person household	Urban	Yes
16	2	ALC	University	Unemployed	Single, one person household	Urban	Yes

ADHD attention-deficit/hyperactivity disorder, *ALC* autistic-like condition (pervasive developmental disorder not otherwise specified; PDD NOS), *AS* Asperger's disorder, *AD* autistic disorder, *AA* atypical autism, *DCD* Developmental Coordination Disorder coach and in the recruitment process at one of the study centres, she did not perform interviews with participants from her own clinic. Ten interviews were conducted by the second author (BHA), a senior female researcher with no previous contact or connection with any of the participants or involved clinics. The interviews had a median duration of 22 min. All interviews were anonymized, recorded and transcribed verbatim by professionals. Transcriptions were proof listened and read by the original interviewer to ensure the accuracy of the transcripts.

Data analysis

Qualitative content analysis was used to analyze the interview data. This method lends itself well to the analysis and interpretation of the meaning in text and uses a systematic way of uncovering underlying patterns and themes [45]. It is also a flexible, inductive method, well suited for exploring participants' perspectives regarding a specific research topic [46, 47]. The process involves dividing the text into meaning units that will then be condensed and abstracted into codes that label and capture the content. Codes are compared and interpreted into themes and subthemes. During the entire process, the text as a whole is to be considered [45, 47, 48].

The analysis started with the first author reading all transcribed interviews several times to provide a sense of the whole data. Then a stepwise process of dividing text into meaning units, codes and larger themes and sub-themes started. The qualitative software program NVivo v.10 was used as a complement to organize data. The analysis was an iterative process of cross-checking and testing categories against new data, revising them if necessary, while re-reading the original interviews ensuring that the initial meaning of a statement was preserved. Citations were chosen that were considered representative of themes and subthemes as well as including a range of participants. The first and second author continuously discussed the analysis process and the relevance of codes and the emerging themes, as well as together revising the analysis. In the case of discrepancy in interpretation, codes and themes were negotiated until agreement was reached. Finally, the codes under the different themes were counted in order to see if any specific diagnostic category completely dominated a certain theme or code. No such tendency was encountered. Examples of how the themes, sub-themes and codes were derived from the meaning units are shown in Table 2.

Ethics approval and consent to participate

The study was approved by the Regional Ethical Review Board at the University of Gothenburg, Sweden (Dnr: 013–08; T364–10; T645–11; T436–12). For ethical considerations the guidelines of the World Medical Association Declaration of Helsinki (2008) were applied. Participants were given written and verbal information about the study. Written informed consent was obtained from all participants before the interview. All participants were deemed as ethically capable and of a level of maturity required for providing consent for themselves. All participants could easily and at any time during the interview receive support or medical supervision from their home clinic. None of the participants needed this.

Results

Findings yielded three themes with a total of ten subthemes of relevance for the aims of this study (see Table 3). The themes were 1) Deciding to participate, with the subthemes *Reflecting personal motives* and *Defining necessary requirements for support;* 2) Taking part in the coaching process, with the subthemes *Defining coaching, Talking it through and receiving advice, Perceived short-term and long-term consequences;* 3) The significance of format, with the subthemes *Making support simple and accessible, Communicating through the written word, Being in one's own home, A feeling of immediacy* and *Shortcomings and suggestions.*

Deciding to participate

This theme describes the participants´ individual reasons for joining the study as well as reflections before participating.

Reflecting personal motives

Participants mentioned curiosity about a novel model as a main motive for participating. The model was seen as positive and progressive, the chat-format appealing to them as technologically familiar from their everyday life. It was also sometimes expected to be better suited to their situation;

> *I thought being able to get in touch through the internet seemed particularly helpful as I experience face-to-face interactions as quite hard due to my Asperger-diagnosis. (Participant 1)*

Wanting to contribute to science and to the development of new "treatment" options that could benefit others were also mentioned, even when the intervention was judged as less relevant on a personal level. Furthermore, a need for support or help with issues specifically pertaining to one's diagnosis or daily life problems, as well as simply wanting someone to talk to, were revealed as motives. The latter was often previously unfulfilled by for instance health care or family. Not having to travel to seek help was mentioned as a key motive.

Table 2 Exemplification of the analysis and how the themes, sub-themes and codes were derived from meaning units

Theme	*Sub-theme*	Code	*Meaning unit*
Deciding to participate	Reflecting personal motives	Curiosity	*Interviewer: What did you think about the opportunity to receive internet-based support and coaching when you decided to participate in the project? From the start, when you decided to join… What did you think about it then, do you remember?* *Participant 7: Wow. I thought it was really exciting to be able to participate in something like this, and… and I thought it sounded really exciting, to be able to try something new, an alternative to going to a clinic like you usually do *pauses*… that I thought was really exciting.*
Taking part in the coaching process	Perceived short-term and long-term consequences	Improved self-confidence	*Interviewer: Is there anything … is there an area where you think "this works very well in my daily life"* *Participant 1: Yes, there is. Since I took part in this chat-project…* *Interviewer: Mmm…* *Participant 1: … I have become much more self-confident. I know that's its okay to kind of withdraw when you feel that it's all too much.*
The significance of format	Communicating through the written word	Missing personal interaction	*Participant 3: I think I felt the same about it then, as I feel about it now really. I felt that for me, for myself, I prefer it more personal. To sort of meet up and talk to each other.* *Interviewer: Mm* *Participant 3: I think you get more out of that.*

Defining necessary requirements for support

Participants mentioned several requirements that were important in order to feel secure in the interaction with coaches and make participation feel meaningful. The necessity of receiving adequate information on the structure of the intervention and the chat-program was brought up, as was secure data transmission. A visual image of the person on the receiving end, along with meeting and getting acquainted with the coach were important so as to be able to share innermost thoughts and feelings. The principle of confidentiality between coaches and participants was also essential.

The coaches' competence and knowledge were considered crucial. Formal training in health care and specific knowledge and experience of working with people with ASD and/or ADHD were viewed as ensuring understanding and trustworthiness, and was essential for asking questions concerning their disability. Participants hoped that the high competence level would avoid a repetition of previously negative experiences due to lack of understanding from others.

> *I believe that people who don't have knowledge about neuropsychiatry, don't have as much of an understanding about the kind of problems you can experience, and therefore can't really respond in a way that you need, especially if you're going to receive coaching... I think most people who don't have that kind of knowledge would be quite useless as coaches for people with neuropsychiatric problems, actually. (Participant 8).*

There were however exceptions to this where a committed, genuinely interested coach was viewed as more important than a high level of training, if this enabled wider availability of support in the future.

Table 3 Themes and subthemes

Themes	Subthemes
Deciding to participate	*Reflecting personal motives* *Defining necessary requirements for support*
Taking part in the coaching process	*Defining coaching* *Talking it through and receiving advice* *Perceived short-term and long-term consequences*
The significance of format	*Making support simple and accessible* *Communicating through the written word* *Being in one's own home* *A feeling of immediacy* *Shortcomings and suggestions*

Taking part in the coaching process

This theme reflects the participant's thoughts on what they actually received in terms of support and coaching, what questions they discussed with their coach and reflections on which effects and consequences they experienced as a result of the process.

Defining coaching

"Coaching" was perceived as guidance in handling everyday issues. The coach was seen as an advisor who would help the participant with practical problem-solving, forming strategies, and reaching a better understanding of social interactions and how the outside world functioned.

> *It means that somebody is with you all the way, showing you how to do something, telling you "this is how to do it" - whatever it is about (...) life, football or*

even reading the newspaper. It's like somebody taking you by the hand and guiding you. (Participant 9).

Although terms like "treatment" or "rehabilitation" were sometimes mentioned, there was a reluctance among participants to use such terms, emphasizing instead the more easy-going and supportive character of coaching, seeing the coach more as a helpful social contact.

I don't consider it a treatment, it's more like someone helping you in general in your daily life. Like a friend that you don't have a personal connection to. (Participant 6).

Talking it through and receiving advice

Despite selecting subjects in advance, participants felt they could choose the chat-topic freely, sometimes preparing themselves by memorizing or writing down occurrences during the week. Participants mentioned talking through previous life experiences as well as more recent events. Help and advice were sought and received in the areas of planning and organization, problem-solving, and interpretation and management of social situations or conflicts. Some also discussed practical subjects such as medication. Topics were often related, directly or indirectly, to the participant's diagnosis. The use of the support for processing feelings of insecurity and worry associated with a recent diagnosis of ASD or ADHD was mentioned.

It came to be a lot about how I function in my everyday life. I need to piece myself together with what the diagnosis means and still keep track of who I am in the middle of everything. (Participant 4).

Perceived short-term and long-term consequences

In the short term, always having someone "there" to turn to with thoughts and questions was reassuring. This was particularly valuable where it did not exist in one's own network or where the individual was hesitant to seek support elsewhere, for example from healthcare.

Fairly often it felt like you had something you wanted to ask about, that you didn't really want to call someone and ask about. (....) I don't call anyone, ever. (...) I really don't like to talk at all. (Participant 15).

Furthermore, chatting with someone had a calming effect on emotions;

You could vent your anger, she listened to me. These things that (others) didn't want to listen to, I got to talk about them there. And then, I must say, it helped to keep a more even mood. (Participant 12).

The set-up of the intervention was described as lending itself to other areas of life, providing structure and valuable everyday reminders.

Long term consequences included improved planning skills and self-confidence, a sense of empowerment both in general and in social situations, and a better balance in life that is to say less stress and fatigue. Taking part in the project could also lead to learning to use writing as a general way of processing feelings and experiences.

Participants expressed being relatively satisfied with the intervention as a whole after the 8 weeks of the study, including length and frequency of chat sessions. Participants brought up having appreciated being offered IBSC in the future, that continuous support probably would have resulted in a greater effect. Difficulties in implementing advice, and doubting that the intervention had any lasting effects were also mentioned.

The significance of format

The theme refers to how the participants perceived that the format and specific characteristics of the intervention impacted on their experiences of taking part in the study, as well as suggestions for improvements.

Making support simple and accessible

The flexibility and accessibility of the support were generally experienced as very positive. The simplicity of the program was appreciated and using a chat-program was a familiar form of communication. Time and effort were minimized compared for instance to taking time off work and travelling to a clinic. This was considered less troublesome, and enabled more frequent meetings.

You don't have to schedule a meeting, or travel to (the clinic) all the time - that type of thing. Given the fact that I have ADD, even getting here is quite a strain. It was simply a relief, being able to just sit down and start talking. (Participant 9).

The same aspects were sometimes described as negative, leading to less commitment than to a physical meeting and even to forgetting about sessions. Views were also voiced that it was unimportant which form the support took, and that the special internet-based features could just as well have been replaced entirely by meetings or telephone calls.

Communicating through the written word

Communication through the written word was perceived as more accurate and precise, reducing the common concern of misunderstandings. Having the time to think things through and gather one's thoughts stood out as particularly important.

You can take your time and think about how to express yourself, and not be as worried about being misunderstood all the time. It made me feel considerably safer. (Participant 15).

In contrast to the spoken word which was seen as fleeting and imprecise, what was written remained available on the screen for both parties, which also eliminated memory issues. Using the text-based format both in the preparation process (writing down questions or experiences) and in chat-sessions was perceived as simplifying. It was mentioned that it was sometimes easier to express oneself and to write down sensitive things rather than voicing them. However, a dislike of the text-based form of communication was also expressed and a feeling that an important part of the personal non-verbal interaction was lost.

Being in your own home

Being able to communicate in the privacy of one's own home was seen as an advantage, alleviating stress and anxiety resulting from face-to-face meetings, social pressure and/or unfamiliar surroundings. This promoted better focus on the desired subject of discussion.

Another effect of not having to leave home was enabling communication even when feeling particularly tired or sad, or having a hard time going anywhere, thus reducing the risk of missed sessions or cancelled appointments.

If I have a bad day I cancel the appointment, and it just doesn't happen. But now I didn't want to cancel, for me it wasn't that difficult to use the chat-program. (Participant 4).

However, chat-sessions were seen as a complement to, not a replacement for face-to-face interaction. A common view was that having to meet at a clinic was also innately worthwhile, even when one would rather stay at home.

A feeling of immediacy

Participants expressed a positive feeling of immediacy in relation to the intervention. This seemed to be an effect both of the higher frequency (two sessions a week) and of the e-mail function as a complement to chat-sessions. Participants experienced that they could reach their coach at almost any time without going through intermediaries e.g. a telephone operator. Communicating feelings immediately as for example in an e-mail was perceived as a great advantage despite the response being delayed, making it feel worthwhile and easier to stay on topic, and reducing the risk of forgetting. Furthermore, the higher frequency sometimes facilitated rapid implementation of given advice into daily life, knowing someone would soon follow up on what had been discussed.

You were able to convey your thoughts and reflections in an email, in the exact same moment as you were thinking it. It's not that easy to remember when you're an "ADHD-kid", you forget all the time (Participant 13).

However, participants also expressed a wish for a more individually tailored chat schedule, varying the weekly frequency or cancelling scheduled sessions if they had nothing to discuss, thus avoiding frustrating "small-talk".

Shortcomings and suggestions

Failing technology was a problem. Server malfunction without notification was confusing for the participants and led to some chat-sessions being cancelled, shorter than planned or carried out with difficulty. Such problems were often handled by means of a phone call from the coach and scheduling of a new session. Many, although frustrated, were tolerant about this as they knew that the program was under development.

Participants suggested automatically updated information about server-status. Furthermore, access to chat-logs between sessions would make it easier to remember and process what had been discussed. A smart-phone application was suggested in order to enable use in any situation, further increasing accessibility. An "on call"-chat service would also have been appreciated.

Participants felt that engaging in activities outside of one's home was important and would presumably result in better effect, offering situations for challenging themselves or practicing skills.

If you had a few more daily activities (..), I think it would be an even better help. Because then you get a little more exposure to things you maybe don't like and so on, (...) and then I think it could result in an even better effect (....) given you simply have more to process (Participant 10).

There was a wish to be able to vary the form of communication between live meetings, chat sessions, email-conversations, video conversations or even group-chat sessions, the latter being helpful when more than one profession was needed or as a way of gathering people with similar problems for discussions. Also mentioned as having been appreciated was help in informing other concerned parties about the program (for example an employer) so as to minimize disruptions.

Discussion

Using a qualitative methodology, this study aimed to gather in-depth information about how adolescents and adults with ADHD and/or ASD experienced an 8-week internet-based support and coaching model. It also aimed to consider how such a format could benefit individuals that often struggle with traditional and existing support options. A number of interesting findings emerged, showing how specific qualities of the intervention corresponded to the needs of this particular group of patients, both in terms of the internet-based format as well as their experienced need for support in general. Findings also highlighted important requirements for receiving support and suggestions for improvements.

The first theme, *"Deciding to participate"*, showed reasons for participating including expecting the internet-based model to be better suited to their situation in the light of an ASD and/or ADHD diagnosis. However, motives could also be related to previously unmet needs for support or wanting to discuss issues pertaining to living with such a disorder. Prior studies suggest that an experience of insufficient support might be common among individuals with both ASD and ADHD, especially when it comes to non-medical alternatives [16, 17, 49, 50]. Participants further felt that coaches' knowledge and experience of these disorders were pivotal and a necessary requirement in deciding to participate. This stemmed largely from prior negative experiences both in health care and in daily life. Such negative experiences have been recognized previously in studies concerning individuals with both ASD and ADHD, often resulting in perceived stigma and a strong desire for more knowledge and raised awareness within these contexts [16, 51–53]. College students with ADHD have described experiencing a lack of knowledge about their disorder among service providers and faculty, these also being perceived as ill equipped to meet their needs [18]. This further stresses the importance of specific knowledge and experience among professionals delivering this kind of support [18].

Findings relating to the theme, *"Taking part in the coaching process"*, showed that participants defined coaching as easy going, as a social contact and as guidance to everyday life concerns. They were also reluctant to the use of terms such as "treatment". In a study by Lefler, Saccetti and Del Carlo [18] students with ADHD showed a preference towards receiving help in the form of coaching as compared to when the term "therapy" was used. This could mean that IBSC might be a more appealing form of support for this kind of individual. Our participants also largely utilized the support to discuss issues directly or indirectly related to their diagnosis. Defining coaching as guidance on issues relating to ASD and/or ADHD corresponds well with the original intentions when developing the IBSC model [12]. Viewing it as a social contact could imply that it was unclear for participants what differentiated the professional support from more informal help. The expressed importance of education and knowledge among coaches however partly contradicts this. Findings further made it apparent that participants appreciated and experienced a need for this kind of support after recently undergoing a neuropsychiatric evaluation as this could raise feelings of worry or uncertainty. A diagnosis of ADHD in adulthood can have great emotional impact, raising concerns about one's identity [54, 55]. Psychoeducation, with the development of compensational strategies, is an important intervention in these cases [56] as in several other psychiatric disorders [57]. Receiving psychoeducation has also been shown to be a strong predictor for overall satisfaction with treatment in ADHD [58]. The intention with IBSC was to offer personalized support and coaching, as well as individualized psychoeducation in order to aid participants in creating a better understanding of their functioning connected to a diagnosis of ADHD and/or ASD. IBSC might thus be a helpful option after newly receiving a diagnosis of ASD or ADHD.

There was an expressed threshold among participants for seeking help from health care or in their own social network. This is in line with a qualitative study in which young adults with ADHD hesitated to seek and receive help as an effect of perceived stigma [18]. Problems for individuals with ASD in initiating social interactions could also contribute to this [59] as well as more general problems with initiative in ADHD [60]. Hence, a valued effect of the intervention was the reassurance of having "someone to turn to" with thoughts and questions. In relation to this there was a tendency to report mostly short-term effects, such as emotional comfort and "on-tap" reassurance. Behaviors resulting in short term relief of anxiety or worry can often maintain such problems in the long run and are therefore not always advisable [61]. On the other hand, the aim of IBSC was primarily information and help with basic strategies related to living with ASD and ADHD, targeting a lack of adaptive skills more prominent in these populations. The intervention can also be considered valuable as an option for reaching these individuals at all, considering the various and shared difficulties and obstacles to seeking and receiving help. Some long term positive consequences as a result of the intervention were mentioned, namely improved planning proficiency, self-confidence and less stress and fatigue. These were in line with results from the pilot study [12].

The theme *"The significance of format"* revealed that participants viewed communication through the written word as largely helpful, offering time to think things through, promoting precision and reducing the risk of misunderstandings. Two previous qualitative studies have highlighted the aspect of writing as a helpful way of communicating for adults with ASD [10, 59]. The ASD-characteristic of slow processing speed has also been shown to present problems in face-to-face communication for these individuals [10], suggesting that written communication could be useful for them. Memory issues during an ongoing chat-session were likewise alleviated, an important advantage considering the fact that working memory-deficits are a problem for individuals with ADHD [62]. Written communication was moreover seen as helpful for disclosing sensitive issues, as shown in previous studies of internet -based treatment [63].

Being in the privacy in one's own home was experienced by our participants as reducing social pressure and anxiety, and promoting better focus on the subject at hand. Although not specifically mentioned, it is not unlikely that sensory issues can in part have contributed to this result. Nicolaidis et al. [10] found that sensory sensitivities such as being disturbed by the lighting or having difficulties filtering out background noises were a prominent problem for adults with ASD within a traditional health care situation. This can be alleviated by home based IBSC. In our study, being able to communicate from one's home was further found to lead to fewer appointment cancellations due to for example having "a bad day". In adolescents and adults with ADHD, difficulties with initiative, planning and memory can affect treatment adherence and high dropout rates are common [35, 36]. Individuals with ASD have furthermore been shown to experience unpredictable and variable mood swings which sometimes present a complete barrier to their activities [52, 64]. In such circumstances, having the possibility to communicate from home is probably an advantage. However, whilst appreciating the home aspect, participants saw meeting face-to-face as valuable and health promoting and online support as a complement to, not a replacement for this. This is in line with results in the pilot study [12]. Responses also indicated that participants felt that some kind of parallel activity outside of the program was important in order to practice skills or challenge themselves to boost the effect. Practicing skills and exercises promoting behavior change are recognized as important components in for example cognitive behavior therapy [61] and social skills training for autism [65] and could thus be important to consider.

The simplicity and accessibility of the support, along with perceived immediacy in contact with the coach, were appreciated features and have been recognized as hallmarks of internet-based solutions [63]. In individuals with ADHD, immediacy and ease in receiving support might generally be key factors in promoting adherence. Also valued was the higher contact frequency facilitating rapid implementation of advice and reducing the risk of forgetting. However, it was also mentioned how the simplicity of the support could in some instances lead to less commitment and not taking the intervention as seriously as would a clinic appointment, which is also consistent with previous knowledge [63].

Disadvantages with the IBSC included experiencing incomplete personal interaction. Also, failing technology was a problem and is important to manage before using the model on a wider scale. Difficulties in implementing advice were voiced, although for some participants the high session frequency seemed to facilitate this. It is unclear if problems of this kind are specific to this support format. Finally, suggestions from participants in the present study included a greater flexibility in support frequency, chat-support "on demand", and being able to vary the form of communication between for example live-meetings, chat, email, video, and group-chat. A desire for practical support on hand has been voiced in previous qualitative articles, where participants suggested that a helpline would be useful to handle unexpected situations and difficult emotions [10, 52]. However, this was tried out in part when developing the original IBSC model with less success [12].

Trustworthiness and limitations

To ensure trustworthiness in this qualitative study certain aspects were important to consider, especially the concepts of credibility and transferability [46]. Credibility refers to how well the method and research process is suited to and answers the research question, making the results believable [66, 67]. To attain credibility in this study we strove to provide a detailed, clear and transparent description of the whole research process, including the gathering of data, the process of analysis and subsequent results. To clarify relations between results and the original data, representative citations were chosen. There was a consistent dialogue between co-researchers during the whole process. Transferability describes to which degree the results can be transferred to other settings [46, 66, 67]. In this study detailed information on the context, participants and interview questions were disclosed to ensure transferability.

In relation to our results the following limitations need to be considered. Firstly, the analysis was carried out including all diagnostic categories (ADHD, ASD or ADHD and ASD in combination). Hence, it does not lend itself well to distinguishing issues or responses that differentiate the ADHD/ASD groups and how specific characteristics of IBSC suited one or the other diagnostic category. However, we also know that there is a considerable overlap between the disorders, that there are often sub-clinical ASD or ADHD-traits present and that there are shared cognitive difficulties in several domains between disorders [7, 68–70]. This questions the value of a separate analysis procedure. Although the current study does not have a quantitative approach, when results were final a count was performed to see if any specific diagnostic group completely dominated a certain code or theme. No such tendency was found.

Another limitation is that for some of the participants, a significant amount of time had elapsed between receiving the intervention and taking part in the interview. This was due to the intervention taking place between the autumn of 2010 and winter 2014, and the decision to carry out an additional qualitative interview study being made in 2012. This could affect how well some participants remembered certain aspects. However, research has shown that adults with

ADHD can in fact accurately recall childhood ADHD symptoms, which could imply that recollection might not be that affected [71]. Also, the aim of this study was not to render accurate or true remembrance but rather the meaning and significance of the participants' experiences.

The first author had previously been involved as a coach and in recruiting participants at one of the study centres. No interviews were for this reason conducted by the first author at this site. There remains a possibility that preconceptions could affect the analysis phase. On the other hand, in qualitative research this does not necessarily equal bias as long as the researcher attends to it and fosters a process of reflexivity, i.e. regarding the effect of the researcher and how knowledge is constructed during the different phases of the research process [72]. It can then contribute to a likewise valid understanding of the subject of research. To promote reflexivity the data was also cross-examined by the second author during the whole process.

Not all participants wanted to go through with the interview unfortunately, but all of them did get the opportunity; hence it was not a convenience sample. This is, however, the first time that the participants themselves get to voice their opinions about the intervention (IBSC) described in the pilot study [12].

Conclusions

This qualitative study provides in-depth data about the experiences of adolescents and young adults with ADHD and/or ASD taking part in an internet-based support and coaching model. The findings highlight an appreciation for the IBSC model and demonstrate that it was in many ways a helpful method of communication for these individuals, as well as offering them support in handling daily life problems. It was not however seen as a substitute for face-to face interaction. The findings imply that IBSC has specific advantages for adolescents and young adults with ASD and/or ADHD. It could therefore be an important complement to standard treatment and support options, especially regarding increased adherence to offered support and as a way of reaching those who experience thresholds for seeking and receiving help.

Abbreviations

ADD: Attention Deficit Disorder; ADHD: Attention deficit hyperactivity disorder; ASD: autism spectrum disorder; DSM: Diagnostic and Statistical Manual of Mental Disorders; ESSENCE: Early Symptomatic Syndromes Eliciting Neurodevelopmental Clinical Examinations; IBSC: internet-based support and coaching

Acknowledgements

We would like to thank the young people who participated for sharing their important experiences with us. We also wish to thank Ingrid Bertilsson and Lena Johannesson for their invaluable assistance during this study. Finally, we would like to thank Dr. Sally Sehlin for language editing and proof reading the article.

Funding

Funding was provided by The Health and Medical Care Committee of the Regional Executive Board, Region Västra Götaland, The Health and Medical Care Committee of the Regional Executive Board, Region Halland, The Vårdal Institute, the Swedish Institute for Health Sciences, Fredrik and Ingrid Thurings Foundation and The Department of Health Sciences at University West.

Authors' contribution

EW initiated the idea for the study, developed the IBCS model and secured funding and ethical approval. EW, BHA and HS developed the interview, administered the study, and recruited participants. H.S and B.H.A collected the data. H.S analyzed data as well as interpreted results with help and significant input from BHA HS was the primary author of the manuscript, to which EW, BHA and GA made important contributions, revised and finally approved. All authors read and approved the final manuscript.

Authors' information

H.S was a clinical psychologist at one of the two involved study-centres during the first phase of recruiting and interviewing, a clinical psychologist at the Clinic of Adult Psychiatry, Department of Psychiatry, Region Halland, Sweden during the analysis phase. When the manuscript was written she was a PhD student at Gillberg Neuropsychiatry Centre, Gothenburg University. B.H A is RN, RNT, MNSc, PhD, Associate Professor, Department of Health Sciences, University West, Trollhättan. G.A is PhD, Professor at the Department of Behavioral Sciences and Learning, Linköping University, Linköping, Sweden; Department of Clinical Neuroscience, Karolinska Institute, Stockholm. E.W is PhD, Associate Professor, senior consultant psychiatrist and Director of Gillberg Neuropsychiatry Centre, Gothenburg University, Sweden.

Consent for publication

Not applicable.

Competing interests

The authors declare that they have no competing interests.

Author details

[1]Gillberg Neuropsychiatry Centre, Institute of Neuroscience and Physiology, University of Gothenburg, Gothenburg, Sweden. [2]Kungsbacka Clinic of Adult Psychiatry, Department of Psychiatry, Kungsbacka, Region Halland, Sweden. [3]Department of Health Sciences, University West, Trollhättan, Sweden. [4]Department of Behavioral Sciences and Learning, Linköping University, Linköping, Sweden. [5]Department of Clinical Neuroscience, Karolinska Institute, Stockholm, Sweden.

References

1. Gillberg C. The ESSENCE in child psychiatry: early symptomatic syndromes eliciting neurodevelopmental clinical examinations. Res Dev Disabil. 2010;31(6):1543–51.
2. Simon V, Czobor P, Balint S, Meszaros A, Bitter I. Prevalence and correlates of adult attention-deficit hyperactivity disorder: meta-analysis. Br J Psychiatry. 2009;194(3):204–11.
3. Faraone SV, Biederman J, Mick E. The age-dependent decline of attention deficit hyperactivity disorder: a meta-analysis of follow-up studies. Psychol Med. 2006;36(2):159–65.
4. Rosler M, Casas M, Konofal E, Buitelaar J. Attention deficit hyperactivity disorder in adults. World J Biol Psychiatry. 2010;11(5):684–98.
5. Fayyad J, De Graaf R, Kessler R, Alonso J, Angermeyer M, Demyttenaere K, et al. Cross-national prevalence and correlates of adult attention-deficit hyperactivity disorder. Br J Psychiatry. 2007;190:402–9.

6. Brugha TS, McManus S, Bankart J, Scott F, Purdon S, Smith J, et al. Epidemiology of autism spectrum disorders in adults in the community in England. Arch Gen Psychiatry. 2011;68(5):459–65.
7. Nyden A, Niklasson L, Stahlberg O, Anckarsater H, Wentz E, Rastam M, et al. Adults with autism spectrum disorders and ADHD neuropsychological aspects. Res Dev Disabil. 2010;31(6):1659–68.
8. American Psychiatric Association. Diagnostic and Statistical Manual of Mental Disorders. 5th ed. Washington DC 2013.
9. Shattuck PT, Roux AM, Hudson LE, Taylor JL, Maenner MJ, Trani JF. Services for adults with an autism spectrum disorder. Can J Psychiatry. 2012;57(5): 284–91.
10. Nicolaidis C, Raymaker DM, Ashkenazy E, KE MD, Dern S, Baggs AE, et al. "Respect the way I need to communicate with you": healthcare experiences of adults on the autism spectrum. Autism. 2015;19(7):824–31.
11. Uchida M, Spencer TJ, Faraone SV, Biederman J. Adult outcome of ADHD: an overview of results from the MGH longitudinal family studies of Pediatrically and psychiatrically referred youth with and without ADHD of both sexes. J Atten Disord. 2015;
12. Wentz E, Nyden A, Krevers B. Development of an internet-based support and coaching model for adolescents and young adults with ADHD and autism spectrum disorders: a pilot study. Eur Child Adolesc Psychiatry. 2012;21(11):611–22.
13. Weyandt LL, Oster DR, Marraccini ME, Gudmundsdottir BG, Munro BA, Zavras BM, et al. Pharmacological interventions for adolescents and adults with ADHD: stimulant and nonstimulant medications and misuse of prescription stimulants. Psychol Res Behav Manag. 2014;7:223–49.
14. Vidal-Estrada R, Bosch-Munso R, Nogueira-Morais M, Casas-Brugue M, Ramos-Quiroga JA. Psychological Treatment of attention deficit hyperactivity disorder in adults: a systematic review. Actas Esp Psiquiatr. 2012;40(3):147–54.
15. Rabito-Alcon MF, Correas-Lauffer J. Treatment Guidelines for attention deficit and hyperactivity disorder: a critical review. Actas Esp Psiquiatr. 2014;42(6):315–24.
16. Matheson L, Asherson P, Wong IC, Hodgkins P, Setyawan J, Sasane R, et al. Adult ADHD patient experiences of impairment, service provision and clinical management in England: a qualitative study. BMC Health Serv Res. 2013;13(184)
17. Sikirica V, Flood E, Dietrich CN, Quintero J, Harpin V, Hodgkins P, et al. Unmet needs associated with attention-deficit/hyperactivity disorder in eight European countries as reported by caregivers and adolescents: results from qualitative research. The patient. 2015;8(3):269–81.
18. Lefler EK, Sacchetti GM, Del Carlo DI. ADHD in college: a qualitative analysis. Atten Defic Hyperact Disord. 2016;8(2):79–93.
19. Lerner MD, White SW, JC MP. Mechanisms of change in psychosocial interventions for autism spectrum disorders. Dialogues Clin Neurosci. 2012;14(3):307–18.
20. Murphy K, Ratey N, Maynard S, Sussman S, Wright SD. Coaching for ADHD. J Atten Disord. 2010;13(5):546–52.
21. Sleeper-Triplett J. The effectiveness of coaching for children and teens with AD/HD. Pediatr Nurs. 2008;34(5):433–5.
22. Goudreau SB, Knight M. Executive function coaching: assisting with transitioning from secondary to postsecondary education. J Atten Disord. 2015;
23. Murphy K. Psychosocial treatments for ADHD in teens and adults: a practice-friendly review. J Clin Psychol. 2005;61(5):607–19.
24. Parker DR, Boutelle K. Executive function coaching for college students with learning disabilities and ADHD: a new approach for fostering self-determination. Learning Disabilities Research & Practice. 2009;24(4):204–15.
25. Kubik JA. Efficacy of ADHD coaching for adults with ADHD. J Atten Disord. 2010;13(5):442–53.
26. Swartz SL, Prevatt F, Proctor BE. A coaching intervention for college students with attention deficit/hyperactivity disorder. Psychol Sch. 2005;42(6):647–56.
27. Zwart LM, Kallemeyn LM. Peer-Based coaching for college students with ADHD and learning disabilities. J Postsecond Educ Disabil. 2001;15(1):1–15.
28. Mesibov GB. Social skills training with verbal autistic adolescents and adults: a program model. J Autism Dev Disord. 1984;14(4):395–404.
29. Weiss AL, Rohland P. Implementing a communication coaching program for students with autism spectrum disorders in postsecondary education. Top Lang Disord. 2015;35(4):345–61.
30. Andersson G, Ljotsson B, Weise C. Internet-delivered Treatment to promote health. Curr Opin Psychiatry. 2011;24(2):168–72.
31. Barak A, Grohol JM. Current and future trends in internet-supported mental health interventions. J Technol Hum Serv. 2011;29(3):155–96.
32. Andersson G. The internet and CBT: a clinical guide. Boca Raton, FL: CRC Press; 2014.
33. Nadig A, Lee I, Singh L, Bosshart K, Ozonoff S. How does the topic of conversation affect verbal exchange and eye gaze? A comparison between typical development and high-functioning autism. Neuropsychologia. 2010;48(9):2730–9.
34. Evolution JCJ. Of autism support and understanding via the world wide web. Intellect Dev Disabil. 2010;48(3):220–7.
35. McCarthy S, Asherson P, Coghill D, Hollis C, Murray M, Potts L, et al. Attention-deficit hyperactivity disorder: treatment discontinuation in adolescents and young adults. Br J Psychiatry. 2009;194(3):273–7.
36. Young S, Murphy CM, Coghill D. Avoiding the 'twilight zone': recommendations for the transition of services from adolescence to adulthood for young people with ADHD. BMC Psychiatry. 2011;11(174)
37. Pettersson R, Soderstrom S, Edlund-Soderstrom K, Nilsson KW. Internet-based cognitive behavioral therapy for adults with ADHD in outpatient psychiatric care. J Atten Disord. 2017;21(6):508–21.
38. Wolf LE. College Students with ADHD and other hidden disabilities. Outcomes and interventions. Ann N Y Acad Sci. 2001;931:385–95.
39. Weyandt LL, DuPaul G. ADHD in college students. J Atten Disord. 2006;10(1):9–19.
40. Parker DR, Benedict KB. Assessment and intervention: promoting successful transitions for college students with ADHD. Assess Eff Interv. 2002;27(3):3–24.
41. Bolic Baric V, Hellberg K, Kjellberg A, Hemmingsson H. Support For learning goes beyond academic support: voices of students with Asperger's disorder and attention deficit hyperactivity disorder. Autism : the international journal of research and practice. 2016;20(2):183–95.
42. Altmaier EM, Hansen J-IC, Morgan ML, Vera EM. Prevention and psychoeducation in counseling psychology. In: Morgan M, Vera E, editors. The Oxford. Handbook of Counseling Psychology: Oxford University Press; 2011.
43. First MBSR, Gibbon M, Williams JBW. Structured clinical interview for DSM-IV Axis I disorders-patient edition (SCID-I/P, version 2.0, 4/97 revision). New York: Biometrics Research Department; 1997.
44. FirstMB GM, Spitzer RL, Williams JBW, Benjamin L. Structured clinical interview for DSM-IV Axis II personality disorders (SCID-II). Washington DC: American Psychiatric Association; 1997.
45. Krippendorff K. Content analysis. An introduction to its methodology. 3rd ed. Los Angeles. London: Sage Publications; 2013.
46. Hsieh HF, Shannon SE. Three approaches to qualitative content analysis. Qual Health Res. 2005;15(9):1277–88.
47. White MDM, E. E.. Content analysis: a flexible methodology. Library Trends. 2006;55(1):22–45.
48. Baxter LA. Studying Interpersonal Interaction. In: Montgomery BM, Duck S, editors. Content Analysis. New York: Guilford Press; 1991. p. 239–54.
49. Nicolaidis C, Raymaker D, McDonald K, Dern S, Boisclair WC, Ashkenazy E, et al. Comparison of healthcare experiences in autistic and non-autistic adults: a cross-sectional online survey facilitated by an academic-community partnership. J Gen Intern Med. 2013;28(6):761–9.
50. Cheung KK, Wong IC, Ip P, Chan PK, Lin CH, Wong LY, et al. Experiences of adolescents and young adults with ADHD in Hong Kong: treatment services and clinical management. BMC Psychiatry. 2015;15(95)
51. Mueller AK, Fuermaier AB, Koerts J, Tucha L. Stigma In attention deficit hyperactivity disorder. Atten Defic Hyperact Disord. 2012;4(3):101–14.
52. Griffith GM, Totsika V, Nash S, Hastings RP. 'I just don't fit anywhere': support experiences and future support needs of individuals with Asperger syndrome in middle adulthood. Autism. 2012;16(5):532–46.
53. Mitchell W, Beresford B. Young people with high-functioning autism and Asperger's syndrome planning for and anticipating the move to college: what supports a positive transition? British Journal of Special Education. 2014;41(2):151–71.
54. Hansson Hallerod SL, Anckarsater H, Rastam M, Hansson Scherman M. Experienced consequences of being diagnosed with ADHD as an adult - a qualitative study. BMC Psychiatry. 2015;15(31)
55. Young S, Bramham J, Gray K, Rose E. The experience of receiving a diagnosis and treatment of ADHD in adulthood: a qualitative study of clinically referred patients using interpretative phenomenological analysis. J Atten Disord. 2008;11(4):493–503.

56. Hirvikoski T, Waaler E, Lindstrom T, Bolte S, Jokinen J. Cognitive behavior therapy-based psychoeducational groups for adults with ADHD and their significant others (PEGASUS): an open clinical feasibility trial. Atten Defic Hyperact Disord. 2015;7(1):89–99.
57. Murray-Swank AB, Dixon L. Family psychoeducation as an evidence-based practice. CNS Spectr. 2004;9(12):905–12.
58. Solberg BS, Haavik J, Halmoy A. Health Care Services for Adults With ADHD: Patient Satisfaction and the Role of Psycho-Education. J Atten Disord. Forthcoming 2015. Available from: https://doi.org/10.1177/1087054715587941
59. Muller E, Schuler A, Yates GB. Social Challenges and supports from the perspective of individuals with Asperger syndrome and other autism spectrum disabilities. Autism. 2008;12(2):173–90.
60. Barkley RA. Differential diagnosis of adults with ADHD: the role of executive function and self-regulation. J Clin Psychiatry. 2010;71(7):e17.
61. Clinical BDH. Handbook of psychological disorders: a step by step treatment manual. 4th ed. New York: Guilford Press; 2008.
62. Ehlis AC, Bahne CG, Jacob CP, Herrmann MJ, Fallgatter AJ. Reduced lateral prefrontal activation in adult patients with attention-deficit/hyperactivity disorder (ADHD) during a working memory task: a functional near-infrared spectroscopy (fNIRS) study. J Psychiatr Res. 2008;42(13):1060–7.
63. Tate DF, Zabinski MF. Computer and internet applications for psychological treatment: update for clinicians. J Clin Psychol. 2004;60(2):209–20.
64. Laurent AC, Rubin E. Challenges in emotional regulation in Asperger syndrome and high-functioning autism. Top Lang Disord. 2004;24(4):286–97.
65. Vernon TW, Miller AR, Ko JA, Wu VL. Social tools and rules for teens (the START program): program description and preliminary outcomes of an experiential socialization intervention for adolescents with autism Spectrum disorder. J Autism Dev Disord. 2016;46(5):1806–23.
66. Graneheim UH, Lundman B. Qualitative content analysis in nursing research: concepts, procedures and measures to achieve trustworthiness. Nurse Educ Today. 2004;24(2):105–12.
67. Elo S, Kyngas H. The qualitative content analysis process. J Adv Nurs. 2008;62(1):107–15.
68. Taylor MJ, Charman T, Robinson EB, Plomin R, Happe F, Asherson P, et al. Developmental associations between traits of autism spectrum disorder and attention deficit hyperactivity disorder: a genetically informative, longitudinal twin study. Psychol Med. 2013;43(8):1735–46.
69. Taurines R, Schwenck C, Westerwald E, Sachse M, Siniatchkin M, Freitag C. ADHD and autism: differential diagnosis or overlapping traits? A selective review. Atten Defic Hyperact Disord. 2012;4(3):115–39.
70. Gillberg C, Gillberg C, Anckarsäter H, Råstam M. Overlap between ADHD and autism spectrum disorder in adults. In: Biutelaar JK, Kaan CC, Ascherson P, editors. ADHD in adults -characterization, diagnosis and treatment. Cambridge: Cambridge University Press; 2011. p. 157–67.
71. Murphy P, Schachar R. Use Of self-ratings in the assessment of symptoms of attention deficit hyperactivity disorder in adults. Am J Psychiatry. 2000;157(7):1156–9.
72. Malterud K. Qualitative research: standards, challenges, and guidelines. Lancet. 2001;358(9280):483–8.

21

Associations among maternal pre-pregnancy body mass index, gestational weight gain and risk of autism in the Han Chinese population

Yidong Shen[1], Huixi Dong[1], Xiaozi Lu[2], Nan Lian[3], Guanglei Xun[4], Lijuan Shi[5], Lu Xiao[1], Jingping Zhao[1*] and Jianjun Ou[1*]

Abstract

Background: Autism is a neurodevelopmental disorder with an unclear etiology. Pre-pregnancy body mass index (BMI) and gestational weight gain (GWG) have been suggested to play a role in the etiology of autism. The current study explores the associations among maternal pre-pregnancy BMI, GWG and the risk of autism in the Han Chinese population.

Methods: Demographic information, a basic medical history and information regarding maternal pre-pregnancy and pregnancy conditions were collected from the parents of 705 Han Chinese children with autism and 2236 unrelated typically developing children. Binary logistic regressions were conducted to calculate the odds ratio (OR) for the relationship among pre-pregnancy BMI, GWG and the occurrence of autism. The interaction between pre-pregnancy BMI and GWG was analyzed by performing stratification analyses using a logistic model.

Results: After adjusting for the children's gender, parental age and family annual income, excessive GWG was associated with autism risk in the entire sample (OR = 1.327, 95% CI: 1.021–1.725), whereas the relationship between maternal pre-pregnancy BMI and autism was not significant. According to the stratification analyses, excessive GWG increased the risk of autism in overweight/obese mothers (OR = 2.468, 95% CI: 1.102–5.526) but not in underweight or normal weight mothers.

Conclusions: The maternal pre-pregnancy BMI might not be independently associated with autism risk. However, excessive GWG might increase the autism risk of offspring of overweight and obese mothers.

Keywords: Autism, Gestational weight gain, Body mass index, Pregnancy

Background

Autism is a neurodevelopmental disorder characterized by impairments in social interactions and communication skills and stereotyped behaviors and interests [1]. According to the most recent epidemiological study, the prevalence of Autism Spectrum Disorder (ASD is 1.46% (1 per 68 persons) in the US [2]. The increasing prevalence of autism calls for further investigations of its unclear etiology [3].

An aberrant maternal pre-pregnancy body mass index (BMI) and gestational weight gain (GWG) have been suggested to increase the autism risk among offspring [4–7]. Although the relevant mechanism is not fully understood, maternal nutritional balance has been shown to be important to the fetus and directly influence fetal neurodevelopment [8]. Additionally, maternal metabolic status may also exert indirect influences on neurodevelopment via the immune or endocrine system [9, 10]. Thus, maternal metabolism before and during pregnancy may be involved in the etiology of autism.

* Correspondence: zhaojingping@csu.edu.cn; oujianjun@csu.edu.cn
[1]Institute of Mental Health, The Second Xiangya Hospital, Central South University; National Clinical Research Center on Mental Disorders, The National Technology Institute on Mental disorders; Hunan Key Laboratory of Psychiatry and Mental Health, Changsha, China

In addition to the unclear mechanism, many other questions remain unanswered regarding the associations between autism and BMI/GWG. For example, although several studies enrolled a large number of participants, the number of studies examining this association is limited, and the findings were not always consistent, indicating that more replication studies are needed. Furthermore, in some US population- based cohort studies, clear ethnic differences in BMI and GWG have been observed in individuals with different genetic backgrounds, living environments and lifestyles [11, 12]. Similarly, different classes of BMI might be related to GWG values that vary by ethnicity [13]. Hence, replicated and verified the associations of autism risk with BMI and GWG in different ethnic populations are necessary. To the best of our knowledge, few studies have focused on this issue in the Han Chinese population. This study explored the possible associations among maternal pre-pregnancy BMI, GWG and the risk of autism in the Han Chinese population.

Methods

Subjects

This study was a part of a larger research project that was approved by the Human Ethics Committee of the Second Xiangya Hospital of Central South University.

Study subjects in the autism group were recruited by the Outpatient Department of the Mental Health Institute at the Second Xiangya Hospital of Central South University, Changsha, Hunan Province and at Elim Training Center for Children with Autism, Qingdao, Shandong Province. After obtaining written informed consent from the children's parents or legal guardians, the children, who were aged 2–9 years, were independently diagnosed by two senior psychiatric doctors according to the DSM-IV-TR criteria for autistic disorder. Children with organic diseases of the nervous system or other psychiatric disorders, such as childhood schizophrenia, were excluded. Patients with a chromosomal abnormality were also excluded. Children with autism whose mothers experienced preterm labor (less than 37 gestational weeks) or multiple pregnancies were excluded from our study because these mothers' GWG values may differ from those of mothers with a single fetus and a full-term birth.

In the control group, typically developing (TD) children within the same age range were recruited by adapting a network survey questionnaire based on the most popular real-name social networking platforms in China mainland. The exclusion criteria were the same as the criteria used for the autism group. Additionally, the children were excluded if their parents reported a suspected developmental problem. In total, 2499 children who had never been diagnosed with a psychiatric or developmental disorder and did not have siblings with autism were recruited; the parents of 119 (4.8%) recruited children expressed concerns regarding their child's development. In addition, 154 (6.2%) children were preterm or multiple births and were excluded from the study based on the exclusion criteria.

Ultimately, 705 children with autism and 2236 unrelated TD children were enrolled for the subsequent data analyses. All subjects were Han Chinese.

Data collection

The parents of the children enrolled in the autism group were asked to complete a self-administered structured questionnaire that included family demographic information, basic medical history and information regarding the maternal pre-pregnancy and pregnancy conditions.

The parents of the children in the control group were solicited through a link to our website. The front page of the website contained a brief explanation of the study. If the parents agreed to participate in the study, they were asked to complete an online questionnaire that contained the same information as the paper questionnaire and included the parents' general impression of their child's development.

BMI and GWG

Pre-pregnancy BMI was calculated as weight (kg) divided by height (m) squared and was categorized into the following four groups according to the adult BMI classification standards for the Chinese population [14]: lean (<18.5 kg/m^2), normal (18.5 kg/m^2 to 24.0 kg/m^2), overweight (24.0 kg/m^2 to 28.0 kg/m^2) and obese (≥28.0 kg/m^2).

The Institute of Medicine (IOM) recommendation for GWG may not be suitable for Chinese women, and no official GWG recommendation is available in China. However, several studies have attempted to provide a Chinese GWG recommendation. In the current study, we adopted the criteria used by Yang [15], who calculated the quartile values from data obtained from a large general population (85,729 pregnant women and their children) and defined adequate GWG as follows: 15–22 kg for lean individuals, 13–21 kg for normal individuals, 10–18 kg for overweight individuals and 9.5–17.0 kg for obese individuals. Values lower than this range were defined as inadequate GWG, and values above this range were defined as excessive GWG.

Other covariates

Several variables, including the child's gender, child age (continuous variable),parental age (continuous variable), maternal history of alcoholism/drug use during pregnancy (coded as yes or no) and family annual income (coded as low, medium and high; the classification standard is shown in Table 1), were chosen as potential confounders.

Statistical analysis

Statistical analyses were conducted using IBM SPSS Statistics, Version 22.0 (Armonk, NY). Prior to the analysis, we used box-plots (case and control groups were analyzed separately) to identify and remove the outliers in the maternal pre-pregnancy BMI and GWG values, and 4 children with autism and 26 TD children were removed from the subsequent analyses. Additionally, four children with autism and 10 TD children were removed from further analysis because their mothers reported losing weight during pregnancy. These children were removed because of their small proportion, and weight lost during pregnancy may be caused by problems or diseases.

Student's t-test and a Chi-square test were performed to compare the demographic characteristics. Student's t-test was also performed to analyze the differences in BMI and GWG between the case and control groups. Binary logistic regressions were conducted to calculate the odds ratio (OR) for the relationships among pre-pregnancy BMI, GWG and the occurrence of autism in the entire sample. We conducted a stratification analysis and divided the samples into subgroups based on the BMI categories, and a logistic regression was performed to explore the relationship between GWG and autism in different BMI-level samples. The selected potential confounders were entered into the regression function as covariates. The significance level of all tests was $p < 0.05$ (two-tailed).

Sensitivity analysis

Because the data were mostly based on the parents' self-reports, we conducted a sensitivity analysis to address the potential misclassification of GWG and BMI. We adapted the World Health Organization (WHO) BMI classifications [16] and IOM GWG recommendation [17] as different standards in the sensitivity analysis (Additional file 1: Table S1) and then repeated the stratification analysis. The range of the WHO BMI standards for underweight was the same but that for the other classifications was wider than that of the Chinese standards. The range of the IOM recommendations for adequate weight gain was narrower and that for excessive weight gain was wider than that of the Chinese recommendation.

Results

Sample characteristic comparisons

Comparisons of the characteristics of the sample revealed a minor but statistically significant difference in the mean age between the children with autism and the TD children (5.78 years, SD = 2.36 years in the TD children vs. 5.04 years, SD = 1.08 years in the children

Table 1 Comparisons of the characteristics of the enrolled children and mothers in the case and control groups

	Control ($N = 2200$)	Case ($N = 697$)	t/χ^2	df	p
1. Child age (years), mean (SD)	5.78 (2.36)	5.04 (1.08)	11.457	2552[b]	<0.001
2. Paternal age (years), mean (SD)	29.39 (4.48)	30.33 (4.30)	−4.877	2895	<0.001
3. Maternal age (years), mean (SD)	27.06 (3.67)	27.94 (3.37)	−5.890	1262[b]	<0.001
4. Birth weight (kg), mean (SD)	3.35 (0.46)	3.38 (0.45)	−1.527	2895	0.120
5. Child Sex, n (%)					
Male	1187 (54%)	599 (85.9%)	229.037	1	0.001
Female	1013 (46%)	98 (14.1%)			
6. Family annual income (Yuan), n (%)					
low <50,000	347 (15.8%)	296 (42.5%)	274.318	2	<0.001
medium 50,000–100,000	715 (32.5%)	246 (35.3%)			
high >100,000	1138 (51.7%)	155 (22.2%)			
7. Maternal history of daily alcohol use, n (%)					
Yes	9 (0.41%)	4 (0.57%)	0.322	1	0.571
No	2191 (99.59%)	693 (99.43%)			
8. Maternal history of drug use, n (%)[a]					
Yes	0	3 (0.43%)	–	–	0.014
No	2200(100%)	694 (99.57%)			

[a]Fisher's exact test was used
[b]The standard variance was not equal, approximate t-test was adapted and adjusted the df

with autism, $t = 11.457$, df = 2552, $p < 0.001$). Significant differences in gender ($\chi^2 = 229.04$, $p < 0.001$), annual family income ($\chi^2 = 274.32$, $p < 0.001$), paternal age ($t = -4.877$, df = 2895, $p < 0.001$) and maternal age ($t = -5.890$, df = 1262, $p < 0.001$) were also observed between the two groups. No significant difference was observed in the children's birth weight ($t = -1.527$, df = 2895, $p = 0.127$). The detailed characteristics of the sample are shown in Table 1.

Regarding the maternal history of alcoholism/drug use during pregnancy, only 9 (0.41%) mothers in the TD group reported a history of daily alcohol use during pregnancy, and no mothers reported a history of drug use. In the autism group, 4 (0.57%) mothers reported a history of daily alcohol use, and 3 (0.43%) mothers reported a history of drug use but did not report the specific names of the drugs used. Because the proportions of mothers with a history of alcoholism/drug use during pregnancy were very low in both groups, we did not enter these two confounders into the subsequent logistic analyses.

Maternal pre-pregnancy BMI and GWG

The comparisons of maternal pre-pregnancy BMI and GWG are shown in Table 2. The mean BMI of the mothers with TD children was 20.30 kg/m^2 (SD = 2.27 kg/m^2), and the mean BMI of the mothers with children with autism was 20.50 kg/m^2 (SD = 2.25 kg/m^2). In the TD group, 21.2% of the mothers were underweight, 71.8% of the mothers were normal weight, 6.4% of the mothers were overweight, and 0.6% of the mothers were obese according to the Chinese criteria. In the autism group, 17.5% of the mothers with children with autism were underweight, 75.0% of the mothers were normal weight, 7.0% of the mothers were overweight, and 0.5% of the mothers were obese before pregnancy. A significant group difference was observed in maternal pre-pregnancy BMI ($t = -2.015$, df = 2895, $p = 0.044$) but not in the BMI categories ($\chi^2 = 4.841$, $p = 0.184$).

Table 2 Comparisons of maternal pre-pregnancy BMI and GWG between the case and control groups

	Control (*n* = 2200)	Case (*n* = 697)	Value	df	p
1. BMI (kg/m^2), mean (SD)	20.30 (2.27)	20.50 (2.25)	−2.015	2895	0.044
2. BMI categories, n (%)					
Underweight	466 (21.2%)	122 (17.5%)	4.841	3	0.184
Normal	1580 (71.8%)	523 (75.0%)			
Overweight	141 (6.4%)	49 (7.0%)			
Obese	13 (0.6%)	3 (0.5%)			
3. GWG (kg), mean (SD)	15.04(5.81)	15.70 (6.21)	−2.526	2895	0.012
4. GWG categories, n (%)					
Inadequate	793 (36.0%)	226 (32.4%)	7.912	2	0.019
Adequate	344 (15.6%)	139 (19.9%)			
Excessive	1063 (48.4%)	332 (47.7%)			

BMI body mass index, *GWG* gestation weight gain

The mean GWG in the mothers with TD children was 15.04 kg (SD = 5.81 kg), and that in the mothers with children with autism was 15.70 kg (SD = 6.21 kg). In the TD group, 36% of the mothers had an inadequate GWG, 48.3% of the mothers had an adequate GWG and 15.6% of the mothers had an excessive GWG. Among the mothers of children with autism, 32.4% had an inadequate GWG, 47.6% had an adequate GWG, and 19.9% had an excessive GWG. The analyses revealed significant differences in the GWG values ($t = -2.526$, df = 2895, $p = 0.012$) and GWG categories ($\chi^2 = 7.912$, $p = 0.019$).

BMI, GWG and autism risk

A logistic regression was conducted to explore the relationship between pre-pregnancy BMI and autism risk (Table 3). The normal weight class was used as a reference. The obese group was combined with the overweight group to create an overweight/obese group because the number of subjects in this group was limited. The relationship was not significant according to the logistic model (underweight group: OR = 0.958, 95% CI: 0.746–1.231; overweight/obese group: OR = 0.743, 95% CI: 0.515–1.073).

Another logistic regression was conducted to explore the relationship between GWG and autism risk (Table 3). The adequate weight gain group was used as a reference. Excessive weight gain during pregnancy was associated with the risk of autism in the entire sample (OR = 1.327, 95% CI: 1.021–1.725). However, an inadequate gestational weight gain was not significantly associated

Table 3 Odds ratios and 95% confidence intervals for the association among maternal pre-pregnancy BMI, GWG and autism in all subjects

	OR	95% CI	p
Maternal pre-pregnancy BMI[a]			
Underweight	0.958	0.746–1.231	0.738
Overweight/Obese	0.743	0.515–1.073	0.113
Gestational weight gain[b]			
Inadequate weight gain	0.855	0.690–1.060	0.154
Excessive weight gain	1.327	1.021–1.725	0.034
BMI by GWG	1.064	1.009–1.123	0.023

BMI body mass index, *GWG* gestation weight gain
Child's gender, child age, parental age, and family annual income were used as covariates
[a]Normal BMI group was used as a reference
[b]Adequate weight gain group was used as a reference

with the risk of autism (OR = 0.855, 95% CI: 0.690–1.060). The interaction term (BMI × GWG) was also explored by introducing into a logistic equation. The result showed that the interaction effect was significantly associated with autism risk (OR = 1.064, 95% CI: 1.009–1.123).

Then we performed the stratification analyses, logistic regressions were conducted to explore the relationship between GWG and autism risk in each BMI category subgroup (the obese group was combined with the overweight group; details provided in Table 4). In the lean mothers, inadequate (OR = 1.164, 95% CI: 0.726–1.866) and excessive GWG (OR = 1.016, 95% CI: 0.502–2.055) were not significantly associated with the risk of autism. In the normal pre-pregnancy weight mothers, excessive GWG (OR = 1.289, 95% CI: 0.947–1.754) and inadequate GWG (OR = 0.784, 95% CI: 0.609–1.010) were not significantly associated with the risk of autism. In the overweight/obese mothers, excessive GWG significantly and more obviously increases the risk of autism (OR = 2.468, 95% CI: 1.102–5.526). In contrast, inadequate GWG was not significantly associated with the risk of autism in the same group (OR = 0.548, 95% CI: 0.193–1.559).

Sensitivity analysis

The results of the sensitivity analyses are summarized in Additional file 1: Table S2. Adopting a different GWG and BMI standard did not alter the significance or direction of the outcomes.

Discussion

To the best of our knowledge, this study included the largest sample to date to explore the relationship among pre-pregnancy BMI, GWG and autism in the Chinese population. In the present study, we found that being underweight or overweight before pregnancy might not be associated with the risk of autism in offspring. Many other studies have reported similar results in underweight and overweight mothers [4, 18, 19]. Bilder et al. did not identify associations between ASD risk and maternal BMI at the start of pregnancy in a population-based ASD cohort that was compared with age- and gender- matched controls [4]. In a recent published study, Jo H et al. observed an association between the risk of autism/developmental delay and obese class II/III (BMI ≥ 35) mothers but not with underweight or overweight mothers in a general population-based, prospective study (although the pre-pregnancy BMI data were retrospectively collected, as the subjects were enrolled during the third trimester of pregnancy) [18]. Suren P et al. conducted a similar population-based, prospective study involving a Norwegian cohort and reported that only maternal obesity (BMI ≥ 30), but not underweight or overweight, was weakly associated with the risk of ASD (adjusted OR = 1.34, 95% CI: 0.84–2.12) [19]. However, other studies have reported different results [6, 7]. In a population-based, case-control study, Getz K et al. reported a significant U-shaped association between maternal BMI and ASD occurrence, and mothers who were underweight before pregnancy were associated with a significantly increased risk of their offspring developing ASD (OR = 1.43 95% CI: 1.01, 2.04) [7]. In a most recent study involving a Danish national birth cohort consisting of 81,892 mother-child pairs, Andersen CH et al. also reported a U-shaped association between pre-pregnancy BMI and ASD [20]. We suspect that the differences in the socio-demographic characteristics and genetic backgrounds might account for the inconsistency in the results among the studies. For example, recently, Gardner et al. [6] reported that the significant association between maternal BMI and the risk of ASD among offspring disappeared when cases were compared to their unaffected siblings. Several other important but ignored confounders, such as paternal obesity, could be associated with autism through a genetic or epigenetic mechanism [19], which could influence the consistency of the findings.

Another main finding of the current study is that excessive GWG might increase the risk of autism among offspring. To date, only a few studies have explored the role of GWG in the risk of autism, and our findings are consistent with those from most previous studies [4–6]. According to Bilder DA et al., GWG was significantly associated with ASD risk (adjusted OR = 1.17, 95% CI: 1.01 to 1.35) [4]. According to Dodds et al., in children with a low genetic susceptibility, pregnancy weight gain greater than 18 kg, which is an excessive weight gain for all BMI classes according to the IOM criteria, is an independent risk factor for autism (OR = 1.21 95% CI: 1.03–1.47) [5].

Table 4 Odds ratios and 95% confidence intervals for the association between GWG and autism in different maternal pre-pregnancy BMI categories

	OR	95% CI	p
Underweight[a]			
Inadequate weight gain	1.164	0.726–1.866	0.530
Excessive weight gain	1.016	0.502–2.055	0.965
Normal[a]			
Inadequate weight gain	0.784	0.609–1.010	0.059
Excessive weight gain	1.289	0.947–1.754	0.107
Overweight/Obese[a]			
Inadequate weight gain	0.548	0.193–1.559	0.260
Excessive weight gain	2.468	1.102–5.526	0.028

BMI body mass index, *GWG* gestation weight gain
Child's gender, child age, parental age, and family annual income were used as covariates
[a]Adequate weight gain group was used as a reference

However, studies on this topic, including the current study, provide only preliminary evidence and do not explain whether excessive GWG is directly or indirectly associated with autism. Therefore, further studies using a prospective design, larger samples and better matching in clinical characteristics remain needed.

In this study, we also conducted a stratification analysis to further explore the potential interactions between BMI and GWG. An excessive GWG might increase the risk of autism among only offspring with overweight/obese mothers and not those with underweight or normal weight mothers. Thus, the interactions between the BMI and GWG may be related to the risk of autism. Connolly et al. reported a similar interaction in their study. These authors found that maternal obesity was associated with only 1.33-fold increased odds of offspring autism, while in obese mothers and mothers with gestational diabetes mellitus (GDM), the odds ratio increased to 2.53 (95% CI: 1.72–3.73) [21]. Furthermore, our result suggests that pre-pregnancy BMI might provide only a susceptible basis. Thus, GWG, which represents the metabolic process and nutritional status during pregnancy, might play a more important role in the etiology or pathophysiology of autism. Leptin, which is a potential biomarker of autism, is an example of a hormone involved in this process [22], and elevated leptin levels predict placental dysfunction [5]. Plasma leptin levels were recently shown to vary in different pre-pregnancy BMI classes, and higher leptin levels may promote greater maternal weight gain during gestation [23]. Additionally, GWG is positively associated with cord blood leptin levels at delivery [24, 25].

This study has some limitations. First, we did not adopt a reliable method to record gestational diseases, such as GDM or gestational hypertension, in the mothers, and these diseases may be important confounding variables related to the risk of autism [26, 27]. Therefore, as mentioned above, we cannot determine whether GWG is directly associated with autism or is only an indication of other metabolic diseases. The second main limitation of this study is that the proportion of obese mothers was small. We did not separately explore the association between BMI and GWG and the risk of autism among obese mothers because of the low statistical power. However, the metabolic or nutritional disturbances may be more obvious in the obese population. Therefore, the association between BMI and GWG and autism in the Chinese population requires further study. Third, the study design has several drawbacks. For example, the subjects were recruited using two different methods, and standardized assessments were lacking, which may limit the validity of the diagnoses and the comparability and representativeness of the population. Another major methodological limitation is the use of parental retrospective self-reports in a case-control study; although the validity of maternal recall of metabolic conditions has gained some support from other studies [28], a false positive result is likely. Hence, more precise and prospective studies are needed.

Conclusion

This is the largest-scale study investigating this topic in the Chinese Han population. This study adopted a case-control design and provided preliminary evidence about the associations between maternal BMI, GWG and the risk of autism. And the results showed that maternal pre-pregnancy BMI might not be independently associated with the risk of autism, but excessive GWG might increase the risk of autism in offspring of overweight and obese mothers. However, given some limitations of the study, more precise and prospective studies are necessary.

Abbreviations

ASD: Autism Spectrum Disorder; BMI: Body Mass Index; CI: Confidence interval; GWG: Gestational weight gain; OR: Odds Ratio; TD: Typically developing

Acknowledgements

We thank all subjects who participated in this study.

Funding

This study was supported by the National Basic Research Program of China (Grant No. 2012CB517901), the Fundamental Research Funds for the Central Universities of Central South University (grant No. 2016zzts135) and the National Natural Science Foundation of China (Grant No. 81601197).

Authors' contributions

SY, DH, OJ, XG, and ZJ designed the study. SY performed the data analyses and wrote the draft of this manuscript. SY, DH, LX, OJ, LN, SL, XL, and ZJ managed the data collection and contributed to the data input. All authors contributed to the editing of the manuscript and agreed with the final text.

Consent for publication

Not applicable. No individual-level data are presented within this publication.

Competing interests

All authors declare that they have no competing interests.

Author details

[1]Institute of Mental Health, The Second Xiangya Hospital, Central South University; National Clinical Research Center on Mental Disorders, The National Technology Institute on Mental disorders; Hunan Key Laboratory of Psychiatry and Mental Health, Changsha, China. [2]Qingdao Mental Health Center, Qingdao, China. [3]The First Affiliated Hospital of Zhengzhou University, Zhengzhou, China. [4]Mental Health Center of Shandong Province, Jinan, China. [5]Neuropsychology and Applied Cognitive Neuroscience Research Group, Institute of Psychology, Chinese Academy of Sciences, Beijing, China.

References

1. Lai MC, Lombardo MV, Baron-Cohen S. Autism. Lancet. 2014;383(9920): 896–910.
2. Christensen DL, Baio J, Van Naarden BK, Bilder D, Charles J, Constantino JN, Daniels J, Durkin MS, Fitzgerald RT, Kurzius-Spencer M, et al. Prevalence and characteristics of autism Spectrum disorder among children aged 8 years–autism and developmental disabilities monitoring network, 11 sites, United States, 2012. MMWR Surveill Summ. 2016;65(3):1–23.
3. Feng L, Li C, Chiu H, Lee TS, Spencer MD, Wong JC. Autism spectrum disorder in Chinese populations: a brief review. Asia Pac Psychiatry. 2013;5(2):54–60.
4. Bilder DA, Bakian AV, Viskochil J, Clark EA, Botts EL, Smith KR, Pimentel R, McMahon WM, Coon H. Maternal prenatal weight gain and autism spectrum disorders. Pediatrics. 2013;132(5):e1276–83.
5. Dodds L, Fell DB, Shea S, Armson BA, Allen AC, Bryson S. The role of prenatal, obstetric and neonatal factors in the development of autism. J Autism Dev Disord. 2011;41(7):891–902.
6. Gardner RM, Lee BK, Magnusson C, Rai D, Frisell T, Karlsson H, Idring S, Dalman C. Maternal body mass index during early pregnancy, gestational weight gain, and risk of autism spectrum disorders: results from a Swedish total population and discordant sibling study. Int J Epidemiol. 2015;44(3):870–83.
7. Getz KD, Anderka MT, Werler MM, Jick SS. Maternal pre-pregnancy body mass index and autism Spectrum disorder among offspring: a population-based case-control study. Paediatr Perinat Epidemiol. 2016;30(5):479–87.
8. Georgieff MK, Brunette KE, Tran PV. Early life nutrition and neural plasticity. Dev Psychopathol. 2015;27(2):411–23.
9. Sullivan EL, Nousen EK, Chamlou KA. Maternal high fat diet consumption during the perinatal period programs offspring behavior. Physiol Behav. 2014;123:236–42.
10. van der Burg JW, Sen S, Chomitz VR, Seidell JC, Leviton A, Dammann O. The role of systemic inflammation linking maternal BMI to neurodevelopment in children. Pediatr Res. 2016;79(1-1):3–12.
11. Walter S, Mejia-Guevara I, Estrada K, Liu SY, Glymour MM. Association of a Genetic Risk Score with Body Mass Index across Different Birth Cohorts. JAMA. 2016;316(1):63–9.
12. Headen IE, Davis EM, Mujahid MS, Abrams B. Racial-ethnic differences in pregnancy-related weight. Adv Nutr. 2012;3(1):83–94.
13. Headen I, Mujahid MS, Cohen AK, Rehkopf DH, Abrams B. Racial/ethnic disparities in inadequate gestational weight gain differ by pre-pregnancy weight. Matern Child Health J. 2015;19(8):1672–86.
14. Zhou BF. Predictive values of body mass index and waist circumference for risk factors of certain related diseases in Chinese adults–study on optimal cut-off points of body mass index and waist circumference in Chinese adults. Biomed Environ Sci. 2002;15(1):83–96.
15. Yang S, Peng A, Wei S, Wu J, Zhao J, Zhang Y, Wang J, Lu Y, Yu Y, Zhang B. Pre-pregnancy body mass index, gestational weight gain, and birth weight: a cohort study in China. PLoS One. 2015;10(6):e130101.
16. Obesity: preventing and managing the global epidemic. Report of a WHO consultation. World Health Organization technical report series. Geneva, Switzerland. 2000;894:i–xii, 1–253.
17. Guidelines IOMU. Weight gain during pregnancy: reexamining the guidelines. Washington (DC): National Academies Press (US); 2009.
18. Jo H, Schieve LA, Sharma AJ, Hinkle SN, Li R, Lind JN. Maternal prepregnancy body mass index and child psychosocial development at 6 years of age. Pediatrics. 2015;135(5):e1198–209.
19. Suren P, Gunnes N, Roth C, Bresnahan M, Hornig M, Hirtz D, Lie KK, Lipkin WI, Magnus P, Reichborn-Kjennerud T, et al. Parental obesity and risk of autism spectrum disorder. Pediatrics. 2014;133(5):e1128–38.
20. Andersen CH, Thomsen PH, Nohr EA, Lemcke S. Maternal body mass index before pregnancy as a risk factor for ADHD and autism in children. Eur Child Adolesc Psychiatry. 2017. [Epub ahead of print].
21. Connolly N, Anixt J, Manning P, Ping-I LD, Marsolo KA, Bowers K. Maternal metabolic risk factors for autism spectrum disorder-an analysis of electronic medical records and linked birth data. Autism Res. 2016;9(8):829–37.
22. Ashwood P, Kwong C, Hansen R, Hertz-Picciotto I, Croen L, Krakowiak P, Walker W, Pessah IN, Van de Water J. Brief report: plasma leptin levels are elevated in autism: association with early onset phenotype? J Autism Dev Disord. 2008;38(1):169–75.
23. Lacroix M, Battista MC, Doyon M, Moreau J, Patenaude J, Guillemette L, Menard J, Ardilouze JL, Perron P, Hivert MF. Higher maternal leptin levels at second trimester are associated with subsequent greater gestational weight gain in late pregnancy. BMC Pregnancy Childbirth. 2016;16:62.
24. Logan CA, Bornemann R, Koenig W, Reister F, Walter V, Fantuzzi G, Weyermann M, Brenner H, Genuneit J, Rothenbacher D. Gestational weight gain and fetal-maternal Adiponectin, Leptin, and CRP: results of two birth cohorts studies. Sci Rep. 2017;7:41847.
25. Rifas-Shiman SL, Fleisch A, Hivert MF, Mantzoros C, Gillman MW, Oken E. First and second trimester gestational weight gains are most strongly associated with cord blood levels of hormones at delivery important for glycemic control and somatic growth. Metabolism. 2017;69:112–9.
26. Polo-Kantola P, Lampi KM, Hinkka-Yli-Salomaki S, Gissler M, Brown AS, Sourander A. Obstetric risk factors and autism spectrum disorders in Finland. J Pediatr. 2014;164(2):358–65.
27. Xiang AH, Wang X, Martinez MP, Walthall JC, Curry ES, Page K, Buchanan TA, Coleman KJ, Getahun D. Association of maternal diabetes with autism in offspring. JAMA. 2015;313(14):1425–34.
28. Krakowiak P, Walker CK, Tancredi DJ, Hertz-Picciotto I. Maternal recall versus medical Records of Metabolic Conditions from the prenatal period: a validation study. Matern Child Health J. 2015;19(9):1925–35.

22

The economic consequences of attention-deficit hyperactivity disorder in the Scottish prison system

Susan Young[1,2*], Rafael A. González[3], Moshe Fridman[4], Paul Hodgkins[5], Keira Kim[6] and Gisli H. Gudjonsson[2,7]

Abstract

Background: Attention-deficit hyperactivity disorder (ADHD) is highly prevalent amongst prison inmates and the criminal justice system (CJS) likely bears considerable costs for offenders with ADHD. We aimed to examine the relationship between ADHD and health-related quality of life (HRQoL) and quality-adjusted life years (QALY) amongst imprisoned adults; and to estimate the annual expenditure associated with ADHD status in prison.

Methods: An observational study was performed in 2011–2013, at Porterfield Prison, Inverness, United Kingdom (UK). The all male sample included 390 adult prison inmates with capacity to consent and no history of moderate or severe intellectual disability. Participants were interviewed using the Diagnostic Interview for ADHD in Adults 2.0. The Health Utilities Index Mark 3 (HUI3) was used to measure health status, and to calculate attribute specific HRQoL scores and QALY. Health service utilisation was obtained through inspection of medical prison records. Inmates with ADHD were compared with inmates without ADHD.

Results: Inmates with ADHD had significantly lower QALYs, with a clinically significant adjusted difference of 0.13. Psychiatric co-morbidity accounted for the variation of ADHD on the HUI3 emotion domain only. Medical costs for inmates with ADHD were significantly higher; and behaviour-related prison costs were similar to prisoners without ADHD, reflecting a low frequency of recorded critical incidents.

Conclusions: ADHD may directly contribute to adverse health and quality of life through cognitive and executive function deficits, and co-morbid disorders. The extrapolation of conservative cost estimates suggests that the financial burden of medical and behavior-related prison care for inmates with ADHD in the UK is approximately £11.7 million annually. The reported cost estimates are conservative as there is great variability in recorded critical incidents in prisons. In turn, for some prison establishments the prison care costs associated with prisoners with ADHD may be considerably greater.

Keywords: ADHD, Health-related quality of life, Economic evaluation, Quality-adjusted life years, Prison, Costs

Background

Among the general population attention-deficit hyperactivity disorder (ADHD) confers significant financial burden [1, 2] and given the disproportionate prevalence in the prison population, the criminal justice system (CJS) likely bears considerable economic consequences for offenders with ADHD.

ADHD is a childhood onset neurodevelopmental disorder [3] often persisting into adulthood. It is one of the most common mental health disorders in children with recent prevalence estimates ranging between 5.9 and 7.1% [4, 5]. There is recent evidence suggesting late-onset of ADHD, which will require research to better understand its implication [6, 7]. Clinically significant symptoms persist beyond childhood in 65% of cases [8], and may affect as much as 2.8–5.3% of adults worldwide [9, 10]. Its substantial burden of disease is evidenced by an increased likelihood for serious accidents [11], earlier mortality rates [12], substance dependence [13],

* Correspondence: suzyyoung@aol.com
[1]Psychology Services Limited, PO Box 1735, Croydon CR97AE, UK
[2]Reykjavik University, Reykjavik, Iceland

criminality, incarceration, and false confessions [14]. ADHD confers significant impairment [15], and reduced quality of life [16] to those afflicted by it. It is also highly prevalent amongst prison inmates, with a meta-analytical prevalence estimate of 25.5% [17]. Prison inmates with ADHD are reported to be at significant risk for having increased psychiatric co-morbidity and poorer psychosocial adjustment to the prison environment [18–21].

Health economic evaluations have become an essential part of research and provide evidence supporting health interventions [22]. ADHD is consistently linked with substantially elevated costs and with significant economic burden on education [23] and health [2]. Annual service costs linked with ADHD are reportedly £670 million in the UK [24]. Meanwhile, annual ADHD-related healthcare costs are estimated between $21 to $44 billion in the United States [23]. Furthermore, in the US costs associated with accident claims are more than three times higher in adults with ADHD [1].

Despite the disproportionate representation of ADHD within the prison population, the health-related quality of life (HRQoL) and related costs remains unknown.

In this study we aim to examine the impact of ADHD amongst imprisoned adults. We set out to determine prisoners': 1) scope and extent of impaired HRQoL utility scores and quality-adjusted life years (QALY) and 2) service use and costs attributable to ADHD.

Methods

Participants and sample selection

Following approval from the Scottish Prison Service Research Access and Ethics Committee and in accordance with the Declaration of Helsinki written consent was obtained by prisoners who were recruited by opportunity sampling from Porterfield Prison, Inverness, Scotland, UK, over a period of 18 months in 2011–2013. Participants included 390 adult male prisoners who consented to participate. Those with moderate or severe learning difficulties, lack of fluency in the English language, and severe mental illness (as judged by prison officers) were excluded from participating.

Participants in the study were indirectly compensated. The study group deposited £20 per participant into a Prison Common Good Fund, which was managed by a group of prisoners. The fund was then used to purchase items for the common good of all prisoners to enhance prison life.

Prisoners who indicated interest attended an appointment with the researcher where they were given detailed oral and written information about the study and the consent procedures. After obtaining written consent, researchers administered a comprehensive battery of measures, which took approximately 4 h to complete (usually split across 2 or 3 sessions). The researchers received comprehensive training to administer the measures from the Maudsley Hospital Adult ADHD Service. Further details about the comprehensive battery of measures have been published elsewhere [25].

Data related to medical service use were gathered through inspection of prison medical records and medical costs were calculated based on reference costs reported by the (NHS; see details below). Data related to behavioural disturbance incidents were gathered through inspection of prison records and related costs were calculated based on similar reference costs and were reported as prison costs (see details below).

Measures

Health utilities index mark 3 (HUI3)

The HUI3 is a multi-attribute health status classification system that enables researchers to map levels in the following categories: vision, hearing, speech, ambulation, dexterity, emotion, cognition, and pain; using decision tables and coding algorithms, which can be represented in terms of attribute specific HRQoL scores [26, 27]. HRQoL refers to the value assigned to life span when considering impairments and functional states that may be affected by disease, injury, and treatment [28]. The HUI3 scoring system provides HRQoL utility scores ranging from 0.00 (dead) to 1.00 (perfect health), and meets criteria for calculating QALY [26]. Prisoners' were asked to answer HUI3 questions based upon their health status in the 4 weeks prior to the interview. The HUI3 composite score was used to calculate QALY and was extrapolated to 1 year to represent the study health evaluation time frame, as previously applied on cost-effectiveness studies [29]. Estimating beyond this time frame would have introduced a very high degree of uncertainty in estimates.

ADHD diagnosis

All participants underwent a comprehensive evaluation for ADHD and were interviewed using the Diagnostic Interview for ADHD in Adults 2.0 (DIVA-2) [30]. The DIVA-2 is a validated semi-structured clinical interview used to diagnose ADHD in adults based on the 5th edition of Diagnostic and Statistical Manual of Mental Disorders (DSM-5) criteria [3]; and has been used in clinical [31] and law enforcement settings [32]. Questions addressed their current and childhood (ages 5 to 12) presentation of ADHD symptoms and scope of impairment.

Participants were also questioned whether they were previously diagnosed or treated for ADHD or any other psychiatric illness.

Brief symptom inventory (BSI)

The Brief Symptom Inventory (BSI) is a brief psychological self-report scale [33]. The BSI has 9 subscales (Somatization, Obsession-compulsion, Interpersonal sensitivity, Depression, Anxiety, Hostility, Phobic anxiety, Paranoid ideation and Psychoticism), and 3 composite measures (Global Severity Index, Positive Symptom Distress Index, and Positive Symptom Total). We used the BSI depression and anxiety measures as covariates in our health evaluation models because they represent common mental health conditions.

Medical service use and costs

Detailed medical service utilization history was obtained through inspection of participants prison medical records. Data from prisoners' medical charts (covering the 3 months prior to the appointment with the researcher) were abstracted, verified, and entered into a database for analyses. The authors chose to include 3 months of service for practical reasons; and additionally thought this time period fairly represented the medical service use of all prisoners given the variance in prison stays. Data included details from appointments with a general practitioner, physical health nurse, mental health nurse, addiction services nurses, or any other type of nurse, psychiatrist, psychologist, podiatrist, oral health practictioner, or any other type of health related visit such as Well-man clinic or other health clinics, and hospital outpatient visit. Medical costs for these appointments were calculated according to reference costs reported by the NHS Trust [34]. Medication costs were not explicitly collected in the study.

Prison service use and costs

Prisoners' behavioural disturbance incidents were obtained from prison records. Reports of non-attendance to prison activities, being under observation, number of adjudications, and critical incidents were collected and used to calculate the related prison costs. Prison costs were calculated based upon reference costs from the UK Ministry of Justice and HM Prison Service [35], Social Research Unit, Dartington [36], and from direct communication with Scottish Prison Service management.

All reported costs were in Pounds Sterling (£) for the years 2012–2015, and adjusted using the Consumer Price Index (CPI, 2016).

Analytical strategy

Frequencies were reported for all categorical variables, and means with their standard deviation for continuous variables. The median and inter-quartile range was used for all cost related values.

Because of the HUI3 utility scores' interval properties, we used t-tests for unadjusted analyses. To estimate the association between ADHD and HUI3 single attribute and composite utility scores, Type I *Tobit* models were used in favour of traditional ordered logistic regression models. A *Tobit* model is designed to estimate linear relationships between variables when there are ceiling or flooring effects on the outcome [37]. Ignoring the censoring and fitting regression models estimated using OLS would have been systematically biased toward the null hypothesis, whereby type II error is increased. HUI3 single attribute and composite utility scores with the value of one are considered censored.

Considering the highly skewed nature of cost variables we used generalised linear models (GLM) with a gamma distribution and log-link function. This way the natural log is modeled and then the predicted margins are calculated in order to obtain the cost differential for those with ADHD [38]. All cost models were adjusted only for age. HUI3 includes an emotion domain that may be sensitive to coexisting disorders (in addition to ADHD). Therefore, models for all HUI3 variables were further adjusted for co-morbid anxiety and depression standardized symptom scores.

We established a significance level at $p \leq 0.05$ for all statistical tests. All analyses were performed using Stata version 13 (StataCorp) [39].

Results

Descriptive statistics

The all male sample was essentially Caucasian British (99.0%) with an average age of 30.3 years (sd 8.3). Prisoners with ADHD had a significantly lower mean age than those without ADHD (28.2 years (sd 7.5) vs. 31.0 years (sd 8.5,) $p < 0.01$). 18.8% (18/96) prisoners with ADHD reported a prior diagnosis of ADHD and 15.6% (15/96) reported having ever received pharmacological treatment for ADHD.

Out of the total sample of 390 participants, 81 (20.8%) required assistance with reading the questionnaires. For those diagnosed with ADHD, 31/96 (32.3%) required assistance in contrast to 50/294 (17.0%) of the other participants. This difference is significant (Chi^2 (*df* 1) = 10.2, $p = 0.001$; Odds Ratio = 2.3, Confidence Interval 1.3–3.9).

Health status

Table 1 includes the mean and distribution of all HUI3 specific attributes and composite HRQoL utility scores for all inmates. Prisoners' variability noticeably increased in scores for emotion, cognition, pain, and HRQoL.

Independent sample t-tests were estimated for all utility scores and HRQoL (Table 2) comparing prisoners with ADHD with prisoners without ADHD. Inmates with ADHD had significantly lower scores in the following categories: speech ($p < 0.05$), ambulation ($p < 0.01$), emotion ($p < 0.001$), cognition ($p < 0.001$), pain ($p < 0.05$),

Table 1 Distribution of HUI3 Specific Attribute Utility Scores for all Inmates

HUI3 Attributes, $N = 390$	n	Mean score	Standard deviation
Vision	385	0.989	(0.024)
Hearing	387	0.989	(0.061)
Speech	390	0.966	(0.073)
Ambulation	389	0.991	(0.072)
Dexterity	390	0.985	(0.078)
Emotion	370	0.787	(0.274)
Cognition	390	0.837	(0.237)
Pain	390	0.854	(0.278)
HRQoL	362	0.647	(0.307)

Notes: HUI3 data covered the 4 weeks prior to interview
Cost per unit is defined as cost per inmate for each visit. Median medical costs were calculated from data collected from medical records covering the 3 months prior to interview
[a]Includes Hepatitis C, Harm reduction, and Smoking cessation nursing staff
[b]Includes any other recorded health visits, e.g. Well-man clinic
[c]Includes all missed prison therapeutic and other activities per inmate
[d]Calculated by time spent and number of prison staff involved (based on average hourly pay rate)
[e]Calculated by time spent and number of prison staff involved in any adjudication process (estimated 15 min. Per process)

and HRQoL composite ($p < 0.001$). Figure 1 shows the distribution of HRQoL utility scores comparing prisoners without ADHD with those with ADHD.

Table 3 demonstrates that even after adjustment for age, anxiety, depression, and/or without correction for missing values, that censored *Tobit* models were significant in each adjusted model for vision, ambulation, emotion, cognition, and QALY. The inclusion of anxiety and depressive disorders in models 2 and 3, attenuated the associations with emotion, hearing, and pain attributes. Attenuation of the association with hearing and pain should be interpreted with caution, as their unadjusted effect sizes were small. Models 2 and 3 show that prisoners with ADHD have a significant difference in QALY of 0.13 and 0.10, compared to those without ADHD.

25% of all participants had missing values by endorsing 'Don't Know' on several questions of the HUI3. Patterns of missing values were analysed and the most plausible values were imputed using a technique developed by Naeim and colleagues specifically for HUI-3 scores [40].

All 41 questions of the HUI-3 instrument allow respondents to answer 'Don't Know'. Because there are no instructions in the instrument manual for how to manage or score these answers, the 'Don't Know' category interferes with the scoring leading to substantial amounts of missing data. Common methods for imputing data in this scenario may not be as effective or can even be misleading, given that answers to other questions within the same domain (e.g. vision) often help identify a sole correct answer to those marked as 'Don't Know'. The well cited imputation method by Naeim et al. [40] advises inspecting each possible change in attribute score for every answer to the 'Don't Know' missing value, then selecting the most plausible value accordingly.

Furthermore, we performed a sensitivity analysis based only on those with complete HUI3 data to examine any differences in estimates before and after using the inspection and deduction method to account for 'Don't Know' answers.

Service utilization and costs

Table 4 includes all cost model inputs for the total median associated medical and prison costs for all inmates.

Table 5 shows that in terms of medical service utilisation, prisoners with ADHD visited significantly more general practitioners ($p < 0.05$), physical health nurses ($p < 0.05$), and mental health nurses ($p < 0.01$) in the three-month period assessed. No significant associations were observed for any other health services.

Table 6 shows that age adjusted medical costs were significantly greater among inmates with ADHD ($p < 0.05$), but prison costs were not. Cost items were assessed based on a 3 month window, then calculated

Table 2 HUI3 Attribute Utility Scores by ADHD Group ($n = 96$ ADHD, $n = 294$ non-ADHD)

HUI3 Attributes	No ADHD Mean score	ADHD Mean score	t	Effect size (d)	p
Vision	0.991	0.986	1.839	0.218	*0.067*
Hearing	0.992	0.979	1.938	0.229	*0.053*
Speech	0.971	0.952	2.20	0.259	*0.028*
Ambulation	0.997	0.974	2.71	0.319	*0.007*
Dexterity	0.984	0.986	−0.113	−0.013	*0.910*
Emotion	0.817	0.692	3.83	0.466	*< 0.001*
Cognition	0.879	0.709	6.41	0.753	*< 0.001*
Pain	0.874	0.792	2.52	0.296	*0.012*
HUI3 Composite HRQoL	0.699	0.477	6.15	0.759	*< 0.001*

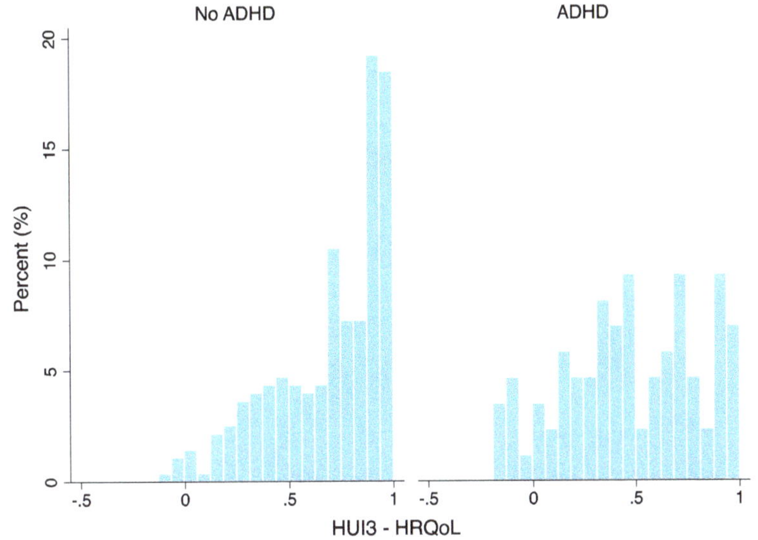

Fig. 1 Distribution of HUI3 Composite HRQoL scores by ADHD group: A greater proportion of inmates without ADHD have HUI composite HRQoL scores above 0.7. There is a greater amount of variability in the HUI composite HRQoL scores among inmates with ADHD

for 1 year assuming similar patterns of health service utilisation and behaviour in prison. Total medical and prison costs for inmates with ADHD were £ 590 more per year than for inmates without ADHD.

Discussion

HUI3 health attributes and QALY

To the best of our knowledge, our study is the first addressing ADHD health status using HUI3 amongst prison inmates. Previous studies documented the relationship between symptom severity and poorer HRQoL, including somatic symptoms [41], whereas a UK cross-sectional study reported that across most health domains, children and adolescents with ADHD had poorer scores when compared with samples of children with diabetes, and a healthy comparison group [42]. These studies highlight the extent that ADHD has on the health impact on affected individuals.

We analysed the role of ADHD on QALY based on a one-year horizon. Notably, the proportion of inmates with a HRQoL over 0.90 (healthy state) was vastly superior amongst those without ADHD. The final adjusted

Table 3 Adjusted Regression Models for HUI3 Attribute Utility Scores for Inmates with ADHD Compared with Inmates without ADHD; ($n = 96$ ADHD, $n = 294$ non-ADHD)

	Model 1	Model 2	Model 3
HUI3 attributes	Beta coef. (se)	Beta coef. (se)	Beta coef. (se)
Vision	−0.04 (0.01)**	− 0.04 (0.01)**	− 0.04 (0.01)**
Hearing	− 0.48 (0.22)*	− 0.30 (0.20)	–
Speech	−0.08 (0.04)	−0.05 (0.05)	− 0.05 (0.05)
Ambulation	−0.51 (0.23)*	− 0.54 (0.25)*	− 0.54 (0.25)*
Dexterity	− 0.06 (0.11)	− 0.03 (0.12)	− 0.03 (0.12)
Emotion	−0.19 (0.04)***	− 0.05 (0.04)	−0.06 (0.04)
Cognition	−0.29 (0.05)***	− 0.20 (0.05)***	− 0.20 (0.05)***
Pain	− 0.15 (0.07)*	− 0.02 (0.07)	−0.02 (0.07)
QALY derived by HUI3[a]	−0.25 (0.04)***	− 0.13(0.04)***	− 0.10 (0.04)*

Note. The first two columns refer to Tobit models using data that was corrected for 'don't know' answers. The third column includes the sensitivity analysis, in which we fitted a similar Tobit model but using only available data without accounting for 'don't know' answers
[a]All tobit models to account for censoring at the upper level of the outcome QALY
Model 1 is adjusted for age
Model 2 is adjusted for age + BSI anxiety + BSI depression
Model 3 is adjusted for age + BSI anxiety + BSI depression and is a sensitivity analysis of the sample without correction for 'don't know' answers
*$p < 0.05$
**$p < 0.01$
***$p < 0.001$

Table 4 Three-month Medical and Prison Costs for All 390 Inmates

	Cost(£)/unit	Median cost over 3 months (£)	Inter-quartile range (£)
Medical costs per inmate			
General practitioner	121	242	242
Physical health nurse	74.3	74.3	74.3
Mental health nurse	78.5	78.5	78.5
Addiction nurse	78.5	78.5	78.5
Nursing other[a]	74.3	0	0
Psychiatrist	148.6	0	0
Psychologist	142.2	0	0
Podiatrist	34	0	0
Oral health	87	0	0
Other health visit[b]	87	0	0
Hospital outpatient	125	0	0
Prison costs per inmate			
Activities non-attendance[c]	38.2	0	76.4
Observation level[d]	13.3	0	0
Adjudications[e]	21.4	0	0
Critical incidents[d]	13.3	0	0
Overall medical costs	–	464.9	488.3
Overall prison costs	–	34.7	76.4
Overall medical and prison costs	–	503.1	532.6

Notes: Cost per unit is defined as cost per inmate for each visit. Median medical costs were calculated from data collected from medical records covering the 3 months prior to interview
[a]Includes Hepatitis C, Harm reduction, and Smoking cessation nursing staff
[b]Includes any other recorded health visits, e.g. Well-man clinic
[c]Includes all missed prison therapeutic and other activities per inmate
[d]Calculated by time spent and number of prison staff involved (based on average hourly pay rate)
[e]Calculated by time spent and number of prison staff involved in any adjudication process (estimated 15 min. Per process)

model that accounted for psychiatric co-morbidity produced a 0.13 difference in QALY, four-fold above the 0.03 clinically relevant threshold estimated by the instrument developers [26]. QALY based on inmates' one-year health utility scores for those with ADHD were significantly lower than those without ADHD. Poorer specific health attribute scores on vision and mobility indicate that inmates with ADHD have significantly compromised health states that go beyond of those more usually expected (such as emotion and cognition) from the disorder. Furthermore, health utilities models adjusted for psychiatric co-morbidity accounted for the variation of ADHD on emotion aspects, but not on the cognition attribute, providing an important insight regarding the contributing factors to impairment amongst inmates with ADHD.

The significantly poorer vision score among the ADHD group may relate to their reading difficulties. In the present study, those diagnosed with ADHD were over two times more likely to require assistance with reading the questionnaires than the other participants. With respect to mobility, the finding that prisoners with ADHD have significantly poorer ambulation problems may reflect that prisoners with ADHD suffer more injuries that hinder their mobility compared with non-ADHD prisoners. Data obtained from the Danish registry reported that the morbidity rate is nearly three times higher if you have ADHD, and that 77.7% of unnatural deaths were accounted for by accidental injury [12]. Additionally, given the higher rates of aggression and violence in the ADHD population [43], there may be mobility problems arising from assault.

ADHD is frequently reported to be associated with a substantial reduction in the quality of life of children [44] and with increased chronic health problems in adults [45]. Study results indicate that ADHD impacts HRQoL with severe effects in emotional and social domains, and at least moderate effects in physical domains [46, 47]. Adult inmates in our sample had an unadjusted HRQoL of less than 0.60. It is likely that undiagnosed and untreated ADHD has a cumulative effect and increases the risk for further health impairments, especially among imprisoned adults with coexisting mental health and social problems.

Table 5 Three-month Medical Service Utilisation for Inmates with ADHD (Compared with Inmates without ADHD; $n = 96$ ADHD, $n = 294$ non-ADHD)

Medical service use	beta coefficient (se)	IRR (95%CI)	p
General practitioner	0.19 (0.09)	1.21 (1.00, 1.45)	0.04
Physical health nurse	0.22 (0.10)	1.25 (1.03, 1.50)	0.02
Mental health nurse[a]	0.61 (0.22)	1.84 (1.19, 2.85)	0.01
Addiction nurse	−0.11 (0.21)	0.90 (0.59, 1.35)	0.60
Other nurse[b]	− 0.18 (0.54)	0.83 (0.29, 2.40)	0.74
Psychiatrist and Psychologist	−0.12 (0.80)	0.89 (0.19, 4.27)	0.89
Oral health	0.93 (1.46)	2.54 (0.14, 44.74)	0.53
Other health related visit[c]	− 1.85 (0.99)	0.16 (0.02, 1.09)	0.06
Hospital outpatient	0.56 (0.54)	1.76 (0.61, 5.04)	0.30

Note: Visits to Podiatrist excluded for $n < 10$
[a]Includes general mental health and psychiatric nursing staff
[b]Includes Hepatitis C, Harm reduction, and Smoking cessation nursing staff
[c]Includes any other recorded health visits, e.g. Well-man clinic

There is evidence to suggest that poor HRQoL in individuals with ADHD may be driven by the existence of co-morbid conditions [48]. In our study, although co-morbidity played a role in the impact of ADHD on HRQoL, the association is not entirely explained by coexisting psychiatric symptoms of anxiety and depression. Moreover, there was no attenuation on the association with the cognitive attribute of the HUI3 on adjusted models, suggesting a domain-specific link. Cognitive dysfunction in the form of difficulties allocating attentional resources [49], response inhibition, and management of reward are hallmarks of the ADHD phenotypic expression. These results denote different paths through which ADHD may impact adverse health and quality of life, directly through cognitive deficits and via co-morbid disorders. We therefore provide evidence of domain-specific and shared contributions to impaired HRQoL in ADHD.

Service use and costs

Health economic studies on the general population report that ADHD (including symptoms of hyperactivity) is associated with significant economic burden [1, 2]; however, studies focusing exclusively on the economic impact of ADHD on adult prisoners were not identified.

A US study of disability claims reported that patients with ADHD had 2.6 more medical claims than those without ADHD and that ADHD imposed a significant financial burden [1]. A recent prospective UK study reported that preschoolers with high levels of hyperactivity had a 17-fold increase in overall costs compared with non-hyperactive controls; costs were mainly driven by mental health, educational, social, and criminal justice system service use [2]. A Danish study reported that the direct medical costs of ADHD patients were relatively high, whereof mental care and inpatient hospitalizations accounted for approximately 60% of the costs and medication use accounted for 13% [50]. Results of one study demonstrated that public costs (due to mental health, school services, and the juvenile justice system) are more than double for youth with ADHD compared with those without ADHD [51].

Hospital inpatient stays are a significant driver of costs attributable to ADHD. A retrospective analysis during a 9 year period reported that median hospital inpatient, hospital outpatient, or ED admission costs for individuals with ADHD were more than double for those without ADHD [52]. Pharmacotherapy costs are also a large part of medical costs attributable to ADHD. Medication costs were reported to account for about 13–38% of total costs [1, 2, 24, 50, 52, 53]. Psychological therapy

Table 6 Average Costs Model Results and Estimated Marginal Predictions for Inmates with ADHD (Compared with Inmates without ADHD; $n = 96$ ADHD, $n = 294$ non-ADHD)

	3 month beta coefficient	3 month Predicted margin	1 year Predicted margin
Medical Costs	0.25*	£ 135.9	£ 543.6
Prison Costs	0.25	£ 11.4	£ 45.6
Total Costs	0.24**	£ 147.5	£ 590

Note: Findings from Generalised Linear Model using gamma error distribution and log link function, adjusted for age
*$p < 0.05$
**$p < 0.01$

(individual or group modalities) is often another common important driver of costs, which was essentially not utilised by the participants of our study.

Our total estimated annual cost of £590 per inmate with ADHD demonstrates that the costs attributable to ADHD are relatively high. But because our estimate did not include costs for hospital stays, medication, and/or psychological treatment, the total cost estimate therefore represents a conservative figure.

In our study, costs associated with ADHD were driven by increased medical service use and not by behavioural disturbance incidents. This may indicate that costs related to behavioural incidents were more generally distributed across the prison sample and due to many other factors besides having a diagnosis of ADHD. Service utilisation patterns were restricted to general medical and nursing services. Low endorsement of engagement with these and other services may have been a true reflection of the patterns of use in our sample, or of the Scottish prison system at large. As many resources were not used, costs remained lower compared with other studies mentioned.

Because the present study found there were significantly greater medical costs but not behaviour-related prison costs, the cost implication seems to be largely for the NHS. While the assignment of prisoner medical costs based on NHS reimbursements may not perfectly represent prisoners medical costs (possibly over- or under-estimated), it helped to estimate and interpret costs using standard more widely used and familiar terms. There may be, however, variability in the recording of critical incident data, which will be a fundamental driver of prison costs, leading to increased number of seclusions, adjudications, injury costs and potentially staff sickness. In a previous study conducted in a large prison in Aberdeen there were highly significant differences found in aggressive critical incidents between an ADHD and a non-ADHD group [43]. Hence for some prison establishments, costs to the prison service may be considerably higher.

Limitations

A key strength of the study is its large sample size and a methodology in which every participant was clinically diagnosed using the DIVA-2. Nonetheless, there are several limitations.

Because of missing data, some bias may be present in our analyses of HUI3 specific attribute scores. However, our models accounted for missing data using a well established and oft cited method and the sensitivity analysis on adjusted models allowed us to have confidence in our methods.

Ethnic minority groups and females did not have representation in this sample, therefore, it remains unclear whether these findings may be fully applicable and generalized to the entire prison population.

ADHD diagnosis was based on self-reported information and we did not include informant (e.g. familial) reports. Recall bias is unaccounted for and may have been a factor in symptom measures and service use. Nevertheless, any bias related to under-reporting was presumed to have similar effects on estimates for both the ADHD and non-ADHD groups. Other studies have reported considerably higher rates of critical incidents [43, 54], and it is likely that prison costs based on these would be considerably inflated compared with the estimates derived from the present data.

Our extrapolation method (using 3 months of data to estimate 1 year) may be limited in its accuracy. We used a one-year horizon for our HRQoL and service use estimates, and more time than this would have conferred too much uncertainty. Future research should address measuring utilities over more time, thereby providing a better foundation of QALY estimates beyond 1 year. Finally, the opportunity sampling method used may have introduced selection bias into the results, limiting their generalizability both within the prison and across other prisons.

Conclusions

Research on HRQoL and costs related to adult ADHD is limited in the general population and is virtually non-existent in the prison population. We addressed this paucity of data on HRQoL, QALY, service utilization, and costs attributable to ADHD based on 1 year in prison. We performed HRQoL and cost analyses for adult prison inmates with ADHD based on a cross-section of the Scottish prison system in the UK.

Our study provides evidence that HRQoL of life is considerably poorer in adult male prison inmates with ADHD, with an adjusted reduction of 0.13 QALY. Affected health attributes extend beyond emotional and cognitive deficits, suggesting chronic effects of ADHD on health over the lifespan. ADHD may contribute to adverse health and quality of life directly through executive function and cognitive deficits; and co-morbid disorders. Combined costs within prison were significantly higher for those with ADHD and were driven by medical expenses. Service utilisation was for the most part limited to general practitioner services and nursing staff visits.

Approximately 80% of inmates considered to have ADHD did not receive a prior diagnosis — indicating that a significant proportion of adult prison inmates are inadequately identified and treated. This has policy implications for both the National Health and the prison service. There is a need for the prison service to develop improved awareness about ADHD in adult prisoners, including the clinical and behavoural presentation of ADHD. There is also a need to introduce a brief and reliable screen on admission, such as the 6-item B-BAARS, which has high sensitivity and specificity [25]. Furthermore, there is a need for the NHS to address the general absence of health service provision for adults with ADHD in prisons, as prisoners continue presenting multiple times for their health problems and seem to remain mis- or undiagnosed.

In 2015 the Ministry of Justice reported a population of 77,472 adult male inmates in the UK. Given the prevalence rate of 25.5% of ADHD among prisoners [55] and our estimated annual total cost per adult inmate with ADHD of £590, we estimate a total cost for medical and behaviour-related prison care of approximately £11.7 million per year. This cost estimate, however, is conservative as it is seemingly driven by general medical expenses and not by critical incidents. There may be variability in the reporting of critical incidents in prisons, and prison care costs associated with behavioural disturbances may be much higher in other establishments.

ADHD is a prevalent mental health disorder, and a known risk factor for a series of adverse health and social outcomes. Population studies report the community (and society at large) bears considerable medical costs associated with ADHD [22, 23]. Although ADHD is disproportionately prevalent in prison, it is understudied and inadequately addressed in this context [55, 56].

Our results provide evidence that adult prisoners with ADHD represent a unique population with unmet needs and high costs. Given the Swedish study of patients showing a 32% reduction in criminality for men and 41% for women during periods when they were receiving ADHD medication [57], effective identification and treatment of ADHD may have important cost implications.

We recommend directing efforts to increase access to effective interventions for adult inmates with ADHD. Setting up provisions for better access to early diagnosis and treatment is likely to improve inmates' HRQoL and decrease impairment related to ADHD symptoms and associated co-morbidities.

Abbreviations

ADHD: Attention-deficit hyperactivity disorder; BSI: Brief Symptom Inventory; CJS: Criminal justice system; CPI: Consumer price index; DIVA-2: Diagnostic interview for ADHD in adults 2.0; DSM-5: 5th edition of Diagnostic and Statistical Manual of Mental Disorders; GLM: Generalised linear models; HRQoL: Health-related quality of life; HUI3: Health Utilities Index Mark 3; NHS: National Health Service; QALY: Quality-adjusted life years

Acknowledgements

We are grateful to Mr. Gordon Morrice, the Scottish Prison Service, and staff at Porterfield Prison in Inverness for their support of the study. We thank Laura Mutch and Isabella Mallet-Lambert for data collection. This study was supported by a grant from Shire Pharmaceutical Development Limited.

Funding

The study was supported by Shire Pharmaceutical Development Limited through a restricted grant. Shire had no role in the design and conduct of the study (collection, management, analysis, and interpretation of the data) or on the preparation, review, or approval of the manuscript, and the decision to submit the manuscript for publication. The research was also supported by the National Institute for Health Research (NIHR) Imperial Biomedical Research Centre.

Authors' contributions

SY, RG, MF, and GG led the planning and scientific input of the study. RG conducted the statistical analysis and wrote the first draft with input from SY and GG. KK critically edited the data tables, figures, and manuscript; and wrote the final draft. All authors have read and approved the final manuscript.

Consent for publication

Not applicable

Competing interests

SY has received honoraria for consultancy, travel, educational talks and/or research from Janssen, Eli Lilly, HB Pharma, and/or Shire. MF consulted for Amgen, CSL Behring, Merck, Novo Nordisk, Shire, and Vertex. GG and RG have no conflicts of interest. PH was an employee of Shire working on ADHD projects from 2009 to 2013. The views expressed are those of the authors and not necessarily those of the NHS, the NIHR or the Department of Health. Aside from KK, none of the authors received funds for their involvement in this manuscript.

Author details

[1]Psychology Services Limited, PO Box 1735, Croydon CR97AE, UK. [2]Reykjavik University, Reykjavik, Iceland. [3]East London NHS Foundation Trust, London, UK. [4]AMF Consulting Inc, Los Angeles, CA, USA. [5]Sage Therapeutics, Cambridge, MA, USA. [6]Indedpendent Medical Writer, San Diego, CA, USA. [7]Institute of Psychiatry, Psychology and Neuroscience, King's College London, London, UK.

References

1. Swensen AR, Birnbaum HG, Secnik K, Marynchenko M, Greenberg P, Claxton A. Attention-deficit/hyperactivity disorder: increased costs for patients and their families. J Am Acad Child Adolesc Psychiatry. 2003;42(12):1415–23.
2. Chorozoglou M, Smith E, Koerting J, Thompson MJ, Sayal K, Sonuga-Barke EJ. Preschool hyperactivity is associated with long-term economic burden: evidence from a longitudinal health economic analysis of costs incurred across childhood, adolescence and young adulthood. J Child Psychol Psychiatry. 2015;56(9):966–75.
3. Diagnostic and statistical manual of mental disorders, 5th ed Washington, D.C.: American Psychiatric Association; 2013.
4. Polanczyk GV, Salum GA, Sugaya LS, Caye A, Rohde LA. Annual research review: a meta-analysis of the worldwide prevalence of mental disorders in children and adolescents. J Child Psychol Psychiatry. 2015;56(3):345–65.
5. Thomas R, Sanders S, Doust J, Beller E, Glasziou P. Prevalence of attention-deficit/hyperactivity disorder: a systematic review and meta-analysis. Pediatrics. 2015;135(4):e994–1001.

6. Moffitt TE, Houts R, Asherson P, Belsky DW, Corcoran DL, Hammerle M, Harrington H, Hogan S, Meier MH, Polanczyk GV, et al. Is adult ADHD a childhood-onset neurodevelopmental disorder? Evidence from a four-decade longitudinal cohort study. Am J Psychiatry. 2015;172(10):967–77.
7. Agnew-Blais JC, Polanczyk GV, Danese A, Wertz J, Moffitt TE, Arseneault L. Evaluation of the persistence, remission, and emergence of attention-deficit/hyperactivity disorder in young adulthood. JAMA Psychiatry. 2016; 73(7):713–20.
8. Faraone SV, Biederman J, Mick E. The age-dependent decline of attention deficit hyperactivity disorder: a meta-analysis of follow-up studies. Psychol Med. 2006;36(2):159–65.
9. Polanczyk G, de Lima MS, Horta BL, Biederman J, Rohde LA. The worldwide prevalence of ADHD: a systematic review and metaregression analysis. Am J of Psychiatry. 2007;164(6):942–8.
10. Simon V, Czobor P, Balint S, Meszaros A, Bitter I. Prevalence and correlates of adult attention-deficit hyperactivity disorder: meta-analysis. British J of Psychiatry. 2009;194(3):204–11.
11. Chang Z, Lichtenstein P, D'onofrio B, Sjölander A, Larsson H. Serious transport accidents in adults with attention-deficit/hyperactivity disorder and the effect of medication: a population-based study. JAMA Psychiatry. 2014;71(3):319–25.
12. Dalsgaard S, Ostergaard SD, Leckman JF, Mortensen PB, Pedersen MG. Mortality in children, adolescents, and adults with attention deficit hyperactivity disorder: a nationwide cohort study. Lancet. 2015;385(9983): 2190–6.
13. van Emmerik-van Oortmerssen K, van de Glind G, van den Brink W, Smit F, Crunelle CL, Swets M, Schoevers RA. Prevalence of attention-deficit hyperactivity disorder in substance use disorder patients: a meta-analysis and meta-regression analysis. Drug Alcohol Depend. 2012; 122(1–2):11–9.
14. Gudjonsson GH, Sigurdsson JF, Sigfusdottir ID, Asgeirsdottir BB, Gonzalez RA, Young S. A national epidemiological study investigating risk factors for police interrogation and false confession among juveniles and young persons. Soc Psychiatry Psychiatr Epidemiol. 2016;51(3):359–67.
15. Shaw M, Hodgkins P, Caci H, Young S, Kahle J, Woods AG, Arnold LE. A systematic review and analysis of long-term outcomes in attention deficit hyperactivity disorder: effects of treatment and non-treatment. BMC Med. 2012;10:99.
16. Danckaerts M, Sonuga-Barke EJ, Banaschewski T, Buitelaar J, Dopfner M, Hollis C, Santosh P, Rothenberger A, Sergeant J, Steinhausen HC, et al. The quality of life of children with attention deficit/hyperactivity disorder: a systematic review. Eur Child Adolesc Psychiatry. 2010;19(2):83–105.
17. Young S, Sedgwick O, Fridman M, Gudjonsson G, Hodgkins P, Lantigua M, Gonzalez RA. Co-morbid psychiatric disorders among incarcerated ADHD populations: a meta-analysis. Psychol Med. 2015;45(12):2499–510.
18. Gonzalez RA, Velez-Pastrana MC, Ruiz Varcarcel JJ, Levin FR, Albizu-Garcia CE. Childhood ADHD symptoms are associated with lifetime and current illicit substance-use disorders and in-site health risk behaviors in a representative sample of Latino prison inmates. J Atten Disord. 2015; 19(4):301–12.
19. Gudjonsson G, Sigurdsson JF, Young S, Newton AK, Peersen M. Attention deficit hyperactivity disorder (ADHD). How do ADHD symptoms relate to personality among prisoners? Personal Individ Differ. 2009;47:64–8.
20. Young S, Wells J, Gudjonsson GH. Predictors of offending among prisoners: the role of attention-deficit hyperactivity disorder and substance use. J Psychopharmacol. 2011;25(11):1524–32.
21. Gregory G, Reddy V, Young C. Identifying children who are at risk of FASD in Peterborough: working in a community clinic without access to gold standard diagnosis. Adoption Fostering. 2015;39(3):225–34.
22. Beecham J. Annual research review: child and adolescent mental health interventions: a review of progress in economic studies across different disorders. J Child Psychol Psychiatry. 2014;55(6):714–32.
23. Doshi JA, Hodgkins P, Kahle J, Sikirica V, Cangelosi MJ, Setyawan J, Erder MH, Neumann PJ. Economic impact of childhood and adult attention-deficit/hyperactivity disorder in the United States. J Am Acad Child Adolesc Psychiatry. 2012;51(10):990–1002. e1002
24. Telford C, Green C, Logan S, Langley K, Thapar A, Ford T. Estimating the costs of ongoing care for adolescents with attention-deficit hyperactivity disorder. Soc Psychiatry Psychiatr Epidemiol. 2013;48(2):337–44.
25. Young S, Gonzalez RA, Mutch L, Mallet-Lambert I, O'Rourke L, Hickey N, Asherson P, Gudjonsson GH. Diagnostic accuracy of a brief screening tool for attention deficit hyperactivity disorder in UK prison inmates. Psychol Med. 2016;46:1449–58.
26. Horsman J, Furlong W, Feeny D, Torrance G. The health utilities index (HUI): concepts, measurement properties and applications. Health Qual Life Outcomes. 2003;1:54.
27. Health Utilities Inc. http://www.healthutilities.com/. Accessed 29 Oct 2017.
28. Patrick DL, Erickson P. Health Status and Health policy: quality of life in health care evaluation and resource allocation. NewYork: Oxford University Press; 1993.
29. Sikirica V, Pliszka SR, Betts KA, Hodgkins P, Samuelson T, Xie J, Erder H, Dammerman R, Robertson B, Wu EQ. Comparative treatment patterns, resource utilization, and costs in stimulant-treated children with ADHD who require subsequent pharmacotherapy with atypical antipsychotics versus non-antipsychotics. J Manag Care Pharm. 2012;18(9):676–89.
30. Kooij JJS. Diagnostic Interview for ADHD in Adults 2.0 (DIVA 2.0). In: Adult ADHD: Diagnostic assessment and treatment. Amsterdam, ND: Pearson Assessment and Information BV; 2010.
31. Deberdt W, Thome J, Lebrec J, Kraemer S, Fregenal I, Ramos-Quiroga JA, Arif M. Prevalence of ADHD in nonpsychotic adult psychiatric care (ADPSYC): a multinational cross-sectional study in Europe. BMC Psychiatry. 2015;15(1):242.
32. Young S, Goodwin EJ, Sedgwick O, Gudjonsson GH. The effectiveness of police custody assessments in identifying suspects with intellectual disabilities and attention deficit hyperactivity disorder. BMC Med. 2013;11:248.
33. Derogatis LR. The Brief Symptom Inventory: Administration, Scoring, and Procedures Manual. 4th ed. Minneapolis, MN: National Computer Systems; 1993.
34. Personal Social Services Research Unit. Unit Costs of Health and Social Care. 2014. http://www.pssru.ac.uk/project-pages/unit-costs/2014/. Accessed 29 Oct 2017.
35. HM Prison Service. Prison population figures. Ministry of Justice. 2016. https://www.gov.uk/government/statistics/prison-population-figures-2016. Accessed 29 Oct 2017.
36. The Social Research Unit at Dartington. Investing in Children: Technical Report. Dartington: Dartington Press; 2013.
37. UCLA Statistical Consulting Group. Introduction to SAS. 2007. http://www.ats.ucla.edu/stat/sas/notes2. Accessed 28 Apr 2016.
38. Wedderburn RWM. Quasi-likelihood functions, generalized linear models, and the gauss Newton method. Biometrika. 1974;61:439–47.
39. StataCorp. Stata Statistical Software: Release 13. College Station, TX: StataCorp LP; 2013.
40. Naeim A, Keeler EB, Mangione CM. Options for handling missing data in the health utilities index mark 3. Med Decis Mak. 2005;25(2):186–98.
41. Riley AW, Spiel G, Coghill D, Dopfner M, Falissard B, Lorenzo MJ, Preuss U, Ralston SJ, Group AS. Factors related to health-related quality of life (HRQoL) among children with ADHD in Europe at entry into treatment. Eur Child Adolesc Psychiatry. 2006;15(Suppl 1):I38–45.
42. Coghill D, Hodgkins P. Health-related quality of life of children with attention-deficit/hyperactivity disorder versus children with diabetes and healthy controls. Eur Child Adolesc Psychiatry. 2015;25(3):261–71.
43. Young S, Gudjonsson GH, Wells J, Asherson P, Theobald D, Oliver B, Scott C, Mooney A. Attention deficit hyperactivity disorder and critical incidents in a Scottish prison population. Personal Individ Differ. 2009;46:265–9.
44. Peasgood T, Bhardwaj A, Biggs K, Brazier JE, Coghill D, Cooper CL, Daley D, De Silva C, Harpin V, Hodgkins P, et al. The impact of ADHD on the health and well-being of ADHD children and their siblings. Eur Child Adolesc Psychiatry. 2016;25(11):1217–31.
45. Erskine HE, Ferrari AJ, Polanczyk GV, Moffitt TE, Murray CJ, Vos T, Whiteford HA, Scott JG. The global burden of conduct disorder and attention-deficit/hyperactivity disorder in 2010. J Child Psychol Psychiatry. 2014;55(4):328–36.
46. Limbers CA, Ripperger-Suhler J, Boutton K, Ransom D, Varni JW. A comparative analysis of health-related quality of life and family impact between children with ADHD treated in a general pediatric clinic and a psychiatric clinic utilizing the PedsQL. J Atten Disord. 2011;15(5):392–402.
47. Lee YC, Yang HJ, Chen VC, Lee WT, Teng MJ, Lin CH, Gossop M. Meta-analysis of quality of life in children and adolescents with ADHD: by both parent proxy-report and child self-report using PedsQL. Res Dev Disabil. 2016;51-52:160–72.
48. Klassen AF, Miller A, Fine S. Health-related quality of life in children and adolescents who have a diagnosis of attention-deficit/hyperactivity disorder. Pediatrics. 2004;114(5):e541–7.
49. Herringa RJ, Birn RM, Ruttle PL, Burghy CA, Stodola DE, Davidson RJ, Essex MJ. Childhood maltreatment is associated with altered fear circuitry and

increased internalizing symptoms by late adolescence. Proc Natl Acad Sci U S A. 2013;110(47):19119–24.

50. Hakkaart-van Roijen L, Zwirs BW, Bouwmans C, Tan SS, Schulpen TW, Vlasveld L, Buitelaar JK. Societal costs and quality of life of children suffering from attention deficient hyperactivity disorder (ADHD). Eur Child Adolesc Psychiatry. 2007;16(5):316–26.
51. Jones DE, Foster EM. Conduct problems prevention research G.: service use patterns for adolescents with ADHD and comorbid conduct disorder. J Behav Health Serv Res. 2009;36(4):436–49.
52. Leibson CL, Katusic SK, Barbaresi WJ, Ransom J, O'Brien PC. Use and costs of medical care for children and adolescents with and without attention-deficit/hyperactivity disorder. JAMA. 2001;285(1):60–6.
53. Wu EQ, Birnbaum HG, Zhang HF, Ivanova JI, Yang E, Mallet D. Health care costs of adults treated for attention-deficit/hyperactivity disorder who received alternative drug therapies. J Manag Care Pharm. 2007;13(7):561–9.
54. Gordon V, Williams DJ, Donnelly PD. Exploring the relationship between ADHD symptoms and prison breaches of discipline amongst youths in four Scottish prisons. Public Health. 2012;126(4):343–8.
55. Young S, Moss D, Sedgwick O, Fridman M, Hodgkins P. A meta-analysis of the prevalence of attention deficit hyperactivity disorder in incarcerated populations. Psychol Med. 2015;45(2):247–58.
56. Young SJ, Adamou M, Bolea B, Gudjonsson G, Muller U, Pitts M, Thome J, Asherson P. The identification and management of ADHD offenders within the criminal justice system: a consensus statement from the UK adult ADHD network and criminal justice agencies. BMC Psychiatry. 2011;11:32.
57. Lichtenstein P, Halldner L, Zetterqvist J, Sjolander A, Serlachius E, Fazel S, Langstrom N, Larsson H. Medication for attention deficit-hyperactivity disorder and criminality. N Engl J Med. 2012;367(21):2006–14.

Permissions

All chapters in this book were first published in PSYCHIATRY, by BioMed Central; hereby published with permission under the Creative Commons Attribution License or equivalent. Every chapter published in this book has been scrutinized by our experts. Their significance has been extensively debated. The topics covered herein carry significant findings which will fuel the growth of the discipline. They may even be implemented as practical applications or may be referred to as a beginning point for another development.

The contributors of this book come from diverse backgrounds, making this book a truly international effort. This book will bring forth new frontiers with its revolutionizing research information and detailed analysis of the nascent developments around the world.

We would like to thank all the contributing authors for lending their expertise to make the book truly unique. They have played a crucial role in the development of this book. Without their invaluable contributions this book wouldn't have been possible. They have made vital efforts to compile up to date information on the varied aspects of this subject to make this book a valuable addition to the collection of many professionals and students.

This book was conceptualized with the vision of imparting up-to-date information and advanced data in this field. To ensure the same, a matchless editorial board was set up. Every individual on the board went through rigorous rounds of assessment to prove their worth. After which they invested a large part of their time researching and compiling the most relevant data for our readers.

The editorial board has been involved in producing this book since its inception. They have spent rigorous hours researching and exploring the diverse topics which have resulted in the successful publishing of this book. They have passed on their knowledge of decades through this book. To expedite this challenging task, the publisher supported the team at every step. A small team of assistant editors was also appointed to further simplify the editing procedure and attain best results for the readers.

Apart from the editorial board, the designing team has also invested a significant amount of their time in understanding the subject and creating the most relevant covers. They scrutinized every image to scout for the most suitable representation of the subject and create an appropriate cover for the book.

The publishing team has been an ardent support to the editorial, designing and production team. Their endless efforts to recruit the best for this project, has resulted in the accomplishment of this book. They are a veteran in the field of academics and their pool of knowledge is as vast as their experience in printing. Their expertise and guidance has proved useful at every step. Their uncompromising quality standards have made this book an exceptional effort. Their encouragement from time to time has been an inspiration for everyone.

The publisher and the editorial board hope that this book will prove to be a valuable piece of knowledge for researchers, students, practitioners and scholars across the globe.

List of Contributors

Arzu Arat and Anders Hjern
Department of Medicine, Karolinska Institute, 171 76, Stockholm, Sweden
Centre for Health Equity Studies (CHESS), Stockholm University/Karolinska Institute, 106 91 Stockholm, Sweden

Viveca Östberg
Centre for Health Equity Studies (CHESS), Stockholm University/Karolinska Institute, 106 91 Stockholm, Sweden

Bo Burström
Department of Public Health Sciences, Karolinska Institute, 171 77 Stockholm, Sweden

Dóra Győri
Institute of Psychology, Eötvös Loránd University, Izabella str. 46, Budapest 1064, Hungary

Judit Balázs
Institute of Psychology, Eötvös Loránd University, Izabella str. 46, Budapest 1064, Hungary
Vadaskert Child and Adolescent Psychiatry Hospital, Budapest, Hungary

Lili Olga Horváth and Dóra Szentiványi
Institute of Psychology, Eötvös Loránd University, Izabella str. 46, Budapest 1064, Hungary
Doctoral School of Psychology, Eötvös Loránd University, Budapest, Hungary

Gergely Mészáros
Vadaskert Child and Adolescent Psychiatry Hospital, Budapest, Hungary
Semmelweis University, School of Ph.D. Studies, Budapest, Hungary

Tobias Arthen, Andreas Riedel, Thomas Fangmeier and Ludger Tebartz van Elst
Department of Psychiatry and Psychotherapy, Medical Center - University of Freiburg, Faculty of Medicine, University of Freiburg, Hauptstraße 5, 79104 Freiburg, Germany

Fabian Frank
Department of Psychiatry and Psychotherapy, Medical Center - University of Freiburg, Faculty of Medicine, University of Freiburg, Hauptstraße 5, 79104 Freiburg, Germany
Department of Social Work, Protestant University of Applied Sciences Freiburg, Bugginger Straße 38, 79114 Freiburg, Germany

Martina Jablotschkin
Department of Psychiatry and Psychotherapy, Medical Center - University of Freiburg, Faculty of Medicine, University of Freiburg, Hauptstraße 5, 79104 Freiburg, Germany
Department of Oncological Rehabilitation - UKF Reha gGmbH, Medical Center - University of Freiburg, Breisacher Straße 117, 79106 Freiburg, Germany

Lars P. Hölzel
Department of Psychiatry and Psychotherapy, Medical Center - University of Freiburg, Faculty of Medicine, University of Freiburg, Hauptstraße 5, 79104 Freiburg, Germany
Parkklinik Wiesbaden Schlangenbad, Rheingauer Straße 47, 65388 Schlangenbad, Germany

Tsubasa Morimoto, Yasuhiro Matsuda, Kiwamu Matsuoka, Fumihiko Yasuno and Toshifumi Kishimoto
Department of Psychiatry, Nara Medical University School of Medicine, 840 Shijo-cho, Kashihara, Nara 634-8522, Japan

Emi Ikebuchi
Department of Psychiatry, Teikyo University School of Medicine, 2-11-1 Kaga, Itabashi-ku, Tokyo 173-8605, Japan

Hiroyuki Kameda
School of Computer Science, Tokyo University of Technology, 1404-1 Katakuramachi, Hachioji City, Tokyo 192-0982, Japan

Toshiaki Taoka
Department of Radiology, Nagoya University Hospital, 65 Tsurumai-cho, Showa-ku, Nagoya, Aichi 466-8550, Japan

Toshiteru Miyasaka and Kimihiko Kichikawa
Department of Radiology, Nara Medical University School of Medicine, 840 Shijo-cho, Kashihara, Nara 634-8522, Japan

Hiroshi Komatsu, Takashi Ono and Yoshihisa Kakuto
Department of Psychiatry, Miyagi Psychiatric Center, Mubanchi, Tekurada, Natori 981-1231, Japan

Masaaki Kato
Department of Neurology, Minami Tohoku Hospital, Iwanuma 989-2483, Japan

Teiko Kinpara
Department of Neurology, Kohnan Hospital, Sendai 982-8523, Japan

Tolesa Fanta, Kibrom Haile and Dessie Abebaw
Amanuel Mental Specialized Hospital Research and Training Department, Addis Ababa, Ethiopia

Dawit Assefa
Amanuel Mental Specialized Hospital, Addis Ababa, Ethiopia

Getahun Hibdye
Amanuel Mental Specialized Hospital Clinical Service Department, Addis Ababa, Ethiopia

Shin Ono
Department of Community Psychiatric Medicine, Niigata University Graduate School of Medical and Dental Sciences, Niigata, Japan
Japanese Society of Clinical Neuropsychopharmacology, Tokyo, Japan

Takuro Sugai, Yutaro Suzuki and Toshiyuki Someya
Japanese Society of Clinical Neuropsychopharmacology, Tokyo, Japan
Department of Psychiatry, Niigata University Graduate School of Medical and Dental Sciences, Niigata, Japan

Kazutaka Shimoda and Yuji Ozeki
Japanese Society of Clinical Neuropsychopharmacology, Tokyo, Japan
Department of Psychiatry, Dokkyo Medical University School of Medicine, Mibu, Japan

Norio Sugawara and Norio Yasui-Furukori
Japanese Society of Clinical Neuropsychopharmacology, Tokyo, Japan
Department of Neuropsychiatry, Hirosaki University School of Medicine, Hirosaki, Japan

Manabu Yamazaki, Takao Mori, Hiroshi Matsuda and Kurefu Okamoto
Japan Psychiatric Hospital Association, Tokyo, Japan

Toyoaki Sagae
Department of Health and Nutrition, Yamagata Prefectural Yonezawa University of Nutrition Sciences Faculty of Health and Nutrition, Yonezawa, Japan

Susan Young
Psychology Services Limited, Croydon CR97AE, UK
Reykjavik University, Reykjavik, Iceland

Gisli H. Gudjonsson
Reykjavik University, Reykjavik, Iceland
Institute of Psychiatry, Psychology and Neuroscience, King's College London, London, UK

Rafael A. González
East London NHS Foundation Trust, East London, UK

Moshe Fridman
AMF Consulting Inc., Los Angeles, CA, USA

Paul Hodgkins
Sage Therapeutics, Cambridge, MA, USA

Keira Kim
Independent Medical Writer, San Diego, CA, USA

Xiacan Chen and Junmei Hu
West China School of Basic Medical Sciences & Forensic Medicine, Sichuan University, Sichuan, China

Jiajun Xu, Bin Li, Wanjun Guo and Jun Zhang
Mental Health Center, West China Hospital, Sichuan University, Sichuan, China

Christian G. Widschwendter, Georg Kemmler, Maria A. Rettenbacher, Nursen Yalcin-Siedentopf and Alex Hofer
Medical University Innsbruck, Department of Psychiatry, Psychotherapy, and Psychosomatics Division of Psychiatry I, Anichstrasse 35, 6020 Innsbruck, Austria

Jennie Hayes, Tamsin Ford, Hateem Rafeeque and Ginny Russell
University of Exeter Medical School, St Luke's Campus, University of Exeter, Exeter EX1 2LU, UK

E. Ahnemark
Shire, Vasagatan 7, SE-111 20 Stockholm, Sweden

M. Di Schiena
Prima Child and Adult Psychiatry AB, Stockholm, Sweden

A.-C. Fredman
Prima Child and Adult Psychiatry AB, Stockholm, Sweden
Psychiatry Centre, Stockholm County Council, Södertälje, Sweden

E. Medin
PAREXEL International, Stockholm, Sweden
Department of Learning, Informatics, Management and Ethics, Karolinska Institute, Stockholm, Sweden

J. K. Söderling
Bell Analytics, Stockholm, Sweden

Y. Ginsberg
Department of Medical Epidemiology and Biostatistics, Karolinska Institute, Stockholm, Sweden
Department of Clinical Neuroscience, Centre for Psychiatry Research, Karolinska Institute, Stockholm, Sweden

Kathrin Nickel, Ludger Tebartz van Elst, Katharina Domschke, Dominique Endres, Simon Maier and Andreas Riedel
Section for Experimental Neuropsychiatry, Department of Psychiatry and Psychotherapy, Medical Center - University of Freiburg, Faculty of Medicine, University of Freiburg, Hauptstraße 5, D-79104 Freiburg, Germany

Birgitta Gläser and Friedrich Stock
Institute of Human Genetics, Medical Center - University of Freiburg, Faculty of Medicine, University of Freiburg, Breisacher Straße 33, D-79106 Freiburg, Germany

Susan Young
Psychology Services Limited, Croydon, UK

Gisli Gudjonsson
Institute of Psychiatry, Psychology and Neuroscience, Department of Psychology, King's College London, London, UK

Prathiba Chitsabesan
Offender Health Research Network, Division of Psychology and Mental Health and Division of Medicine and Health, University of Manchester, Manchester, UK

Sarah Maginn
Kent Prisons, Oxleas NHS Foundation Trust, Dartford, UK

Peter Mason
Cheshire & Wirral Partnership NHS Foundation Trust, The Stein Centre, St Catherine's Hospital, Birkenhead, UK

Caihong Sun, Mingyang Zou, Xuelai Wang, Wei Xia, Yongjuan Ma, Shuang Liang and Lijie Wu
Department of Children's and Adolescent Health, Public Health College, Harbin Medical University, Harbin 150081, China

Yanqiu Hao
Department of Pediatric, The Second Affiliated Hospital, Harbin Medical University, Harbin 150081 China

Songbin Fu
Laboratory of Medical Genetics, Harbin Medical University, Harbin 150081, China

Javier Quintero
Psychiatry Department, Hospital Universitario Infanta Leonor and Psychiatry and Medical Psychology Department, Complutense University, Madrid, Spain

Josep A. Ramos-Quiroga
Department of Psychiatry, Hospital Universitari Vall d'Hebron, Barcelona, Spain; Biomedical Network Research Centre on Mental Health (CIBERSAM), Barcelona, Spain
Department of Psychiatry and Legal Medicine, Universitat Autònoma de Barcelona, Bellaterra, Spain

Javier San Sebastián
Child and Adolescent Psychiatry Department, Hospital Universitario Ramón y Cajal, Madrid, Spain and Psychiatry Department, Universidad de Alcalá, Madrid, Spain

José Martínez-Raga
UDPyPC, Hospital Universitario Dr. Peset and University of Valencia and University CEU-UCH, Valencia, Spain

Marta García Giral
Child and Adolescent Psychiatry and Psychology Department, Institute of Neuroscience, Hospital Clinic, Barcelona, Spain

Ling Qin, Hairun Liu, Hong Zhang, Yanhong Fu and Dandan Li
From the center of Cognitive and Sleeping, The people's hospital of Guangxi Zhuang autonomous region, Nanning 530021, Guangxi, China

Christopher Hautmann
Department of Child and Adolescent Psychiatry, Psychosomatics and Psychotherapy, Medical Faculty of the University of Cologne, Cologne, Germany
School of Child and Adolescent Cognitive Behavioral Therapy (AKiP), University Hospital Cologne, Pohligstraße 9, 50969 Cologne, Germany

Josepha Katzmann
School of Child and Adolescent Cognitive Behavioral Therapy (AKiP), University Hospital Cologne, Pohligstraße 9, 50969 Cologne, Germany

Charlotte Jaite
Department of Child and Adolescent Psychiatry and Psychotherapy, Charité - Universitätsmedizin Berlin, Freie Universität Berlin, Humboldt-Universität zu Berlin, and Berlin Institute of Health (BIH), Berlin, Germany

Christian Jacob
Department of Psychiatry, Psychosomatics and Psychotherapy, Center for Mental Health, University Hospital of Würzburg, Würzburg, Germany
Department of Psychiatry, Psychosomatics and Psychotherapy, Medius Clinic, Kirchheim, Germany

Marina Šagud, Alma Mihaljević-Peleš and Darko Marčinko
School of Medicine, University of Zagreb, Zagreb, Croatia
Department of Psychiatry, University Hospital Center Zagreb, Kišpatićeva 12, 10 000 Zagreb, Croatia

Nenad Jakšić
Department of Psychiatry, University Hospital Center Zagreb, Kišpatićeva 12, 10 000 Zagreb, Croatia

Bjanka Vuksan-Ćusa
Department of Psychiatry, University Hospital Center Zagreb, Kišpatićeva 12, 10 000 Zagreb, Croatia
School of Medicine, University of Osijek, Osijek, Croatia
School of Medicine, University of Mostar, Mostar, Bosnia and Herzegovina

Maja Živković and Suzana Vlatković
Psychiatric Clinic Vrapče, Zagreb, Croatia

Tea Prgić
Department of Psychiatry, General Hospital Vinkovci, Vinkovci, Croatia

Wei Wang
Department of Clinical Psychology and Psychiatry, Zhejiang University College of Medicine, Hangzhou, China

Elisabet Wentz
Gillberg Neuropsychiatry Centre, Institute of Neuroscience and Physiology, University of Gothenburg, Gothenburg, Sweden

Helena Sehlin
Gillberg Neuropsychiatry Centre, Institute of Neuroscience and Physiology, University of Gothenburg, Gothenburg, Sweden
Kungsbacka Clinic of Adult Psychiatry, Department of Psychiatry, Kungsbacka, Region Halland, Sweden

Britt Hedman Ahlström
Department of Health Sciences, University West, Trollhättan, Sweden

Gerhard Andersson
Department of Behavioral Sciences and Learning, Linköping University, Linköping, Sweden
Department of Clinical Neuroscience, Karolinska Institute, Stockholm, Sweden

Yidong Shen, Huixi Dong, Lu Xiao, Jingping Zhao and Jianjun Ou
Institute of Mental Health, The Second Xiangya Hospital, Central South University; National Clinical Research Center on Mental Disorders, The National Technology Institute on Mental disorders; Hunan Key Laboratory of Psychiatry and Mental Health, Changsha, China

Xiaozi Lu
Qingdao Mental Health Center, Qingdao, China

Nan Lian
The First Affiliated Hospital of Zhengzhou University, Zhengzhou, China

Guanglei Xun
Mental Health Center of Shandong Province, Jinan, China

Lijuan Shi
Neuropsychology and Applied Cognitive Neuroscience Research Group, Institute of Psychology, Chinese Academy of Sciences, Beijing, China

Susan Young
Psychology Services Limited, Croydon CR97AE, UK
Reykjavik University, Reykjavik, Iceland

Gisli H. Gudjonsson
Reykjavik University, Reykjavik, Iceland
Institute of Psychiatry, Psychology and Neuroscience, King's College London, London, UK

Rafael A. González
East London NHS Foundation Trust, London, UK

Moshe Fridman
AMF Consulting Inc, Los Angeles, CA, USA

Paul Hodgkins
Sage Therapeutics, Cambridge, MA, USA

Keira Kim
Indedpendent Medical Writer, San Diego, CA, USA

Index